PAIN

A Nursing Approach to Assessment and Analysis

Noreen T. Meinhart, R.N., M.S.
Private Practice, Patients and Families Coping with Catastrophic Illness and Pain, Los Angeles, California; Clinical Nurse Specialist, Division of Medicine, UCLA; Analgesic Research, UCLA School of Medicine

Margo McCaffery, R.N., M.S., F.A.A.N.
Clinician/Unit Manager, Pain
Centinela Hospital Medical Center
Inglewood, California

ACC
APPLETON-CENTURY-CROFTS
Norwalk, Connecticut

0-8385-7703-2

Notice: The author(s) and publisher of this volume have taken care that the information and recommendations contained herein are accurate and compatible with the standards generally accepted at the time of publication.

83 84 85 86 87 88 / 10 9 8 7 6 5 4 3 2 1

Prentice-Hall International, Inc., London
Prentice-Hall of Australia, Pty. Ltd., Sydney
Prentice-Hall Canada, Inc.
Prentice-Hall of India Private Limited, New Delhi
Prentice-Hall of Japan, Inc., Tokyo
Prentice-Hall of Southeast Asia (Pte.) Ltd., Singapore
Whitehall Books Ltd., Wellington, New Zealand
Editora Prentice-Hall do Brasil Ltda., Rio de Janeiro

Library of Congress Cataloging in Publication Data

Meinhart, Noreen T.
Pain, a nursing approach to assessment and analysis.

Bibliography: p.
Includes index.
1. Pain. 2. Pain—Nursing. I. McCaffery, Margo, 1938- II. Title. [DNLM: 1. Pain—Nursing. 2. Nursing process. WB 176 M514p]
RB127.M44 1983 616'.0472 82-22779
ISBN 0-8385-7703-2

Design: Lynn Luchetti

PRINTED IN THE UNITED STATES OF AMERICA

Contents

Preface

PURPOSES OF THIS BOOK

In general clinical practice, pain relief, unfortunately, tends not to be a priority. The detrimental effects of pain are often unnoticed or, if noticed, they may not be treated. Sometimes these effects are attributed to other causes. As an example, postoperative nausea is commonly attributed to the narcotic or anesthetic when quite often the nausea is due to pain. When adequate doses of a narcotic are given both pain and nausea can be alleviated (Andersen & Krogh, 1976), but if the narcotic is withheld, the patient may continue to suffer pain and nausea. When pain continues untreated, or is improperly treated, obviously it may seriously complicate the patient's condition and result in a myriad of additional problems for him or her.

The primary purpose of this book is to help remedy the clinical problems of bodily pain and their associated detrimental effects for the patient by increasing the nurse's responsibility and accountability for pain management. We propose accomplishing this through implementation of the first step in the nursing process, which is the collection of an objective, systematic assessment and analysis of the patient's pain problem. Assessment should recognize the individuality of the pain experience and incorporate all phases of this experience—anticipation, occurrence, and aftermath—and all of the variables which influence it. Thus the content includes information on:

1. Specific behavioral responses to pain and variables which may influence the individual's perception of and response to his pain.
2. Practical methods of assessing the existence and effects of pain on the individual.

PHILOSOPHY OF THIS BOOK

We believe that pain, like death, is one of the most universally frightening experiences not only for those experiencing it but also for those witnessing it. Therefore, it may be avoided by nursing practitioners (McCaffery & Hart, 1976.)

It is our philosophy that failure to treat pain is inhumane and constitutes professional negligence. The Irish adage, "Better the devil ye know than the devil ye don't", contains much wisdom. We believe just confronting the problem of pain through an objective, systematic assessment and analysis will reduce the nursing practitioner's fears, feelings of powerlessness, and consequent alienation from the individual needing her or his expertise. Such an assessment of the patient with a pain problem will also increase the nurse's understanding of pain and suggest how much can be done to eliminate, control, or reduce pain. Thus, pain relief will assume the priority it deserves as a mandate for nursing practice.

AUDIENCE FOR THIS BOOK

This book is primarily addressed to nurses in all areas of practice, including practitioners, administrators, educators, researchers, and nursing students who are concerned with patients anticipating, experiencing, or having experienced bodily pain. However, it should be useful to most individuals working with patients who must cope with pain problems.

FRAMEWORK OF THIS BOOK

This book presents content which is essential in the assessment of the individual experiencing pain: that is, it provides a data base, tools, and methods essential for an accurate nursing diagnosis on which to form one's treatment plan for the patient with pain.

An introductory chapter, Chapter 1, includes information on the historical, social, and legal mandates for the nurse assuming responsibility for assessing and assisting the patient in pain management. The professional rationale for establishing and adhering to standards of nursing practice utilizing the nursing process for patients with pain will also be included. Following this introductory chapter, the content is presented in two major parts, Part A and Part B.

Part A will consider preexisting variables which are fairly stable and sometimes unalterable including the neurophysiology of the pain response, the cultural factors influencing the patient's pain experience, and the psychosocial influences.

Part B provides an overview and description of specific components of the pain experience itself. This includes such factors as the sensation and experience of pain, some of the more common pain syndromes, the effects of pain on the individual, situational factors that influence the patient's pain experience, how the patient communicates about his pain, and finally, methods and tools the nurse may use to assess the patient's pain.

LIMITATIONS OF THIS BOOK

This book is limited to the systematic assessment and analysis of the patient's experience with problems of bodily pain. This book does not offer plans and interventions for the problems of pain and their detrimental effect on the patient and his significant others.*

We recognize that there are many problems of pain which are more mental or emotional in nature. Indeed, physical pain may cause significant mental or emotional pain to an individual. However, for purposes of assessment of bodily pain in this book, mental or emotional pain will be considered only as a psychological variable which may influence the patient's bodily pain. Because of our beliefs about the nature of pain, we will not classify pain in relation to a specific clinical setting such as surgical or obstetrical pain. However, the examples of pain we will use will cut across all clinical divisions, and because there is no one agreed upon conceptual model for nursing practice, we have elected not to preferentially adopt any one model on which to organize the content of this book.

In problem solving, it is often said that half of the battle is in defining the problem. It is to that half of the battle that we address ourselves.

REFERENCES

Andersen R. & Krogh K.: Pain as a major cause of postoperative nausea. Can Anaesth Soc J 23:366–369, 1976.

McCaffery M.: Nursing Management of the Patient with Pain (2 ed.) Philadelphia: J. B. Lippincott, 1979.

McCaffery M. & Hart L.L.: Undertreatment of acute pain with narcotics. AM J Nurs 76:1586–1591, 1976.

---

* *Nursing intervention for patients anticipating and/or experiencing pain is covered in depth in: McCaffery M: Nursing Management of the Patient With Pain (2 ed.) Philadelphia: J. B. Lippincott, 1979.*

Acknowledgments

Although we are very appreciative for the support from all of our significant others, we would particularly like to acknowledge the assistance of three special people: Carol M. Hamcke, who progressed from single vision to bifocals during her repeated readings of our manuscript; Terry Oleson, Ph.D., who graciously and diplomatically critiqued the chapter on the Neurophysiology of Pain, and Antonia Turman, who typed more accurately and rapidly than a sophisticated word processor.

1

The Relationship of the Nursing Diagnosis to the Patient in Pain

Pain may be harmful to one's physical and mental health. Or the need for the nursing diagnosis.

IMPORTANCE AND RELEVANCE OF THE NURSING DIAGNOSIS

Why is the nursing diagnosis critical to the management of the patient in pain? In contrast to other major health problems our society has focused little attention on pain until quite recently. This is in spite of the facts that pain probably affects and/or disables more individuals than any other disease and that the monetary costs of pain are considered a major economic problem. Not only that, sociologists studying the work of health professionals with hospitalized patients with pain have come to the conclusion that, even in hospitals, "the staff is not genuinely accountable for much of its interaction with or behavior towards patients in pain. . . ." This assertion "means not merely the staff's perceived responsibilities, but their actual legal and organizational ones" (Strauss et al., 1974, p. 566). Further, moral values about how one expresses pain and whether or not it should be relieved are as unique to practitioners as they are to the individuals experiencing pain. Moral judgments such as whether pain is "real" and how the patient must express his or her pain for the staff to consider the expression acceptable along with misconceptions, such as exaggerated fears about addiction, often result in the nurse withholding pain relief measures, especially narcotics (Marks & Sachar, 1973; McCaffery & Hart, 1976; Cohen, 1980). When the lack of knowledge about pharmacological agents is coupled with the lack of knowledge about noninvasive pain relief methods, such as guided imagery or distraction, much more of the nurse's effort may be directed at controlling the patient's expression of pain rather than relieving it. Even if the nurse is knowledgeable about pain relief methods, if she or he does not feel responsible for relieving the patient's pain, she or he may not make it a priority to objectively and systematically assess the patient's pain problem, let alone teach the patient some of the noninvasive pain-relief techniques.

One wonders about the lack of accountability by health professionals for pain management. Are we more likely or willing to assume accountability for pain which we have had first-hand experience with such as a headache or dental pain and thus can validate and legitimize, than the more complicated or diagnostically elusive pain problems that we are less likely to have experienced? It is easy to discredit things of which we do not have personal knowledge or of which we are afraid. Does the patient's feelings of fear of his or her pain and powerlessness to control it confront us with our own vulnerability and limitations and trigger a denial of his or her experience?

Diagnostic dilemmas often result in treatment dilemmas. By not diagnosing the patient's pain as a problem, the nurse may both overtly and covertly communicate "grin and bear it" to those suffering individuals. Although the directive for the health team is "Primum, non nocere" ("First of all, do no harm") the nurse's failure to do anything about pain assessment and relief may not only be a great injustice to the patient but may also result in serious harm.

It is incumbent upon the health professional to put a diagnostic label on the patient's problems, preferably prior to instituting treatment. Thus, it is not at all surprising that there is often great difficulty devising a treatment plan for the patient with pain if the diagnosis or etiology is uncertain. This becomes especially problematic if one is even questioning whether or not an individual has pain and if it exists to the degree the patient says it does. With our obvious uncertainty it is little wonder that patients themselves may not have much information about their pain or how to relieve it. The patient may not know whether pain relief is even available for this particular episode of pain. He or she may have no idea of the types of pain relief, how to obtain them, from whom, or to what degree a selected intervention will alleviate the pain. The patient may not know to whom he or she should report the pain, or when. On the other hand, the patient may have some very definite ideas about each of these points. It becomes increasingly clear that an objective accurate nursing assessment of the patient experiencing pain is a nursing imperative.

The primary focus of this chapter is to examine the nurse's clinical work with patients experiencing pain and explain how an accurate nursing diagnosis facilitates accountability and responsibility for pain management. Other areas that are considered in this chapter are the professional and legal mandates for accountability and responsibility for patients with pain. First, we will review some of the current interest in and economics of pain as a major health problem.

RECENT INTEREST IN THE STUDY OF PAIN

Health professionals, scientists, and the lay public have shown increasing interest in algology or dolorogy, the science of pain. Journals of the various health professions have begun to publish many more articles on pain. It is estimated that between 1972 and 1977 over 2400 articles and books related to pain were published (Buckwalter, et al. 1977). This is a dramatic increase in published information on pain as is readily apparent by looking up "pain" in the index of any nursing textbook published in the 1950s or 1960s. There, a few pages will be listed and on those pages only a few sentences will deal with pain relief. Now, some nursing textbooks contain entire chapters on pain, and books devoted to the subject of pain alone are available. Another encouraging indicator of nurses' concern and desire to treat pain as a major health problem was demonstrated in a nationwide survey designed to probe priorities for clinical nursing research. Pain management was identified as being among those topics with the greatest potential value to the profession (Lindeman, 1975).

In 1974, an association devoted to dolorogy was founded, the International Association for the Study of Pain (IASP). Their goals are to foster research, promote education, and facilitate the dissemination of information about pain. Scientists, physicians, nurses, and other health professionals from all over the world who are interested in the objectives of the IASP are eligible for membership (International Association for the Study of Pain, 1974).

It has become increasingly common to see some of the leading authorities on pain as guests on television and radio talk shows. In addition, there have been programs devoted exclusively or in part to discussions about the subject of pain. Indeed, if organizations that assess programming popularity are as influential in determining what is broadcast as we are led to believe, programs about pain fare quite well. Many of the authorities are repeatedly invited back to "guest" and some of the programs are rerun. Some have even reported back on the evolution of an area related to pain, such as a program devoted to an update of the drug dimethyl sulfoxide, DMSO.

In spite of this recent interest in the study of pain, it seems perhaps only the tip of the total pain-problem iceberg is being reached. This comment is based on information presented by the president of the IASP, J. J. Bonica, M.D., D.Sc., on the magnitude and cost of chronic pain (discussed later in this chapter) and his illustration of the attention paid to one major area of chronic pain—the cancer pain syndrome. Bonica says that "even though there are good drug and other pain relief modalities for treating the one million Americans afflicted with cancer pain each year, most of these patients spend their last weeks and months with unrelieved pain, suffering, and disability. This results in depriving these patients of a quality to their lives" (1980, p. 23).

In Table 1.1, Bonica illustrates what he refers to as "a total lack of interest or concern about the problem of cancer pain by oncologists." Of the nearly 9500 pages in ten of the most important textbooks and monographs on cancer less than 18 pages are devoted to the treatment of cancer pain (1980, pp. 24–25).

What about government concern to deal with the major health problem, pain? If there is a correlation between the amount of research funding for a problem and the degree of concern and commitment to solving it, then the situation for advancing algology by our government is very discouraging. Very little money has been allocated for pain-related research. In the 1970s the National Institutes of Health (NIH) spent about $2.2 billion on research, but only $34 million, or 1.5 percent was spent on pain. Research specifically directed to pain as a disease entity was less than $3 million, or about 0.014 percent of the total biomedical research budget (Bonica, 1976).

TABLE 1.1. Discussion of Pain In Oncology Textbooks

Title of Book	Authors	Year of Publication	Total Pages	Pages Devoted to Pain Therapy
Cancer Medicine	Holland & Frei	1974	2,018	13
Clinical Oncology	Horton & Hill	1977	819	2½
Cancer Diagnosis, Treatment and Prognosis	Ackerman & Del Regato	1970	783	None*
Cancer: Manual For Practitioners	Mass. Division Am. Cancer Soc.	1968	408	None
Clinical Oncology: Manual for Students & Doctors	Committee on Professional Education U.I.C.C.	1973	322	1¼
Advances in Cancer Surgery	Najerian & Delaney	1976	608	None
Principles of Surgical Oncology	R. W. Raven (ed)	1976	510	None
Clinical Oncology	U.I.C.C.	1978	304	None
Clinical Oncology for Medical Students and Physicians (3rd ed)	Rubin & Bakemeier Am. Cancer Soc.	1971	429	None
Cancer Vol. 1-6	Becker	1975–1977	3,082	None

*This volume contains brief description of pain associated with different types of cancers but does not discuss pain therapy. *(Bonica, J.J. Pain Research and Therapy: Past and Current Status and Future Needs. In L.K.Y. Ng & J.J. Bonica (Eds.) Pain, Discomfort and Humanitarian Care, Proceedings of the National Conference. Bethesda, MD: National Institutes of Health. February 15-16, 1979. New York: Elsevier/North-Holland, 1980, p. 25, with permission).*

TREATMENT FACILITIES FOR PATIENTS WITH PAIN

Beginning in the early 1970s, numerous pain clinics were established throughout the United States and a few in other countries. The underlying philosophy of most clinics is that almost all patients can receive some assistance in coping with their pain problem. Although theoretically any patient could be treated at a pain clinic, most clinics focus on working with patients with chronic benign pain. Some also treat patients with acute pain, especially those with a diagnosis of cancer. These clinics all differ, but most clinics offer a variety of treatment modalities including invasive measure such as medications, acupuncture, and surgery and noninvasive measures such as biofeedback, self-hypnosis, and nutritional counseling. The clinics may be conducted as either inpatient or outpatient units. While these pain clinics have treated many patients with pain, there is increasing awareness of the fact that there are not nearly enough pain clinics to meet the needs of the vast numbers of patients who could potentially benefit from them. Some pain clinics have waiting lists so long that it will take months, even years, for all of the patients to be seen.

Other options to pain clinics that are receiving increased utilization include hospices, which treat only terminally ill patients, holistic health centers, and individuals who specialize in some service which may benefit the patient with pain, such as acupuncturists, anesthesiologists, and psychologists.

COST OF HAVING AND TREATING PAIN

The monetary cost of pain is a major problem. On the one hand, the occurrence of acute pain can be expensive. For example, recovery from illness or surgery may be delayed when uncontrolled pain prevents the patient from assuming adequate physical activity or nutritional intake. With chronic pain the cost is considerably greater, although the exact amount is unknown. Again in the 1970s, at the National Conference on Pain, Discomfort and Humanitarian Care in February, 1979, Bonica speculated on the incidence and cost of chronic pain. He estimated that over one-third of the American population have persistent or recurrent pain problems necessitating medical intervention. Fifty million of the patients with pain problems are partially, totally, or even permanently disabled *not* by the underlying pathology, such as cancer or arthritis, but by their pain. These pain problems not only preclude the afflicted from carrying out a productive life but are also extremely costly in other ways. Bonica presents statistics that demonstrate that over 700 million work days are lost each year. Combined with other costs this totals nearly $60 billion annually, a figure which equals more than 10 percent of the national budget. This information is summarized in Table 1.2 (Bonica, 1980, pp. 10–11).

TABLE 1.2. Prevalence and Cost of Chronic Pain States in the United States

Pathological Process or Type of Pain	Prevalence (in Millions of Patients)		Disability (Millions of Pts)		Work Days Lost		Health Care Costs $ Billions	Other Costs $ Billions	Total Costs $ Billions
			Partial	Total	No. in Millions	Cost $ Billions			
Chronic back Disorders (including hip and lower extremity)	Low back	17.7	8.0	2.4	240	12.0	4.0	1.6	17.6
	Other	5.3							
	Total	23.0							
	Painful	18.4							
Arthritis[a] Rheumatism Gout	RA	7.0	5.0	0.6	160	8.0	5.2	1.9	15.1
	OA	16.5							
	Other	4.5							
	Total	28.0							
	Painful	19.0							
Other Musculo-skeletal Disorders Myofascial Upper limb	Total	5.0	3.0	—	12	0.6	0.4	0.2	1.2
	Painful	3.0							

Recurrent Headaches[b]								
Migraine Others	M/M21 S/SV 15 M/M40 S/SV 20	4d/yr 2d/yr	—	124	6.2	1.2	—	7.4
Cardiac Pain	Myocardial Infarction 0.5 Ang Pect 2.7 Total 3.2	2.8	0.4	110	5.5	5.6	—	11.1
Cancer Pain[b]	M/M 0.75 S/VS 0.25 Total 1.00	0.6	0.25	?20	1.0[c]	?0.5[c]	0.2[c]	1.7[c]
Other Chronic Pain States Orofacial Neuralgic Visceral Vascular	? 5.0–7.0	?1.2	?0.2	?40	?2.0	?1.8	?0.3	?4.1
Total	Total Disorders 126.2 Painful 86.6	55.6	3.85	706	35.3	18.7	4.2	58.2

[a]RA = rheumatoid arthritis; OA = osteoarthritis: Other = other types

[b]M/M = mild to moderate; S/VS = severe to very severe pain

[c]Estimated cost of pain therapy only. In all other instances, cost also includes health care for underlying process. (*Pain Research and Therapy: Past and Current Status and Future Needs by Bonica J.J. in Ng L.K.Y. & Bonica J.J. (Eds.) Pain, Discomfort and Humanitarian Care, Proceedings of the National Conference. Bethesda, MD: National Institutes of Health, February 15-16, 1979, p. 11*).

On the other hand, a different approach to the treatment of pain is also costly. That is, to attempt to relieve pain more effectively may be expensive. With acute pain, giving a sufficient amount of narcotic to relieve pain after a thoracotomy, for example, may require additional personnel to monitor and administer intravenous doses and to provide artificial ventilation because of the respiratory depressant effects of the narcotic.

The cost per patient for a program to relieve chronic pain will vary considerably, ranging from $200 for outpatient treatment using one or two pain relief methods to $20,000–$25,000 for four to eight weeks of hospitalized nonsurgical multimodality treatment. If surgery is involved, the cost is much greater. Success is not guaranteed regardless of the approach.

SOCIAL AND LEGAL DIRECTIVES TO THE NURSE TO BE ACCOUNTABLE FOR ASSESSING PAIN

In addition to the moral and ethical reasons why nurses are obligated to assess the patient's pain problem, nurses are mandated legally by the consumer through government and court systems and professionally through our own professional organizations. We are informed about what we must do for the patient to meet the minimum standards of acceptable professional practice. In recent years there has been a deluge of information in both professional and lay literature on this subject. One of the early publications which had an impact on the direction of standards for health care was "The Patient's Bill of Rights" (American Hospital Association, 1972). This listed what the patient, as a consumer of health care, had a right to expect from the health care providers such as hospitals and health care professionals. Now, not only are we told what these standards are and how we must meet them, but we are also told what happens to the consumer and to us, as health professionals, if we fail to meet them.

There are several terms currently used synonymously to reflect our responsibilities for an organized system to improve the quality of health care using standards of professional practice as the criterion for evaluation. They include Quality Assurance, Quality Control, Audit, Peer Review, and Professional Standards Review Organizations (PSROs).

Many nurses may think that this structured method of setting standards and evaluation of patient care is a new concept and/or approach. This is far from true. In fact, in 1855, Florence Nightingale presented a paper for discussion at the Statistical Conference entitled "Miss Nightingale's Scheme for Uniform Hospital Statistics." Her objective for collecting statistics was to improve the quality of patient care and to attempt to foster the use of a uniform format for the collection of such statistics (Jensen et al., 1959).

Ernest Codman, M.D. was also concerned with statistics as a method of establishing professional standards. In 1900, he developed a method of evaluation of medical practice known as "end result analysis." This concept was adopted by the American College of Surgeons in 1912. These surgeons attempted to have a uniform format for the medical record instituted to accurately document the patient's clinical progress. In 1918, the American College of Surgeons also developed a Hospital Standardization Program to identify health care facilities committed to the highest ideals of medical practice. The Joint Commission on Accreditation of Hospitals (JCAH) is an outgrowth of Codman's original work and evolved because of the magnitude and expense of monitoring the quality of health care, which could no longer be assumed by the professional organizations which had organized to attempt to accomplish this. Initially, the sole purpose of the JCAH was "to encourage the voluntary attainment of uniformly high standards of institutional medical care" (Joint Commission on Accreditation of Hospitals, 1980, p. x). Today their functions have expanded to include consultation, education, and evaluation (p. xii).

In 1965, when the Medicare Law, Public Law 89–97, was enacted, the Social Security Administration published "Conditions for Participation." In this publication, standards for health care which had been identified by JCAH were identified as those which would be considered as the norms for health care and qualify hospitals to participate in Medicare programs. Hospitals, which had been accredited by JCAH on a voluntary basis, were automatically considered in compliance with the federal regulations for Medicare (Joint Commission on Accreditation of Hospitals, 1980, p. x).

What makes Quality Assurance really seem like a relatively new idea, however, is that in 1972 Congress passed an amendment to the Social Security Act. Two critical and far-reaching directives of this amendment, referred to as Public Law 92–603, influence us as health professionals. First, this law mandated the establishment of Professional Standards Review Organizations to review the quality and cost of health care for Medicare, Medicaid, and Maternal Child Health Programs. As a profession we were told that we must accomplish this by 1976 and our failure to do so would result in the government doing it for us (Marriner, 1979). Second, the law provided for optional, random surveys of all hospitals which had been accredited by JCAH. This provided the Department of Health, Education, and Welfare with its own method of internal control to audit and monitor standards of health care and to respond to complaints. Although one can say that accreditation by JCAH "signifies a professionally motivated voluntary commitment to self-evaluation and self-improvement," very serious and often disastrous consequences await a facility failing to achieve compliance with these standards. Failure to comply with warnings may result in a temporary closure of a department and/or permanent closure of the entire health facility and ineligibility for reimbursement for services from third party payors such as Medicare. Without this financial support many agencies would not be able to survive economically (JCAH, 1980, p. xii).

In addition to these social laws, there are criminal laws that significantly influence professional practice. Most nurses must be aware of the increased incidence of malpractice litigation against health care professionals. These suits result when the consumer of the health care professional's services feels that he or she has incurred damages through criminal negligence by the failure of the health care professional to meet the standards of her or his profession.

Health care providers have responded to social forces, demands, and threats in a variety of ways. Some of these include requiring appropriate licensure, credentialling, and continuing education of their staff. Other facilities offer programs in such things as problem solving, communication skills, and stress-reduction techniques. Still others have developed specialized departments in utilization review, patient education, and patient advocacy or patient relations.

CAN NURSES REALLY INFLUENCE THE DIRECTION OF THE CARE OF THE PATIENT WITH PAIN?

With all of the challenges and obstacles facing the nurse, one may wonder if there is any possibility that the patient with pain can expect to receive the type of nursing expertise he or she needs. A very optimistic note about the potential influence of the nurse is offered by Ramphal (1974). She says "Neither bureaucratic controls nor the medical profession can ensure quality because they do not have any relationship to improvement of the quality of nursing care provided. The introduction of peer review could tip the balance of power since it could increase the strength of nursing to implement its own group decisions and to resist interference in such decisions from groups of nonnurses" (p. 66).

The nurse's responsibility to make a unique contribution to the patient is evident in the American Nurses Association's (ANA) definitions of Nursing Practice and Philosophy of Peer Review. The ANA's Congress for Nursing Practice has defined nursing practice as "a direct service, goal-directed, and adaptable to the needs of the individual, family, and community during health and illness." The Association goes on to state: "Professional practitioners of nursing bear primary responsibility and accountability for the nursing care clients/patients receive. The purpose of Standards of Nursing Practice is to fulfill the profession's obligation to provide and improve this practice . . . through a systematic approach to Nursing Practice" (ANA Standards of Nursing Practice, 1973). Their statement of their philosophy of peer review is that "nursing care affects the outcome of the patient's illness and influences his future health status and even though nursing shares responsibility for patient care with many health disciplines, there exists identifiable outcomes that are primarily attributable to nursing care" (ANA Philosophy of Peer Review, 1974).

Because our responsibilities and accountability are clearly defined by our profession the question, therefore, is not *can* the nurse really influence the direction of the care for the patient with pain but rather *how* can the nurse make a major impact on the care of the patient with pain.

OPERATIONAL DEFINITION OF PAIN AND ITS IMPLICATION FOR NURSING PRACTICE

The primary goal for the nurse in working with the patient with pain is to eliminate the patient's pain if this is possible and desirable. When this is not possible or desirable, the minimal goal becomes one of reducing the patient's pain to a level that enables him to sustain some quality of life and to continue to search for the cause of his pain through assessment and reassessment.

Before the nurse can embark on establishing a nursing diagnosis for the patient with pain she or he must have a clear operational definition of pain. We feel that the only one who can be the real authority on whether an individual is experiencing pain or not is the individual. Our operational definition of pain is "Pain is whatever the experiencing person says it is, existing whenever he [or she] says it does" (McCaffery, 1968, p. 8; 1979, p. 11).

Our philosophy on whether or not and how to assess the patient with pain is consistent with the Rationale for and the First Standard of Nursing Practice developed to provide a basis for the provision and improvement of the quality of our professional nursing service. The Rationale states "Comprehensive care requires complete and ongoing collection of data about the client/patient to determine the nursing care needs of the client/patient. All health status data about the client/patient must be available for all members of the health care team". And the first Standard is that "The collection of data about the health status of the client/patient is systematic and continuous. The data are accessible, communicated, and recorded" (ANA Standards of Nursing Practice, 1973).

POTENTIAL STUMBLING BLOCKS TO AN ACCURATE NURSING DIAGNOSIS

Both the patient's and the nurse's beliefs about pain may preclude an accurate nursing diagnosis of the patient's pain problem. Thus the patient ultimately may not receive adequate treatment for his pain. Some patients deny they have pain. Others cannot report their pain in an understandable way. Others will not report their pain. Still others may feel that the nurse knows their diagnosis and, therefore, whether or not they have pain and that they would do something about it if they felt they could or it were indicated. Because of these beliefs the patient may feel no responsibility for communicating about his pain. The patient may be correct in his assumption about the nurse's knowledge about his pain problem because there are two common areas that nurses often draw their conclusions about a patient's problem from. These are the degree of demonstrated pathophysiology and the patient's verbalizations about his symptoms or problems. The nurse may assume that if a patient has pain and it is troublesome enough to him he would report it. Or the nurse may feel that discussing the patient's pain may precipitate or increase his pain-related behaviors.

Reliance on demonstrated pathophysiology can be misleading in establishing a nursing diagnosis of pain. This often occurs for the patient who is admitted to the hospital for a medical diagnosis of chronic benign pain. Probably no one except the patient can fully realize how misleading this diagnosis is. A common definition of chronic benign pain is pain that is not life-threatening but which persists for six months or more. The medical dictionaries describe benign with such words as "mild" and "not recurrent". An example of such a patient is one who is admitted for diagnosis and treatment of low back pain. This patient may have irreversible musculoskeletal damage from the prolonged muscle spasm, including weakness and atrophy and an endocrine imbalance resulting in weight loss or gain, and sleep disturbances. Other complications that this patient may experience include irritability, depression, feelings of worthlessness and powerlessness, personality changes, decreased motivation, and suicidal ideation. Inability to maintain gainful employment and sustain significant relationships are also common consequences of such a pain problem. Truly, this is a pain-management problem that tends to snowball. Almost all of the complications of the pain problem can be either the cause or the effect of each other. For example, unrelieved pain leads to muscle tension, insomnia, and irritability. Insomnia may result in increased pain, irritability, and muscle tension. The patient with chronic benign pain may have minimal demonstrated pathophysiology yet the complexities of his pain problem may totally destroy the quality of his life and perhaps that of his significant others.

An example of the erroneous beliefs of both a patient and a nurse occurred in a surgical intensive care unit. A patient who had open-heart surgery was visited 24 hours postoperatively by his daughter, a nurse. She asked her father how much pain he had and what had been done to relieve it. He informed her that he imagined he had the expected amount of pain, that no one had asked him about his pain, and that nothing had been done to relieve it. His doctor had informed him, he said, that he would have pain in the postoperative period. He went on to state that the staff knew what was normal in this intensive care unit and if there were anything that they could do they would have done it. His daughter explained why it may be necessary for him to indicate to the staff that he had pain and ask for something to relieve it. In spite of his daughter's explanation this patient neither requested nor received any treatment for pain during his entire hospitalization. Unfortunately, this is not an uncommon occurrence.

Jacox & Stewart (1973) studied patients' expression of pain. Of the 72 patients they studied, approximately two-thirds of the patients stated they tried to remain calm and not show that they were in pain. They also stated that they were reluctant or ambivalent about discussing their pain. Marks & Sachar (1973) studied 37 hospitalized patients experiencing pain. They found that the patient's response to a general question about pain correlated poorly with answers to specific questions about pain. Specific questions resulted in more complete information about the pain problem.

Even if the nurse were correct about her fear that discussing the patient's pain with him may result in an increase in his pain-related behaviors, we agree with Jacox & Stewart (1973) who noted that the assessment of pain would seem to be overall less detrimental than assuming that patients will report pain spontaneously. We believe further that the possible negative effects of a thorough assessment of a patient's pain problem are neither as frequent nor as serious as the nurse may fear. If pain-related behaviors are caused or increased by the nurse's assessment then she may need to alter her method of assessment. No matter what, the nurse must not allow her preconceived notions about pain to inhibit her search for the cause and treatment of the patient's pain problem.

We will now consider establishing the nursing diagnosis for the patient with pain and then look at a possible system for communicating the information we have obtained through our assessment.

ESTABLISHING A NURSING DIAGNOSIS FOR THE PATIENT WITH PAIN

Because patients are reluctant or ambivalent about discussing their pain Jacox & Stewart have suggested that it might be "useful for nurses to assume that all patients are experiencing some type of discomfort or pain" (1973, p. 152). Based on their research, they say that "nurses must encourage patients to discuss their pain, and not simply wait until the patient complains or requests pain medication" (p. 151).

The nursing assessment is a logical sequential method for obtaining such information. It is also the basis on which to establish a nursing diagnosis, set goals, establish plans, interventions and evaluation of the care for the patient with pain.

Gebbie & Lavin (1974) defined a nursing diagnosis as "the identification of those patient problems or concerns most frequently identified by nurses, problems which are usually identified by nurses before they are recognized by other health care workers, and problems which are amenable to some intervention which is available in the present or potential scope of nursing practice" (p. 250). At the American Nurses' Association Biennial Convention (1976) the House of Delegates made a resolution on the classification system of nursing diagnosis. They stated that a "Nursing Diagnosis describes actual or potential health problems which nurses are capable of and licensed to treat". Also, at the second National Conference on Classification of Nursing Diagnoses, "Pain" and "Discomfort" were identified as acceptable diagnostic labels (Gebbie, 1976).

McCaffery (1979) qualified the content for inclusion in the statement of the nursing diagnosis for the patient with pain to include the "(1) type of pain, (2) factors that influence the existence and characteristics of the pain sensation, (3) patient's behavioral responses to the pain experience, and (4) factors that influence the patient's pain sensation" (p. 286). She also recommended as a method of possibly moblizing the health team's energy to treat pain to include a statement about the detrimental effect of pain on the patient. An example of a nursing diagnosis for the patient with pain then might be: "The patient is experiencing acute burning epigastric pain of moderately severe intensity, increased during periods of hunger, nothing by mouth (NPO), and during and after his wife's visits. During the pain episodes the patient's pulse is 110, respirations 30, and blood pressure 140/90. He becomes diaphoretic, cries and moans. He will ask for pain relief measures and obtains 90 percent relief from food or antacids. If he does not experience pain relief his pulse increases to 130, respirations to 40, and blood pressure to 160/100, and he becomes profusely diaphoretic, motionless, and silent."

Reassessment of the patient's pain problem is warranted as long as the patient has pain and is particularly important when pain is poorly relieved. In addition to determining the cause of the pain this continued reassessment may fortify the patient's faith in the health team. Patients with pain who have had difficulty in having a diagnosis for the cause of their pain confirmed may be convinced that no one believes that they have pain or if they do that it is not as severe as they say it is. The sensitive communication utilized in the assessment and diagnosis of the patient's pain problem may provide him with an increased sense of self-respect, dignity and hope that relief and/or a cause which is treatable will be found.

Other reasons that make reassessment very important include the possibility that the patient has changed his goal for his health care and failed to communicate it to the staff. His behavior may be inadvertently mislabelled if he abandons a pain relief measure which was collaboratively planned with him. Also, the patient's pain problem may have been resolved. Notation of this is vital to providing accurate, ongoing diagnosis and treatment. Assessment without proper documentation may be of little value to the patient and, in fact, may extend his diagnostic workup and/or erroneous treatment, causing him further pain and time lost in resolving his pain problem.

RECORDING AND COMMUNICATING THE NURSING ASSESSMENT AND DIAGNOSIS—THE PROBLEM-ORIENTED RECORD

Unfortunately nurses' notes, nursing histories, and nursing care plans receive little attention and are often ridiculed not only by nurses but also by other members of the health team. Nurses often resent complying with the required documentation they must make in nursing notes, nursing care plans, nursing histories, and recording in other sections of the record such as vital sign sheets, and medication records. Reasons frequently cited by the nurses for their resentment include that no one reads their charting, that it is redundant (the same information is recorded in several places), it is time consuming, and it minimizes the time available to provide direct patient care. Not only can the nurse's lack of interest and accurate recording lead to disrespect from other health members but it also can lead to very serious consequences for the patient because all of his signs, symptoms, and other relevant behavior may not be evaluated in relation to his health problems and current status.

Unfortunately, the nurses' feelings about the merits of their charting seem to be well founded. Walker & Selmanoff (1964) and Walker et al. (1965) found that the recording of nurses' notes was, in fact, of little significance to the nursing or medical staff. They suggested the following reasons for this negative attitude toward nurses' notes.

1. The notes did not serve as an effective means of communication. Much information was omitted, and verbal communication had been substituted for written.
2. The former high status accorded to the writing of nurses' notes had diminished as lower levels of nursing personnel began writing in the record.
3. Lack of use by superiors had led to the assumption that the notes had little value.
4. Attempts to omit repetitive or meaningless recordings had resulted in no recording at all.

Healey & McGurk (1966) have also addressed the lack of value of the nurses' notes stating that they are considered repetitive, incomplete, and characterized by statements of procedure rather than by observations of response to care (p. 32).

The use of the patient's record was also viewed as problematic for physicians by Weed (1969). He felt that contributions of other health team members were not always logically accepted by physicians. In addition, he was concerned that the physicians' own use of medical records and charting did not always reflect the fact that each of the patient's problems had been well defined and logically pursued. The method of record keeping used exclusively at this time was known as the "Source Record". This is the traditional style of record, in which the data is organized according to the professional or department generating it, such as nurses' notes, physicians' progress notes, physicians' orders, laboratory reports, and radiology reports. To identify all of the patient's problems and their current status one must repeatedly read the entire record. Weed (1968) states that "there is no evidence that he [the physician] does this reliably and consistently; he and others using the record lose their way and problems get neglected, missed entirely, or treated out of context" (1969, p. 597).

To decrease the fragmentation of patient care and improve the quality of patient care, Weed devised a system of record keeping known as the "Problem Oriented Medical Record" often referred to as POMR or POR. His system attempts to accomplish its goal in two major ways. The first is to focus on the patient as an individual and the second is to collect and document data about the patient in a logical, systematic manner. This system of data collection gives evidence of the collaboration of the entire health team toward the resolution of the patient's problems. All health team members using the patient's record chronologically make entries rather than segregating their contributions by department or profession (pp. 597–599). The acronym for this approach to the patient and his medical record is "SOAP" referring to Subjective, Objective, Assessment, and Plan. Charting of information in this format is referred to as "SOAPING". When nurses use this format for their patient care and records they usually add "IE" for Intervention and Evaluation. Thus their acronym is "SOAPIE" but their charting is still referred to as "SOAPING".

Data collected during the initial assessment of the patient should be detailed and comprehensive. The Subjective data are provided from the patient, the patient's family, and nursing histories. The Objective data are obtained through laboratory tests, x-rays, other specialized test results, and the physical examination. This combined information is referred to as the "Data Base". From this assessment the patient's problems are identified and listed numerically. These problems include not only known diagnosis but symptoms which need to be studied. Therefore, pain from a known source such as trigeminal neuralgia and undiagnosed pain would both be listed as problems. The Problems identified during the initial assessment are used to initiate the "Problem List" which is considered to be the "Table of Contents" for the medical record. Problems are categorized as Active and Inactive with the list being modified as additional data are collected. At the time of the collection of the initial data, data which needs to be monitored regularly are setup and recorded on "Flow Sheets" like vital signs and intake and output sheets. Information on the "Flow Sheets" should include the date, time, the frequency with which the problem is to be monitored, the content to be monitored, and variables which influence it. All information is reported chronologically. (A flow sheet for the patient with pain is presented in the final chapter of this book.) In addition to the documentation of the Subjective and Objective findings of the assessment of the problem, the Plans for the management of that problem are recorded and each problem is numbered (Weed 1969, pp. 597–599). An example of "SOAPING" for the patient in the previous example who had burning epigastric pain might be as follows:

Problem List

1/31/81 10:30 A.M.	#1	Epigastric Pain
	S	continues to c/o burning epigastric pain, mod. severity, $\uparrow$ by hunger, NPO, wife's visits
	O	P 110-130, R 30-40 BP 140/90-160/100, profuse diaphoresis, crying during and after wife's visits
	A	(See previous Nursing Diagnosis)
	P	1. Continue to offer food and antacids prophylactically 2. Discuss social work consult to assess family situation
	I	1. Evaluate crying with patient prior to wife's next visit 2. Involve patient in gaining control to $\downarrow$ stress and pain 3. Nurses to teach Patient-Guided Imagery
	E	90% pain $\downarrow$ from food and/or antacids

Utilization of this format for recording a patient's pain problem would provide a channel for accountability and responsibility not only by the nurse but by the whole health team. Pain certainly would emerge as a problem in need of much more attention than it has received.

Auditing Nursing Practice Through The Nursing Record

As previously discussed, legally, nursing practice must be monitored. The system utilized for monitoring nursing practice is referred to as an audit, and the nursing audit is defined as an objective systematic method based on explicit measurable criteria that can be applied to a number of patients for the purpose of documenting and improving provider performance and the quality of care (Nadolnay, 1979).

There are three types of audit which obtain this data. The first considers the structure, the second the process, and the third the outcome. The purpose of the *structure audit* is to review things which influence the delivery of health care, such as the purpose of the hospital, the method of management, systems of recording patient care, and the qualifications and orientation of employees. The purpose of the *process audit* is to evaluate the functioning and judgment of the nurses while the patient care is being provided. Questions raised to determine this may include: Does the nursing care reflect the use of the nursing process? Does it reflect the rationale for the nurse's interventions? The purpose of the *outcome audit* is to determine the results and effectiveness of the care provided. Questions raised for this type of audit may include: Were the goals achieved? Did the patient's symptoms abate? Did the patient improve? Obviously, all three systems of audit influence each other.

Auditing may be done either concurrently or retrospectively. The concurrent audit occurs while the patient is still in the hospital. Data for the concurrent audit are obtained through direct observation of the staff while they are providing patient care or through interviews with the patients, families, and staff members. Interviewing may be done either individually or in groups. Retrospective auditing is done after the patient is discharged. Although post-questionnaires and interviews may be used, the method most frequently employed is a review of the patient's record and nursing care plans.

One of the problems in auditing nursing records is that the audit basically measures an individual's professional performance. Most hospitals employ nurses with a great variation in their educational preparation and levels of sophistication and experience. This necessitates a team approach to providing nursing care. How can a nurse truly be responsible and accountable for another team member, especially if she or he is not known to the team leader or has just arrived on the unit as a float or from a registry? Other factors which may influence a nurse's performance and ultimately the audit are the physical facility and the type of equipment available. For example, how much time is taken from providing direct nursing care if the nurse must run from one end of the corridor to another for a piece of equipment?

The criteria for the evaluation of patient care cannot be based on an arbitrary current level of practice in a given agency. They must be based on standards for the profession providing the service. The audit criteria are established by reviewing the relevant literature on the subject to be audited and audit criteria on the subject which have been developed by others. The audit process itself should generate much valuable information for establishing new criteria in addition to providing direct benefits both to patients with pain and to the staff caring for them. Documentation of pain problems and pain relief strategies can be more easily and clearly monitored and evaluated for effectiveness, quality, and frequency. Areas of strength and weakness can be elucidated by the gap between what is ideal and what is really occurring in professional practice. Specifically for the patient with pain, this information could lead to increasing the quality and streamlining the assessment process, modifications and revisions of pain relief strategies, and determining the staffing patterns and the education and experience required of the staff to adequately assess and intervene with patients with pain.

SUBSEQUENT CHAPTERS

The focus of the subsequent chapters of this book will be limited to the first step of the nursing process, which is to establish a sound data base through a systematic nursing assessment. Both preexisting factors and specific components of the pain experience itself will be discussed. The purpose of examining these variables in depth is to help foster in those working with a patient in pain an understanding and acceptance of the unique manner in which a person may express pain. Another important goal is to help people realize that an individual may express the same type of pain in a different manner from time to time and may express different types of pain in different manners. For example, a football player may be willing to endure considerable pain from a football injury on the football field and exhibit almost no expression of pain. Yet, he may vehemently complain about a headache between games.

The information in the following chapters is divided into two parts, Part A and Part B. Part A takes a look at preexisting factors that affect the person's highly personal experience with pain. These factors cannot be viewed as having a predictable or specific relationship to the patient's response to pain. As yet, there is no agreement about cause and effect. However, these factors often seem to be associated with similarities and differences and reactions to the pain experience. Part A is divided into three chapters, beginning with Chapter 2. Chapter 2 deals with the neurophysiology of pain. Content discussed includes the basic organization and functional components of the nervous system specifically related to pain perception, how information is transmitted and processed, and major theories of pain mechanisms. Chapter 3 presents information on the major cultural variables which may influence the patient's pain experience. There is a dearth of such information in the literature and the available studies are often controversial. However, in an attempt to encourage the nurse to appreciate how cultural diversity may affect the patient's perception and response to pain, how her own culture and that of her colleagues may influence the patient's pain experience, and to provide the nurse with some rationale for her nursing interventions, the major findings of studies related to culture and pain will be reviewed. In Chapter 4, preexisting factors which influence one's pain experience and pain syndromes which are usually considered to be psychogenic will be reviewed. Some of the information presented includes algesic types, differences between introverts and extroverts, cognitive processes, level of vigilance, and past experiences with pain.

Part B, the assessment of the patient in pain, is divided into six chapters. The first chapter, Chapter 5, classifies the pain experience. The focus is on the type of pain in relation to the cause and duration, the phase of the pain experience (anticipation, presence, or aftermath), and how the patient has adjusted to the pain experience. Chapter 5 details the characteristics of the pain experience including onset, duration, location, intensity, quality, and variations which may occur at different times of the pain experience. Chapter 6 presents information on some of the more common pain syndromes, both those of pathological pain and pain from pathology. Chapter 7 views the effects of the pain experience on the patient. Topics to be considered will include the patient's response to pain. What does the patient do or not do that indicates he or she is in pain? Does he cry? Does blood pressure increase or decrease? What does the patient feel the pain does to his normal life style? Is the patient motivated to obtain pain relief? Why? Chapter 8 considers situational factors that influence the patient's pain experience. The patient's knowledge and understanding about the pain experience, the presence and attitudes of others and their effect on the patient, the influences of the environment on the patient, and possible secondary gains will be identified. Chapter 9 concerns the communication of pain. Topics addressed include the patient's ability and willingness to communicate about pain and how to enhance one's assessment through other resources when the patient is unwilling or unable to do so. In the final chapter, Chapter 10, methods and tools for the assessment of the patient's pain will be presented. Specific areas to be considered include tasks which the nurse may do in working with the patient in pain, general guidelines for assessment of the patient with pain, methods for ongoing specific and overall assessment, assessment tools, considerations when pain relief strategies do not result in pain relief, and for the more difficult pain problems, possible resources to which a patient may be referred.

The purpose of presenting this detailed information on the assessment of the patient in pain is to foster an understanding and acceptance of the possibility that the person with pain may respond in a variety of ways, that his or her response may vary with different types of pain and also with the same type of pain at different times. Even though some of the reasons for these variations among patients cannot necessarily be changed by the nurse, her or his understanding and accountability may facilitate a more constructive and supportive approach to the patient experiencing pain.

How then can we begin to understand what happens when we must work with patients who have pain or with those upon whom we inflict pain in the process of attempting to diagnose and treat the individual? The answer in part is an objective systematic assessment of the individual's pain.

REFERENCES

American Hospital Association: The Patient's Bill of Rights, Chicago: American Hospital Association, 1972.

American Nurses' Association: The American Nurse. Kansas City, MO: American Nurses' Association, September 1, 1976, (Vol. 8), No. 11, p. 9.

American Nurses' Association: Philosophy of Peer Review. Kansas City, MO: American Nurses' Association, 1974.

American Nurses' Association Congress for Nursing Practice: Standards of Nursing Practice. Kansas City, MO.: American Nurses' Association, 1973.

Bonica, J.J. Introduction to the First World Congress on Pain: Goals of IASP and the World Congress. In J.J. Bonica, & D. Albe-Fessard, (Eds.), Advances in Pain Research and Therapy (Vol 1). New York: Raven Press, 1976, pp. xxvii–xxxix.

Bonica, J.J. Pain research and therapy: Past and current status and future needs. In L.K.Y. Ng, & J.J. Bonica, (Eds.), Pain Discomfort and Humanitarian Care, Proceedings of the National Conference, National Institute of Health: Bethesda, MD., Feb. 15–16, 1979. New York: Elsevier/North-Holland, 1980.

Buckwalter, K.C., Rains, J.W. & Daniels, J.S. Annotated bibliography of pain literature. In A.K. Jacox, (Ed.). Pain: A Source Book for Nurses and Other Health Professionals. Boston: Little, Brown, 1977.

Cohen, F.L. Postsurgical Pain Relief: Patient's Status and Nurses' Medication Choices. Pain, 9, 265–274, 1980.

Gebbie, K.M. (Ed.). Summary of the Second National Conference: Classification of Nursing Diagnosis. St. Louis: Clearinghouse—National Group for Classification of Nursing Diagnosis, 1976.

Gebbie, K. & Lavin, M.A. Classifying nursing diagnosis. Amer J Nurs 74: 250–253, 1974.

Healy, E.E. & McGurk, W. Effectiveness and acceptance of nurses' notes. Nurs Outlook 14, (3): 32–34, 1966.

International Association for the Study of Pain: Articles of Incorporation and Bylaws. May 9, 1974, Washington, D.C.

Jacox, A.K. & Stewart, M. Psychosocial Contingencies of the Pain Experience. Iowa City, IA: University of Iowa, College of Nursing, 1973.

Jensen, D.M., Spalding, J.F., & Cady, E.L. History and Trends of Professional Nursing. St. Louis: C.V. Mosby, 1959.

Joint Commission on Accreditation of Hospitals: Accreditation Manual for hospitals, AMH (1981 ed.). Chicago: Joint commission on Accreditation of Hospitals, 1980.

Lindeman, C.A. Priorities in clinical nursing research. Nurs Outlook. 23: 693-698, 1975.

Marks, R.M., & Sachar, E.J. Undertreatment of medical inpatients with narcotic analgesics. Ann Intern Med 78: 173-181, 1973.

Marriner, A. The research process in quality assurance. Amer J Nurs 79: 2158-2161, 1979.

McCaffery, M. Cognition, Bodily Pain, and Man-environment Interactions. Los Angeles: University of California Student Store, 1967, (out of print).

McCaffery, M. Nursing Management of the Patient with Pain (2nd, ed.), New York: J.B. Lippincott, 1979.

McCaffery, M., & Hart, L.L. Undertreatment of acute pain with narcotics. Amer J Nurs 76: 1586-1591, 1976.

Nadolnay, M.D. The patient care audit. Hosp Topics November/December: 30-33, 1979.

Ramphal, M. Peer review. Amer J Nurs, 74: 63-67, 1974.

Strauss, A., Fagerhaugh, S.Y., & Glaser, B. Pain: An organizational-work-interactional perspective. Nurs Outlook, 22: 560-566, 1974.

U.S. Public Law 89-97.

U.S. Public Law 92-603.

Walker, V.H., McReynolds, D.A., & Patrick, E. A care plan for ailing nurses' notes. Amer J Nurs 65: 74-76, 1965.

Walker, V.H., & Selmanoff, E.D. A study of the nature and uses of nurses' notes. Nurs Res 13 (2): 113-121, 1964.

Weed, L. Medical records that guide and teach. New Eng J Med 278, (11): 593-600, 1968.

SUGGESTED READINGS

Aspinal, M.J. Nursing diagnosis—The weak link. Nurs Outlook, 24: 433-437, 1976.

Blount, M., Green, S.S., Harmony, A., et al. Documenting with the problem-oriented record system. Amer J Nurs 78: 1539-1542, 1978.

Bullough, B. The Medicare-Medicaid Amendments. Amer J Nurs 73: 1926-1929, 1973.

Campbell, C. Nursing Diagnosis and Intervention in Nursing Practice. New York: John Wiley, 1978.

Donabedian, A. Some issues in evaluating the quality of nursing care. Amer J Public Health 69: 1833-1836, 1969.

Glennin, C. Formulation of standards of nursing practice using a nursing model. In J.P. Riehl & C. Roy, (Eds.). Conceptual Models for Nursing Practice. New York: Appleton-Century-Crofts, 1974, pp. 234-246.

Gordon, M. Nursing diagnosis and the diagnostic process. Amer J Nurs 76: 1298-1300, 1976.

Haussman, R.K., & Hegyvary, S.T. Monitoring quality of nursing care, Pt. III, Professional review for nursing: An empirical investigation. DHEW publication no. HRA 77-70. Hyattsville, MD: U.S. Department of Health, Education, and Welfare, Public Health Service, Health Resources Administration, Bureau of Health Manpower, Division of Nursing, August, 1977.

Howe, J. The nursing process and standards of nursing practice. In M. Armstrong, et al. (Eds.). McGraw-Hill Handbook of Clinical Nursing. New York: McGraw-Hill, 1979.

Laros, J. Deriving outcome criteria from a conceptual model. Nurs Outlook 25: 333-336, 1977.

Lesnik, M.J. & Anderson, B.E. Nursing practice and the law (2nd ed.). Philadelphia: J.B. Lippincott, 1976.

Luckman, J. & Sorenson, K C. Medical-Surgical-Nursing, a Psychophysiologic Approach (2nd ed.), Philadelphia: W.B. Saunders, 1980, pp. 12-22.

Mitchell, P.H. A systematic nursing progress record-The problem-oriented approach. Nurs Forum XII (2): 187-210, 1973.

Phaneuf, M.C. The Nursing Audit: Profile for Excellence. New York: Appleton-Century-Crofts, 1972.

Phaneuf, M.C. Quality Assurance: A nursing view. Hospitals 47: 62-68, 1973.

Phaneuf, M.C., & Wandelt, M.A. Quality assurance in nursing. Nurs Forum, XIII (4): 329-345, 1974.

Vengrowski, S.M. Peer review in quality assurance. Amer J Nurs 78: 2094-2096, 1978.

PART A

Preexisting Factors That Influence the Individual's Pain Experience

2

Neurophysiological Aspects

The somewhat disconcerting fact is that there is no agreement about nociception, that is, what actually causes a sensation to be perceived as painful. Not only are there questions about the cultural and psychological influences on pain, but there is considerable controversy and lack of knowledge about how a stimulus is transformed into an awareness of pain. The anatomy and physiology involved in the reception, transmission, and perception of pain are extremely complex.

Although the patient and the nurse may equate the degree of pain with the seriousness of the patient's condition, this supposition often is not an accurate one. For example, cancer, frequently a life-threatening disease, rarely causes pain in its early stages. Therefore, pain is not listed by the American Cancer Society as an early warning sign of cancer. In contrast, a minor localized inflammation from an ingrown nail may produce significant pain as an early symptom. Few diseases or conditions do not have pain associated with some phase of their course. Indeed, pain is usually cited as nature's earliest sign of disease and the symptom which most frequently motivates the individual to seek medical care.

Because pain is a subjective experience, there is no direct relationship between stimulus and response. Even when significant metastatic bone lesions exist on x-ray examination, patients will not necessarily report higher degrees of pain sensation than the patients with less extensive lesions, nor will patients with comparable lesions report comparable pain sensations. In fact, the expectation that they will may lead to overkill or underkill prescriptions for the treatment of their pain problem. In addition, one's perception of one's pain, and the meaning one attributes to it and the disease may markedly influence the treatment an individual will seek and accept.

Initially, pain must be viewed as a symptom and its physical etiology pursued. Interventions for pain done prior to an accurate assessment may mask the true cause of the patient's pain thus causing further suffering and possibly even death by allowing the progression of signs, symptoms, and the disease process. A thorough assessment provides the opportunity of ascribing the accurate meaning to a given set of behaviors and variables such as a pain pattern.

Only after all physiological causes which are treatable by traditional medical and surgical techniques are ruled out does one treat pain as a disease entity. Even when pain becomes a treatable disease, vigilance must be maintained for *any changes and new symptoms*. Additional information may provide a more accurate diagnosis, therefore, possibly, a different treatment plan will be devised. One patient with severe pain illustrates this point. Two years prior to his referral to a pain clinic for intractable pain, this patient had received a diagnosis of cancer of the pancreas and had been treated with ongoing chemotherapy. This was done without a confirming tissue diagnosis. Because cancer of the pancreas is a difficult disease to diagnose, the algoloist believed it was essential to have a definitive tissue diagnosis to establish an accurate treatment plan for this patient's pain problem. However, by the time the patient had received this suggestion, he and his family felt that he had already suffered excessively. They were very reluctant to expose him to any further procedures which may result in additional pain and physical deterioration, let alone death. With much encouragement, the patient underwent diagnostic surgery. The tissue diagnosis was chronic pancreatitis, a treatable condition requiring a different treatment for the concommitant pain.

All pain is interpreted as such in the brain. Pain cannot exist unless impulses reach the higher cortical centers of a conscious individual. An unconscious person does not have pain. Pain does not exist in the tissues in which it is felt; the brain identifies the existence and location of pain. Although many exciting discoveries relating to pain have been made in recent years, the route by which impulses arrive in the brain is very complex and still not entirely known. Certain anatomical structures and physiological events are known to be associated with the transmission and processing of impulses that are eventually perceived by the individual as painful. The fact that specific chemical changes or nerves are involved in the transformation of a stimulus into felt pain does not necessarily explain how the sensation of pain is produced. That is, knowing *what* is involved is not the same as knowing *how* it all works together.

Following a brief overview of the anatomy and physiology associated with pain perception and response, theories about the mechanisms underlying the production of pain are discussed. For more detailed descriptions of current information on the anatomy and physiology of nociception, the reader is referred to Guyton (1981), Melzack (1973) Mountcastle (1980), and Ruch & Patton (1979).

ANATOMY AND PHYSIOLOGY OF NOCICEPTION

The body is coordinated, regulated, and integrated by two systems—the nervous system and the endocrine or hormonal system. Neither system functions independently nor is their function mutually exclusive. Through the transmission and processing of information from both the internal and external environments, the *nervous system* achieves its major function of modulating the physiological and psychological responses of the body. Processing by the central nervous system (CNS) involves channeling, comparing, averaging, and responding in a coordinated manner to the sensory input. In addition, the CNS is the substrate of conscious perception allowing the mind to become aware of information so that it can use it in a meaningful way. Other functions of the CNS include abstract thinking, reasoning, language expression, and emotion. The peripheral nervous system exerts primary control over such functions as muscular contraction, both skeletal and smooth, and endocrine and exocrine glandular functions through somatic and autonomic functional components.

The *endocrine system* exerts its control in response to other chemicals in the body or as a direct response to nervous system control. It does so by secreting hormones into body fluids. These hormones are composed of protein (large polypeptides) or protein derivatives (amino acids). Some hormones exert their effect locally, called *local hormones*, such as the kinins. Others have a more general effect, called *general hormones* like neurotransmitters such as ephinephrine. General hormones exert their influence at more distant sites and may do so by effecting all tissues of the body. Other hormones such as estrogen effect only specific tissues, called *target tissues*. Hormones exert their control by altering chemical reactions in the cells, changing the permeability of cell membranes, activating cellular mechanisms such as muscle contraction, increasing the cellular transportation of certain substances, and increasing enzymatic action of proteins.

Some nerve cells secrete chemical substances into the blood, thus extending the usual sensory, motor, and integrative functions of the nervous system to include a hormonal one. Neurons which possess both neurologic and endocrine functions are referred to as the *neuroendocrine system*. The general use of the word *neuroendocrine* pertains to the anatomic or functional relationship of the nervous and endocrine systems.

The Nervous System

Basic Organization The neuron with all of its processes, shown in Figure 2.1, is the anatomical and functional unit of the nervous system. The connective matrix of neurons is called *neuroglia* (nerve glue). *Afferent* neurons are nerve fibers which receive sensory stimuli from the outside environment and transmit them toward the *soma* (cell body) of the neuron and then through it to the axon. The fine freely branching afferent nerve fibers are called *dendrites* or *receptors*. They form an intricate network throughout the body in the skin, blood vessels, muscles, and viscera. *Efferent* fibers or *axons* have fewer branches and conduct impulses away from the

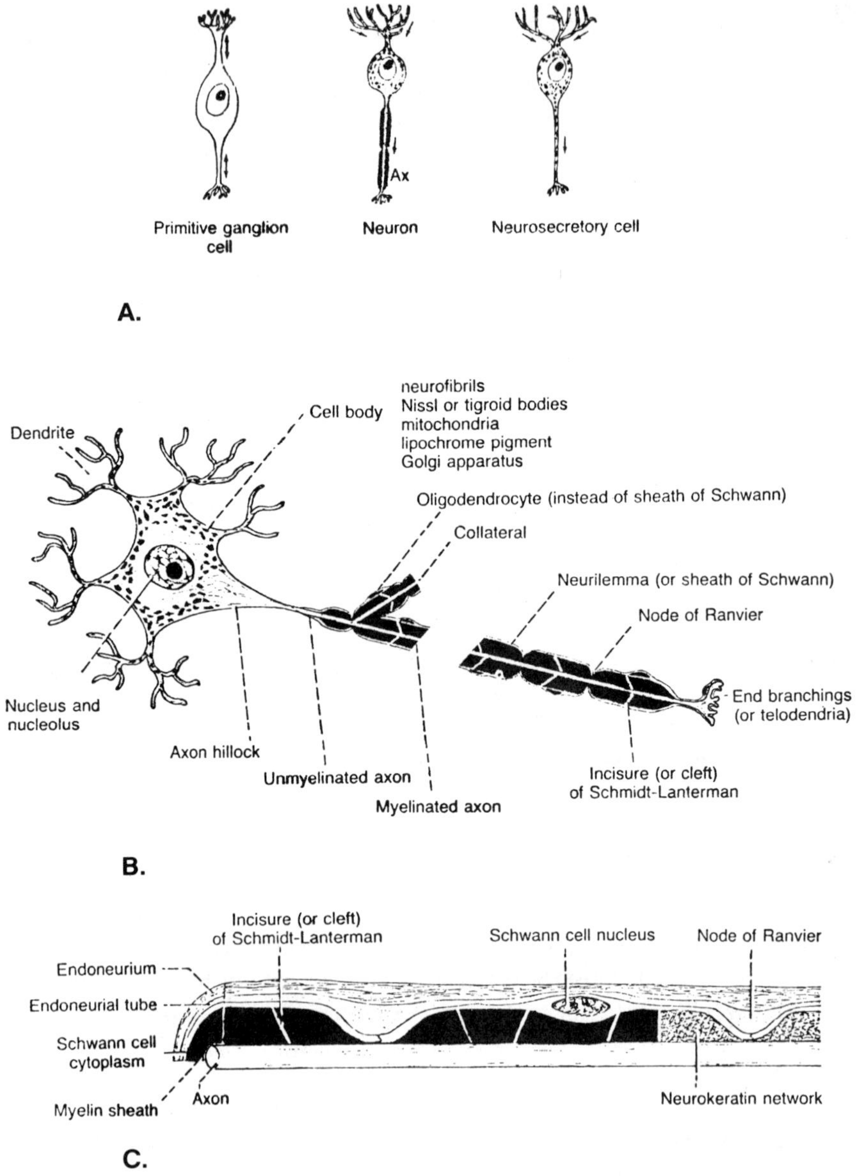

Figure 2.1. Diagram of (**A**) nerve cells, (**B**) a typical neuron, and (**C**) sheaths of a nerve fiber. *(Bossy, J. Atlas of Neuroanatomy and special sense organs. Philadelphia: W.B. Saunders, 1970, p. 5. (Modified from Ham, A.W. Histology (5th ed.) Philadelphia: J.B. Lippincott, 1965, p. 554.)*

soma of the neuron to the dendrite of another neuron, or to *effector* structures such as muscles and glands.

All nerve cells are encased in two discrete membranes called the *plasmalemma* and the *neurilemma*, or *sheath of Schwann (Schwann cells)*. Larger fibers are further encased in another membrane which lies between the plasmalemma and the neurilemma called the myelin sheath. The major function of Schwann cells is for nutrition of the cells and to insulate them so that there is minimal in-and-out movement of ions. However, for conduction of impulses along the sheath of Schwann, between every two successive Schwann cells there are uninsulated areas called *Nodes of Ranvier* where the electrical transmission of nerve impulses occurs in myelinated nerve fibers. After a peripheral nerve has been injured or destroyed, the Schwann cells proliferate and the axons sprout randomly out of a nerve ending. Some cross the transected area and enter the neurilemma of both sensory and motor terminals. If good fortune prevails, the proliferating cells may connect with a motor end-plate and function will be restored. Fibers in the central nervous system, brain, and spinal cord do not regenerate effectively.

There are three classes of nociceptive afferents, sensory nerve fibers which transmit information about pain. They are: 1) *nociceptive-specific* neurons, 2) *wide-dynamic range* neurons, and 3) *low-threshold mechanoreceptors*. *Nociceptive-specific neurons* respond to intense mechanical or thermal stimuli and may be activated by nonnoxious pressure. *Wide-dynamic range neurons* are activated by weak mechanical stimuli and hair movement. *Low-threshold mechanoreceptors* respond only to light touch, pressure, and hair movement.

The central nervous system is made up of aggregates of neurons called *neuronal pools* (see Figure 2.2). These pools vary in size and complexity, each having specific characteristics that account for the various functions of the nervous system. For example, the cerebral cortex is one large neuronal pool and the sensory gray matter of the spinal cord is a smaller one. Each neuronal pool has both afferent and efferent connections with other neuronal pools.

In addition to afferent and efferent neurons there is another type of neuron, the *interneuron* also referred to as the *association* or *internuncial* neuron. These neurons are found in the brain and spinal cord and conduct impulses from the primary afferent neuron to the final efferent motor neuron. Interneurons are located in all areas of the gray matter of the spinal cord. Most signals from the spinal cord and the brain are processed by the interneurons before they stimulate the efferent neurons. Interneurons often interconnect with each other in the same neuronal pool. They are highly excitable and fire rapidly. Because of their high degree of efficiency in processing information, only a few of the incoming sensory signals actually evoke a motor response. The reason for this will be explained later in this chapter.

Groups of nerve fibers are organized into *tracts*. These tracts are named by forming a word which contains the name of the site of origin followed by the name of the site of termination. For example, nerves in the spinothalamic tract originate in the spinal cord and terminate in the thalamus. The

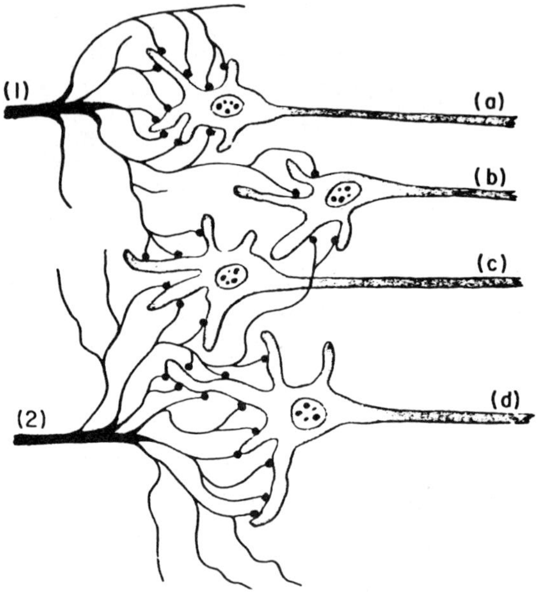

Figure 2.2. Schematic diagram of the basic organization of a neuronal pool. Input fibers, (1) and (2) are on the left. Output fibers (a), (b), (c), and (d) are on the right. Note that each input fiber divides hundreds to thousands of times providing an average of a thousand or more terminal fibrils that spread over a large area in the pool to synapse with the dendrites or cell bodies of the neurons in the pool. The dendrites of some of the neurons also arborize and spread in the pool. *(Guyton, A.C. Textbook of Medical Physiology, 6th ed. Philadelphia: W.B. Saunders, 1981, Figure 47.4 p. 579, with permission.)*

spatial organization of nerve fibers into tracts occurs throughout the entire nervous system from periphery to the somesthetic cortex and back down to the periphery. This spatial organization allows an individual to perceive and localize various types of both afferent and efferent sensory information, all with a reasonable degree of accuracy.

Nerves from the peripheral nervous system innervate segments of skin which are referred to as *dermatomes*. Dermatomes correspond to the segment of the body from which the viscera developed embryonically. For example, the heart developed in the neck and upper thorax. Thus, cardiac pain results from innervation of spinal segments from C-3 to T-5. On a diagram, the anatomical distribution appears discrete. In reality, however, the boundaries are only approximate. Dermatomes will be presented and illustrated as they relate to the sensation and referral of pain in Chapter 5 and to pain syndromes in Chapter 6.

The entire nervous system may be divided into two functional components: the peripheral nervous system and the central nervous system. We will now consider these more specifically in relation to pain. First, the peripheral nervous system will be discussed because acute pain usually is initiated here. Then we will consider the central nervous system, where the information about pain is transmitted and processed. Next, interactional systems which account for the dimensions of pain will be discussed.

The following section will present information on the transmission and processing of information in the nervous system such as electrical and chemical transmission including the neurotransmitters and neumodulators—the endorphins and other influencing factors of transmission. Finally, we will consider theories of mechanisms which produce pain as they relate to information known at this time.

Functional Components

The Peripheral Nervous System The *peripheral nervous system (PNS)* is composed of all the cranial and spinal nerves and their associated ganglia and as previously mentioned is divided into somatic and autonomic components. *Ganglia* are nerve cell bodies located outside the central nervous system in contrast to *nuclei* or nerve cell bodies within the central nervous system. Tissues and organs are linked to the CNS by sensory and motor spinal nerves of the PNS. The major components of a spinal nerve are illustrated on the left side of Figure 2.3. The anatomy of the spinal cord and transverse sections of the spinal cord at various levels are illustrated in Figure 2.4. Although sensory fibers conducting pain stimuli enter the spinal cord primarily through the dorsal roots and transmit signals to the central nervous system, it has now been found that some pain impulses are transmitted by ventral roots. The cell bodies of nociceptors from both the dorsal and ventral roots lie in the dorsal root ganglia. *Motor fibers* leave the central nervous system by way of the ventral roots of the spinal cord. There are two types of motor fibers, somatic and autonomic. *Somatic fibers* innervate skeletal muscles. *Autonomic fibers* innervate glands, cardiac muscle, and smooth muscles.

Information about pain is gleaned through five major categories of sensory receptors; the nociceptors, mechanoreceptors, thermoreceptors, chemoreceptors, and electromagnetic receptors. This information is communicated through the *special senses* of sight, hearing, taste, smell, equilibrium, and the somatic senses. The somatic senses include the mechanoreceptive somatic senses, thermoreceptive senses, and pain, the nociceptive sense.

The *mechanoreceptors* provide information about distortion of the receptor itself and/or adjacent cells. It does so through the kinesthetic sense (muscle sense) and the tactile senses—touch, pressure, and vibration. The somatic sensations may be grouped together as exteroreceptors, propricep-

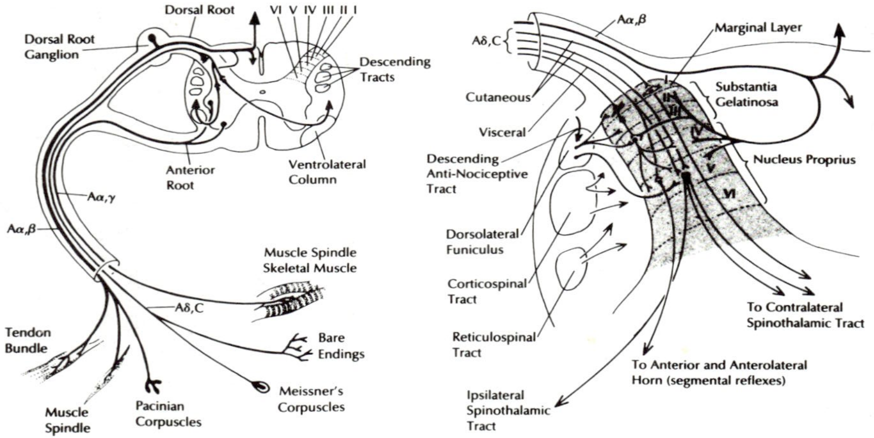

Figure 2.3. Transmission of nociceptive information in the A delta and C fibers with projection onto the laminae. In this schematization of nociceptive and other anatomically related afferent and efferent pathways in a spinal nerve and the dorsal horn, the left-hand drawing shows the fibers of a typical nerve and their distribution in the cord. Focus for purpose of this discussion should be on small, thinly myelinated A delta and on the small unmyelinated C fibers, a significant number of which transmit nociceptive impulses and project onto the laminae. In the more detailed drawing (right), it is seen that the small A delta and C fibers synapse primarily with cells in lamina V, but also synapse in laminae IV and VI. Convergence of cutaneous and visceral fibers in V are probably the basis for referred pain. Laminae I and V cells, and probably IV and VI cells, send most of the axons to the contralateral spinothalamic tract, although some ascend ipsilaterally. The supraspinal descending tracts connect with dorsal, ventral, and ventrolateral horn cells, with modulation of their output. Descending inhibitory fibers of the dorsolateral funiculus make contact with cells in laminae I, II, and V, and they impair or block nociceptive transmission. *(Bonica, J.J. Management of Acute and Chronic Pain—An Introduction. Proceedings: Recent Advances In the Management of Acute and Chronic Pain, a symposium held in conjunction with the Second World Congress on Pain, Montreal Canada, August 26, 1978. New York: HP Publishing Co., 1979. Sponsored by Pfizer Laboratories Division, Pfizer, Inc., New York, with permission.)* Figure 2, p. 6.

tors, visceral sensations, and deep sensations. The *exteroreceptors* provide information from the body surfaces. The *proprioceptors* provide information relative to the physical state of the body. This includes *kinesthetic* sensations which provide an awareness of movement and position sense of the body parts, equilibrium (sometimes considered a special sense itself), possible tendon and muscle sensations, and the sensation from pressure on the bottom of the feet. *Visceral sensations* refer to those sensations from the internal organs. *Deep sensations* are those which come from tissues located deep in the body, including bone and fascia. Sensations provided are mainly deep pressure, vibration, and pain.

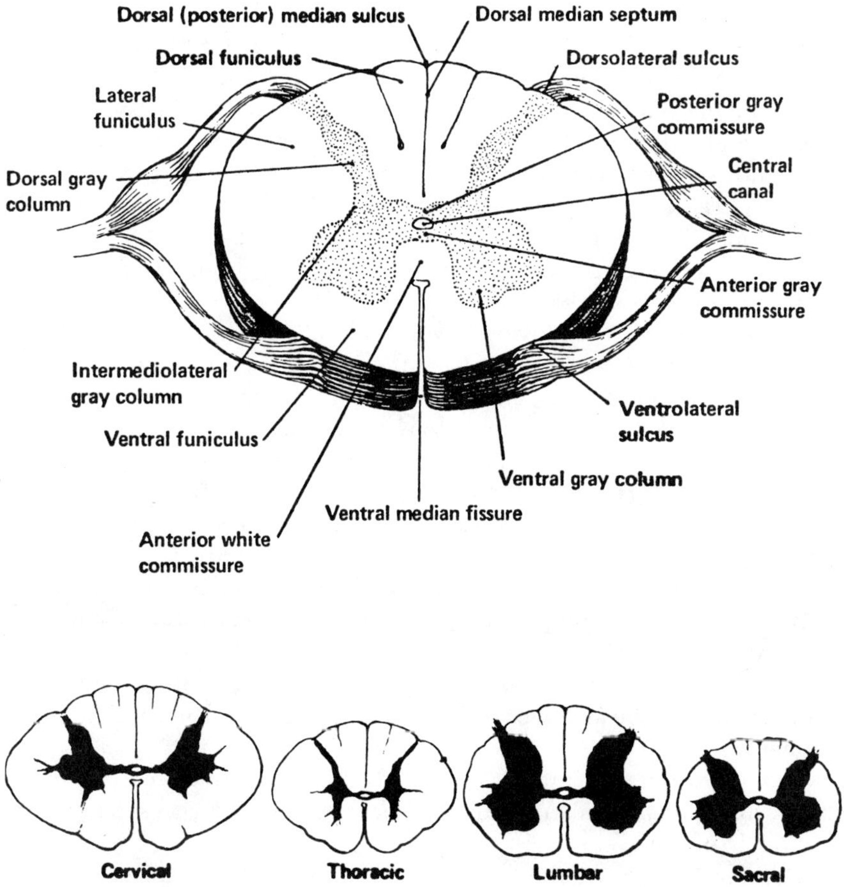

Figure 2.4. The anatomy of the spinal cord and transverse sections of the spinal cord at various levels. (*Chusid, J.G. Correlative neuroanatomy and functional neurology (17th ed.). Los Altos, CA: Lange Medical Publications, 1979, Figure 2.2, p. 66.)*

In addition to the tactile receptors that we will now consider, it is believed that there are many others. *Free nerve endings* are receptors found in all areas of the skin and many other tissues. They detect touch and pressure. The *Meissner's corpuscles* are stimulated by large myelinated sensory fibers that adapt rapidly. They are found in areas of the skin such as the fingertips and lips which discern the spatial characteristics of touch. The Meissner's corpuscles are particularly involved with light touch and low frequency vibration. As such, they can identify the exact point at which the body is touched and the texture of the object touching it. *Merkel's discs* subserve the same structures as Meissner's corpuscles but differ functionally in adaptability. Merkel's discs are believed to provide the steady state of signals allowing for one to determine continuous touch of objects against the skin. *Hair end-organs* are composed of the hair and its basal nerve and are rapidly adapting. They detect any slow movement of a hair and provide information about movement on the surface of the body. *Ruffini's end-organs* are found in deep layers of the skin and deeper tissues of the body such as joint capsules. Because they adapt very little, they provide information of continuous states such as pressure and heavy continuous touch. The *Pacinian corpuscles* are present in deep tissues and beneath the skin. They are rapidly adapting receptors and respond to rapid movement of the skin and deep tissues. They provide information about changes in the mechanical states of tissues such as vibration.

The *thermoreceptors* provide information about temperature. *Thermal gradations* are subserved by at least three types of sensory afferents: cold receptors, warm receptors, and pain receptors. Nociceptors are stimulated only by extremes of heat or cold. As with pain, at this time no specialized receptors for cold or warmth have been identified. There are only a few free nerve endings for cold and warmth making it difficult to evaluate gradations when only a small area is stimulated. When larger areas are stimulated the thermal signals summate from the entire area stimulated. For example, when one is fully clothed and out in the sun after awhile one may be aware of getting a sunburn on the face. If, on the other hand, one were to change into a bathing suit, a much greater portion of the body surface would be exposed and stimulated all at once. Consequently, the individual would be aware of the thermal stimulation from the sun much sooner.

Chemoreceptors detect taste, smell, and information relative to the metabolic activity and chemistry in tissues. *Electromagnetic receptors* detect light on the retina of the eye.

As far as is known, there are no specific end organs for pain. *Nociceptors* are tree nerve endings which detect both physical and chemical damage to tissues. They just end in the tissues. All areas of the body do not possess receptors capable of transmitting pain signals. For example, pain is identified by the brain, but the brain itself does not feel pain from ordinary tissue damage such as cutting. Although the brain parenchyma is insensitive to pain, many structures near the brain such as the scalp and arteries are pain sensitive. Similarly, the parenchyma of the liver and alveoli of the lungs are almost insensitive to pain, yet the liver capsule and bronchi are very sensitive to pain.

There are two specific sets of peripheral nerve fibers which transmit and process pain sensations separately, the A-delta fibers and the C fibers, illustrated in Figure 2.3. The *A-delta* fibers are small myelinated fibers typically found in the spinal nerves. These fibers transmit information rapidly, detect fine gradations of intensity, and discretely localize the information. Pain produced by A-delta fibers is called pricking or epicritic pain.

The *C fibers* are very small unmyelinated nerve fibers and constitute over two-thirds of the fibers in the peripheral nerves. They transmit information which needs slower processing, less specificity in gradation of intensity, and localization. Even though they conduct impulses very slowly in comparison to the A-delta fibers, the multiplicity of these fibers allows for conduction of vast amounts of information. The C fibers are primarily responsible for conducting the slow burning *"second"* or *"C fiber pain."* Although the intensity of this type of pain is weak, the characteristic that makes it often seem intolerable is the summation of impulses over long periods of time. Summation will be discussed later in this chapter. Patients often report that this type of pain "just wears them down."

An example of the difference in the transmission of A-delta and C fiber pain has been experienced by most people. When one bumps one's elbow, one feels a sharp pain immediately, the A-delta pain. Shortly thereafter, the individual experiences a dull, more aching, C fiber pain. This later type of aching or burning pain, which is considered more difficult to endure, is the type of pain that most patients with chronic pain syndromes experience.

In the midst of experiencing pain, it often is difficult for one to see the protective role that the pain may serve. However, if an individual did not receive the information from the initial injury in the above example, he would not have had the opportunity to respond by protective withdrawal of the injured part. Thus, he may have incurred irreversible damage. A simple reflex arc having its center in the spinal cord is illustrated in Figure 2.5. Because of the interactional components of the pain experience, a simple reflex arc is doubtful. This reflex is particularly important in certain types of nerve damage. For instance, if there is injury to spinal nerves the spinal cord or parts of the brain, a person may not be capable of perceiving pain. This is a fairly common problem for patients who have been paralyzed. When sitting for a prolonged period of time, one normally becomes uncom-

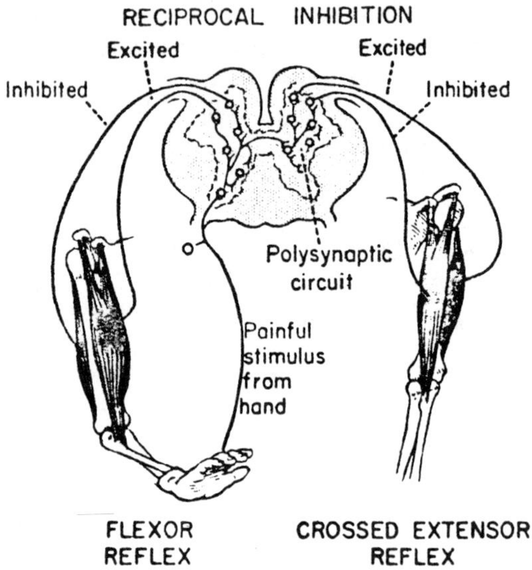

Figure 2.5. The flexor reflex, the crossed extensor reflex, and reciprocal inhibition. *(Guyton, A.C. Textbook of medical physiology (6th ed.). Philadelphia: W.B. Saunders, 1981, Figure 51.8, p. 634.)*

fortable and unconsciously shifts one's weight. Because of the absence of discomfort or pain perception, the paralyzed individual must constantly be vigilant of the need to shift weight. If he or she forgets or is asleep, the prolonged pressure and venous stasis will result in tissue necrosis and ulceration of the dependent anatomical structures, such as heels, elbows, and buttocks.

Autonomic nerve fibers were previously mentioned as the other component of the peripheral nervous system. These *ganglia* (nerve cell bodies are usually located in groups outside of the brain and spinal cord) are referred to as the *autonomic nervous system (ANS)* which is illustrated in Figure 2.6. The autonomic nervous system is sometimes referred to as the *vegetative nervous system* or *involuntary nervous system*. It functions at a subconscious level and is responsible for maintaining a stable internal environment by regulation of viscera and control of circulation. Although the autonomic nervous system acts somewhat independently, it is integrated with the rest of the body and is primarily regulated by the hypothalamus. This descending control system will be discussed later in this chapter. The autonomic nervous system is subdivided into the sympathetic and parasympathetic systems. These divisions act in a reciprocal manner. Stimulation of one produces the same general result as inhibition of the other. Stimulation of the *sympathetic nervous system* results in mobilization of the body's resources for fight or flight. Stimulation of the *parasympathetic nervous system* results in maintenance of the body's vegetative functions.

The Central Nervous System The brain and the spinal cord constitute the

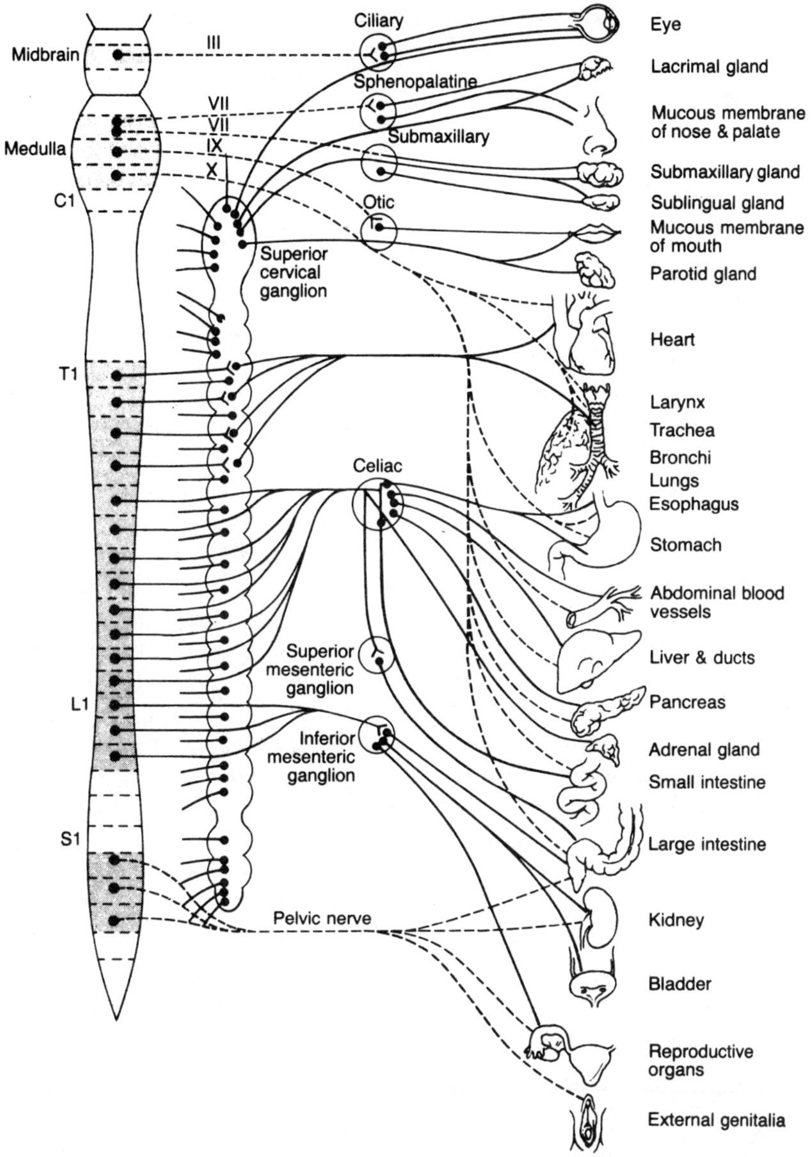

Figure 2.6. Autonomic nervous system. The visceral afferent fibers mediating pain travel with the sympathetic nerves, except for those from the pelvic organs which follow the parasympathetics of the pelvic nerve. Sympathetics are represented here by solid lines; parasympathetics by dashed lines. *(Sawyers, J.L. Abdominal Pain. Proceedings of the Symposium, the Management of Pain in Surgical Practice—Postoperative Pain, Boston, Sept. 22–23, 1978 by Chirurgecom, Div. Appleton-Century-Crofts, Copyright, Pfizer, Inc., 1979, Fig. 2, p. 21. Adapted from Way, L. Abdominal pain. In Sleisinger, M.H. & Fordtran, J.S. (eds.) Gastrointestinal Disease—Pathophysiology, Diagnosis and Management. Philadelphia: W.B. Saunders, 1973, p. 327, with permission.)*

functional units of the central nervous system, which is composed of hundreds of neuronal pools and neuroglia.

Both the A-delta and C peripheral sensory nerves have their cell bodies in the *dorsal root ganglia*. These ganglia are made up of several layers called laminae shown in Figure 2.3. Although the exact source of input and output of each laminae is not entirely known, their specialized function is. Lamina 1 neurons receive information from A-delta and C fibers from skin that is burned or crushed. Some of the lamina 1 cells project directly to higher levels of the spinal cord. The substantia gelatinosa is comprised of cells from lamina 2 and 3, and many peripheral nerve terminals from the skin and lower lamina. The axons of many of the lamina 2 and 3 cells project to the brain. It has been proposed that the substantia gelatinosa acts to modulate between peripheral fibers and spinal cells. Lamina 4 cells are made up of many cutaneous receptors that selectively respond to gentle pressure to the skin. Their response does not increase when the skin is pinched or crushed. Lamina 4 cells project ipsilaterally (on the same side) to the dorsolateral pathway. Lamina 5 cells have a wide-dynamic range and are particularly responsive to noxious stimuli. Their receptive fields are very complex in organization. Lamina 5 cells receive input from multiple cells including the small myelinated and unmyelinated fibers from the skin, blood vessels, muscles, and viscera. They probably received this input from lamina 4. Also, not only do the cells in the lamina 5 respond to a wide range of intensity but each cell in lamina 5 has a three-zone receptive field. Zone 1, the center of the field, is excited by a full range of mechanical stimuli. As the intensity of the stimulus is increased, so is the firing rate. Its discharges become repetitive and prolonged. Facilitation follows intense stimulation and inhibition follows gentle stimulation. In zone 2, which surrounds zone 1, intense stimulation of small fibers produces excitation and some facilitation whereas tactile and electrical stimulation of large fibers result in inhibition. Zone 2 is surrounded by zone 3. In zone 3 natural stimuli inhibit the firing of lamina 5 cells.

Both the A-delta and C peripheral sensory afferents enter the spinal cord through the dorsal roots of a spinal nerve, and travel upward from one-to-six segments and downward from one-to-four segments in the tract of Lissauer where they synapse in the substantia gelatinosa of the tip of dorsal horn of the spinal cord. In the dorsal roots the impulses pass through one or more other neurons and cross immediately in the anterior white commisure and ascend contralaterally to the cortex by the long fibers of the dorsal column system and the spinothalamic systems. Figure 2.7 illustrates the position of these and other tracts in the spinal cord. Figure 2.8 illustrates the ascending systems from the spinal cord to the brain for the transmission of pain and temperature.

The *dorsal column system* is made up of the fasciculi cuneatus and the fasciculi gracilis. The *fasciculi cuneatus* receives fibers from the cervical and

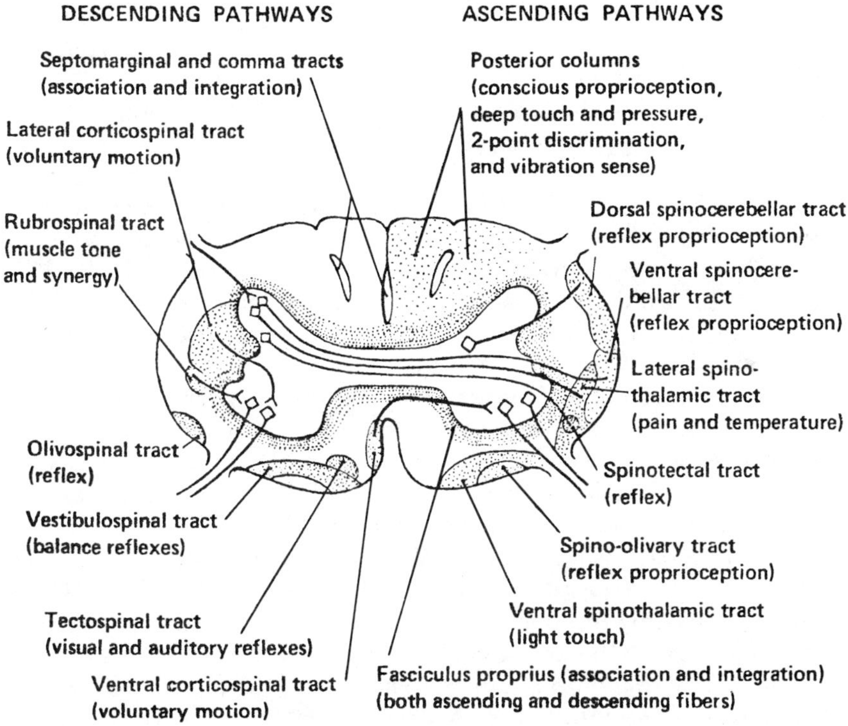

Figure 2.7. Cross-section of the lower cervical region of the spinal cord showing the ascending pathways on the right and the descending pathways on the left. *(Chusid, J.G. Correlative Neuroanatomy & Functional Neurology, 17th ed. Los Altos, CA.: Lange Medical Pub. 1979, Figure 2.3, p. 67, with permission.)*

upper thoracic ganglia innervating the upper trunk, neck, and upper extremities. The *fasciculi gracilis* receive fibers from the dorsal ganglia of the lower thoracic, sacral, and lumbar regions which innervate the legs and lower extremities. These dorsal root fibers enter the dorsal columns, ascend, and terminate in the medulla. They are called *first-order neurons*. *Second-order neurons* originate from the terminations of the fasciculi cuneatus and gracilis in the medulla and form the internal arcuate fibers which cross in the medial lemniscus and ascend through the pons and midbrain, terminating in the ventral posterolateral nucleus of the thalamus. There, the *third-order neurons* relay the information to the sensory areas of the cortex. The major functions of the dorsal column system are in relation to mechanoreceptive sensory input. It transmits information requiring rapid and accurate processing, fine gradations of intensity, and discrete localization. Functions which it subserves are those of fine touch and pressure, vibration, and the kinesthetic, or muscle sense.

The *spinothalamic tract* is referred to as the pain tract because it has sometimes been surgically sectioned in an attempt to provide pain relief by performing an anterolateral cordotomy. The spinothalamic tract is divided into three pathways: the ventral spinothalamic tract, the lateral spinothalamic tract, and the spinoreticular tract.

Most A-delta fibers project onto the superficial layers of the dorsal horn of the spinal cord, *trigeminal nucleus caudalis.* On entering the spinal cord, they immediately enter the dorsal columns and ascend the entire length of the cord to the second-order neurons of the dorsal horns of the medulla and synapse in the dorsal column nuclei. Here these fibers decussate (cross in the form of an X). The *ventral spinothalamic* tract arises after the spinothalamic and dorsal column fibers decussate and it ascends, and terminates in the ventrobasal complex of the thalamus. The *ventrobasal complex*, sometimes referred to as the *neospinothalamic tract,* projects contralaterally onto the *somesthetic (somatic sensory) cortex.* The ventral spinothalamic tract subserves the functions of crude touch and pressure which require little intensity discrimination and localization on the body surface.

The *lateral spinothalamic tract* is primarily formed by the long fibers which conduct pain and temperature, particularly the A-delta and C fibers. These fibers, after passing through one or more local neurons cross in the anterior commisure of the gray matter of the dorsal horn and pass to the opposite lateral column. The lateral spinothalamic tract terminates in the intralaminar nuclei of the thalamus. This area of the thalamus is sometimes referred to as the *paleospinothalamic tract.* The lateral spinothalamic tract primarily transmits signals for intolerable aching and burning pain and thermal sensations.

The *spinoreticular tract* is composed primarily of the small C fibers and, therefore, is exclusively or almost exclusively concerned with the transmission of pain signals. After the fibers leave the dorsal horn they ascend and terminate in the reticular substance of the bulbar and mesencephalic areas of the midbrain which constitute the spinoreticular tract. After synapsing with one or more successive neurons, they ascend to the intralaminar nuclei of the thalamus and terminate. Signals are then transmitted to other parts of the thalamus, hypothalamus, and cortex. The intralaminar nuclei of the thalamus and the reticular formation in the brain stem are parts of the *reticular activating system.*

The *limbic system* is an umbrella term for the subcortical structures in the basal regions of the brain. Subsummed under this term are the anterior nuclei of the thalamus, hypothalamus, mesencephalon, periventricular structure, portions of the basal ganglia, the hypocampus, and the amygdala. All of these structures are believed to play an important role in pain modulation. The thalamus and hypothalamus are believed to subserve the fight or defense reaction. Some researchers believe that the flight reaction also is evoked in these areas. The limbic system and the hypothalamus are

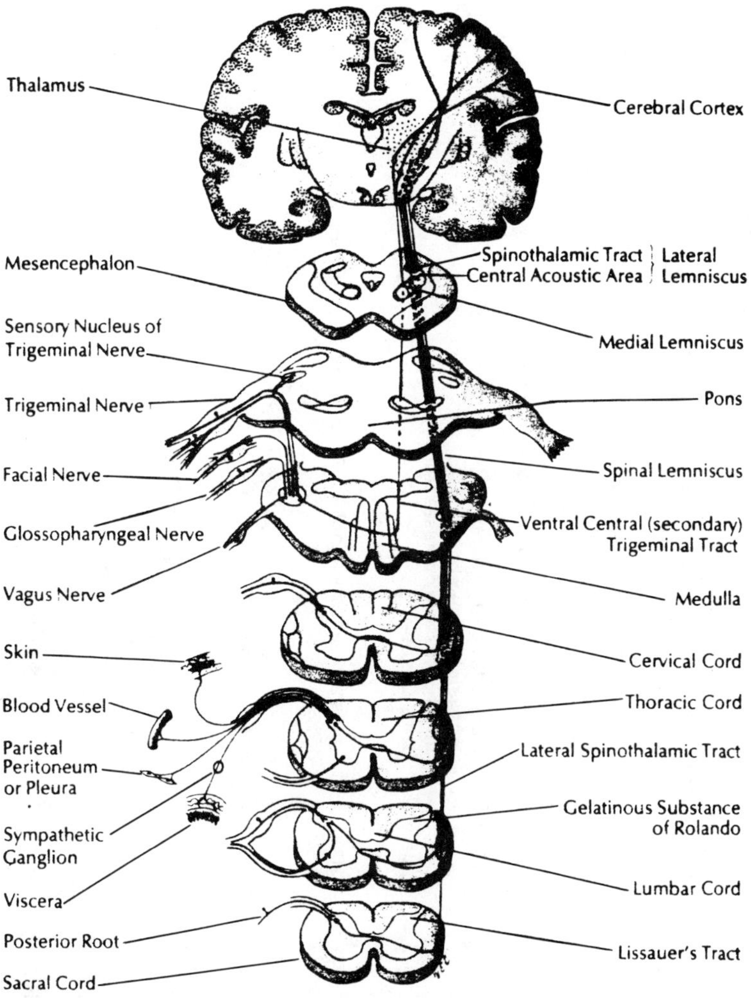

Figure 2.8. Pain conduction—periphery to brain. *(Bonica, J.J. Pathophysiology of pain. In: Current concepts in postoperative pain. New York: H.P. Publishing Inc., 1978, p. 6.)*

involved in certain autonomic functions, biologic rhythms, sexual behavior, motivated behavior, and the emotions of fear and rage.

The periaqueductal gray (PAG) of the midbrain contains neurons which have opiate receptors. When the PAG is electrically stimulated these receptors lead to the reduction of pain. This is a neurosurgical procedure sometimes used as a "last resort" intervention for pain relief. The PAG projects through neurons in and around the midline of the caudal pons and the rostral medulla. This area is called the region of raphe. The descending

TABLE 2.1. Principal Ascending and Descending Tracts of the Spinal Cord.

Name of Tract or Bundle[a]	Location in Cord (column)	Major Functions[b]
A. Ascending (sensory) tracts		
1. Fasciculus gracilis (tract of Goll)	Posterior	Pathway for tactile sensations, position sense, passive movement, spatial discrimination, two-point discrimination, and "vibration"
2. Fasciculus cuneatus (tract of Burdach)	Posterior	Same as above
3. Fasciculus posterolateralis (dorsolateral fasciculus, tract of Lissauer)	Lateral	Pathway for pain and thermal sensations
4. Dorsal (posterior) spinocerebellar tract (direct cerebellar tract, tract of Flechsig)	Lateral	Transmits sensory impulses from proprioceptors of muscles, tendons, and joints to cerebellum, i.e., reflex proprioception; also conveys touch, pressure impulses from skin
5. Ventral (anterior) spinocerebellar tract (indirect cerebellar tract, tract of Gowers)	Lateral	Same as above
6. Dorsal (posterior) spinothalamic tract (anterolateral spinothalamic tract)	Lateral	Transmits sensory impulses underlying pain and thermal sensations
7. Spinotectal tract	Lateral	Sensory pathway for visuospinal reflexes (?); nociceptive impulses (?)
8. Ventral (anterior) spinothalamic tract	Anterior	Sensory pathway for touch and tactile localization
B. Descending (motor) tracts		
1. Lateral corticospinal tract (crossed pyramidal tract)	Lateral	Transmits motor impulses to skeletal muscles; underlies voluntary movements of body
2. Rubrospinal tract (tract of Monakow)	Lateral	Transmits motor impulses underlying muscle tone and synergistic contractions of skeletal muscle
3. Dorsal (posterior or lateral) vestibulospinal tract	Lateral	Transmits motor impulses underlying postural and balance reflexes
4. Olivospinal tract (Helwig's bundle)	Lateral	Functions unknown; possibly mediates thalamospinal reflexes
5. Reticulospinal tract	Anterior	Transmits motor impulses underlying muscle tone; controls activity of autonomic nervous system; regulates threshold of peripheral end-organs, e.g., sensory pathways and muscle spindles

6.	Ventral (anterior) vestibulospinal tract	Anterior	Transmits motor impulses underlying postural and balance reflexes
7.	Tectospinal tract	Anterior	Transmits motor impulses underlying visuospinal and audiospinal reflexes
8.	Ventral (anterolateral) corticospinal tract (direct pyramidal tract)	Anterior	Transmits motor impulses to skeletal muscles; underlies voluntary movements
C	Ascending plus descending fibers fasciculi proprii)		
OB	Oval bundle (fasciculus septo-marginalis	Dorsal	
CT	Comma tract of Schultze (fasciculus interfascicularis)	Dorsal	
PGB	Posterior ground bundle (posterior intersegmental fasciculus)	Dorsal	The fasciculi proprii collectively form intrinsic pathways within the spinal cord for the unconscious coordination of spinal reflexes, e.g., during voluntary movement and postural adjustments that are initiated by higher centers. Also concerned with integration of reflex activities within the cord, and with coordinating reflex functions at different levels within the cord per se
LGB	Lateral ground bundle (lateral inter-segmental fasciculus)	Lateral	
AGB	Anterior ground bundle (anterior intersegmental or su comarginal fasciculus)	Anterior	

[a]Alternative names for these structures are given in parentheses. The long (projection) tracts are summarized under headings A and B in the table, whereas the short (association or intersegmental) tracts (collectively known as the fasciculi proprii) are summarized in part C.

[b]A mnemonic device for recalling the general functional and anatomic relationships within the spinal cord, as well as the spinal nerves, is: Sensory Afferent, Motor Efferent = SAME; Dorsal Afferent, Ventral Efferent = DAVE. *(Jensen, D. The Human Nervous System. New York: Appleton-Century-Crofts, 1980, Table 2.1, p. 44, with permission.)*

axons of the raphe magnus travel via the dorsolateral columns to the regions of the trigeminal nucleus and dorsal horn of the spinal cord.

There are other ascending sensory tracts but their functions are not as important to the pain experience. All of the ascending sensory tracts are summarized in relation to their location and function in Table 2.1.

The somesthetic cortex is divided into two areas, somatic sensory area I and somatic sensory area II (Fig. 2.9). Somatic sensory area I is considered much more important to the sensory functions of the body. When the somesthetic cortex is referred to, it most often refers to somatic sensory area I. In somatic sensory area I, there are specific areas where sensory information from different parts of the body is received (Fig. 2.10). The amount of space in this homologus of the body is relative to the number of specialized sensory receptors in the areas of the body region represented. Somatic sensory area II has been suggested as the terminus of pain information and some complex body movements.

The primary motor cortex, seen in Figure 2.11, is a mirror image of the somatic sensory cortex. It is the highest level in the nervous system responsible for precise integration and control of voluntary muscular con-

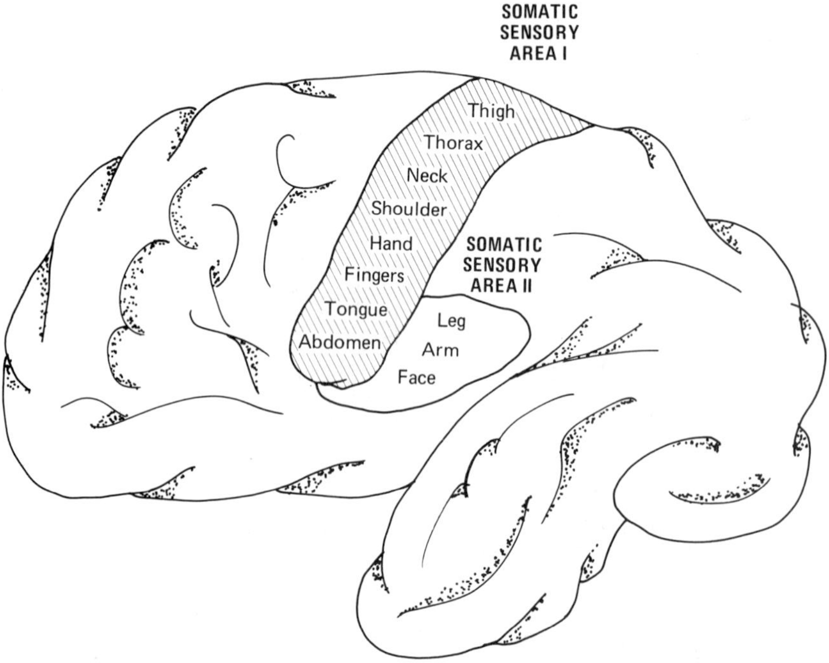

Figure 2.9. Somesthetic cortex illustrating somatic sensory area I and somatic sensory area II. *(Guyton, A. Textbook of Medical Physiology (6th ed.). Philadelphia: W.B. Saunders, 1981, Fig. 49-5, p. 603, with permission.)*

The 3RD Sensory Neurones (conveying information from the opposite side of the body) synapse with cells in the POST-CENTRAL GYRUS of the PARIETAL LOBE of the CEREBRAL CORTEX. The exact points on this Gyrus at which impulses coming from the different regions of the skin surface terminate are indicated on this coronal view of the Gyrus

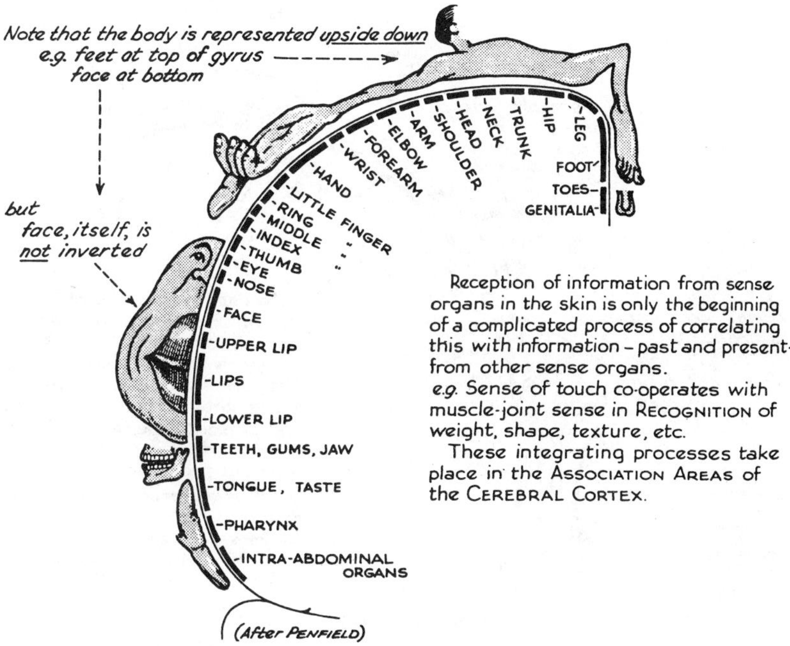

Note the relatively large area devoted to FACE (especially lips) and to HAND (especially thumb and index finger) while trunk representation is very small.

Figure 2.10. Sensory cortex. *(McNaught, A.B. & Callander, R. Illustrated Physiology. New York: Churchill Livingstone, 1975, p. 250, with permission.)*

traction. Figure 2.12 illustrates the relationship of the motor cortex to the somesthetic cortex.

Nociceptive information descends from the cortex by the lateral and ventral pyramidal (corticospinal) and extrapyramidal tracts. Extrapyramidal tracts refer to all descending tracts except the pyramidal tract. They include, the rubrospinal, vestibulospinal, reticulospinal, tectospinal and tectobulbar, medial longitudinal fasciculus, autonomic pathways, and the

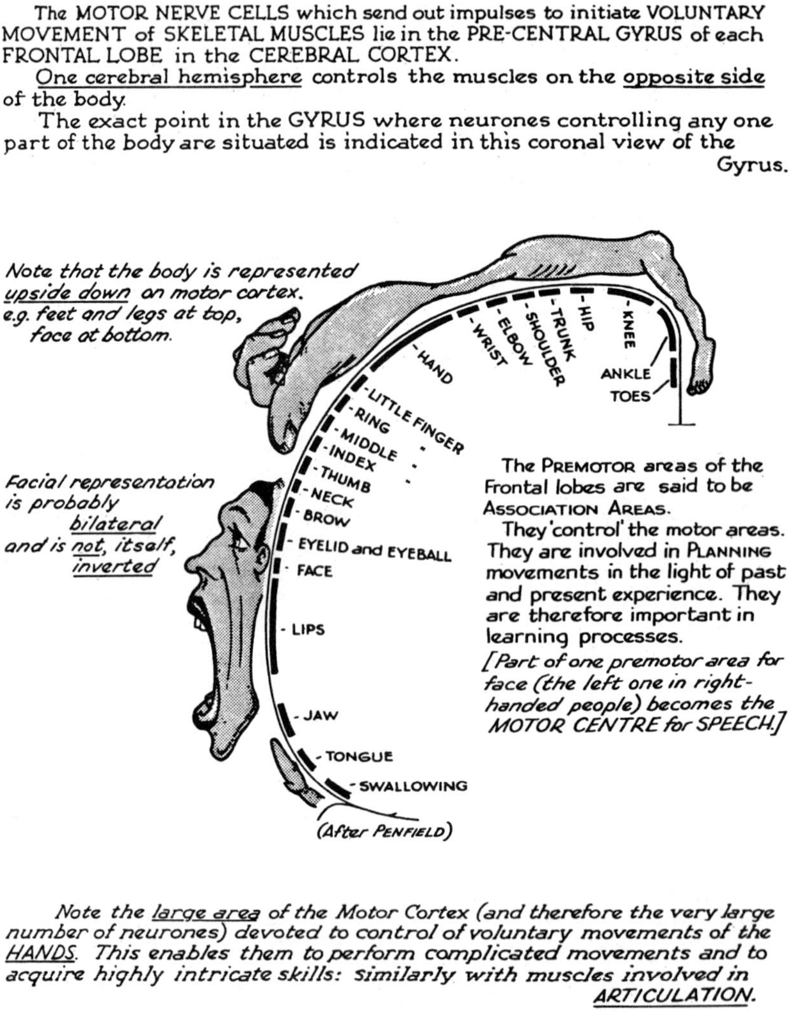

Figure 2.11. Motor cortex. *(McNaught, A.B. & Callander, R. Illustrated Physiology. New York: Churchill Livingstone, 1975, p. 251, with permission.)*

fasciculi propii. The long descending motor tracts are illustrated in Figures 2.13 A and B. Table 2.1 summarizes their location and function.

The largest and most important descending motor system is the pyramidal tracts. All of the fibers of the motor region of the precentral gyrus in the cerebral cortex exit by the corona radiata, descend through the internal capsule, crus cerebri, and pons, and enter the medulla where they

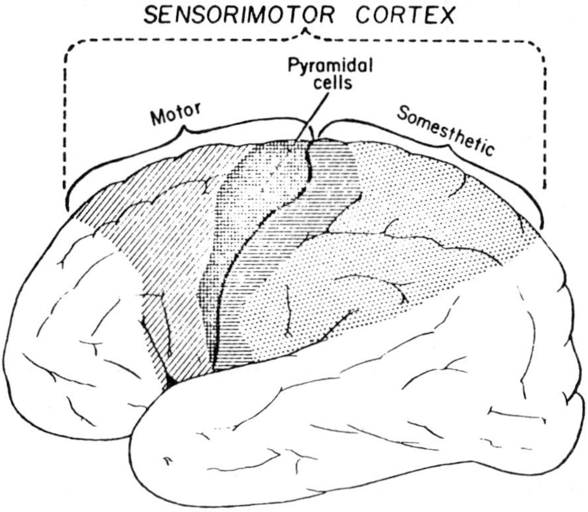

Figure 2.12. Relationship of the motor cortex to the somesthetic cortex. *(Guyton, A.C. Textbook of Medical Physiology, 6th ed. Philadelphia: W.B. Saunders, 1981, Figure 53.1, p. 653, with permission.)*

emerge on the surface like pyramids. At the junction of the medulla and the spinal cord 75–90 percent of the pyramidal fibers incompletely decussate. When they do, they divide into three tracts, the lateral (crossed) corticospinal, anterior uncrossed corticospinal, and a small lateral uncrossed corticospinal tract. The decussed fibers travel in the posterior area of the lateral funiculus down the cord as the large lateral crossed corticospinal tract. As they continue their descent, 55 percent of the pyramidal fibers terminate in the cervical spinal cord, 20 percent in the thoracic area, and 25 percent in the lumbosacral segments. The Bundle of Türck, the uncrossed ventral pyramidal tract, innervates the muscles of the upper extremities and the neck. It usually descends only to the upper thoracic segments of the spinal cord. The tract of Barnes, the anterolateral pyramidal tract, is comprised of the rest of the uncrossed fibers and descends more anteriorly in the lateral funiculus.

All three corticospinal tracts enter the dorsolateral area of the gray matter of the spinal cord and terminate on the interneurons or the anterior horn motorneurons. The function of the corticospinal or pyramidal tracts is to transmit impulses to the skeletal muscles. The strength of the muscle contraction is directly proportional to the amount of energy transmitted in these tracts.

The extrapyramidal descending fibers act in a collaborative fashion with those of the pyramidal descending tracts. The lower motorneuron or common final pathway is where the axons which provide motor innerva-

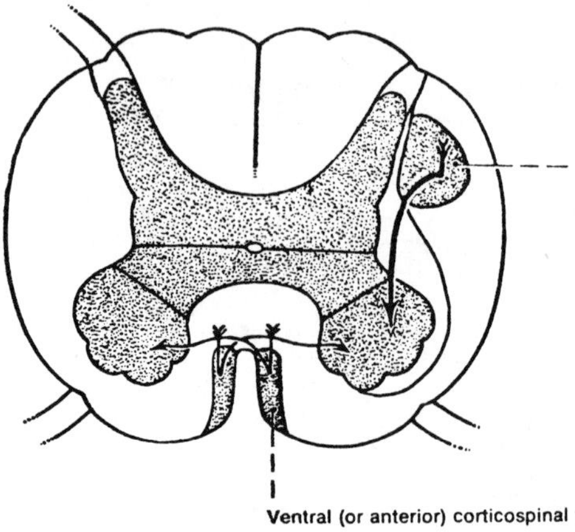

A.

The anterolateral pyramidal tract of Barnes, not represented on this drawing, is formed by uncrossed and fine corticospinal fibers.

The majority of pyramidal fibers are projected upon the anterior horn cells through internuncial cells.

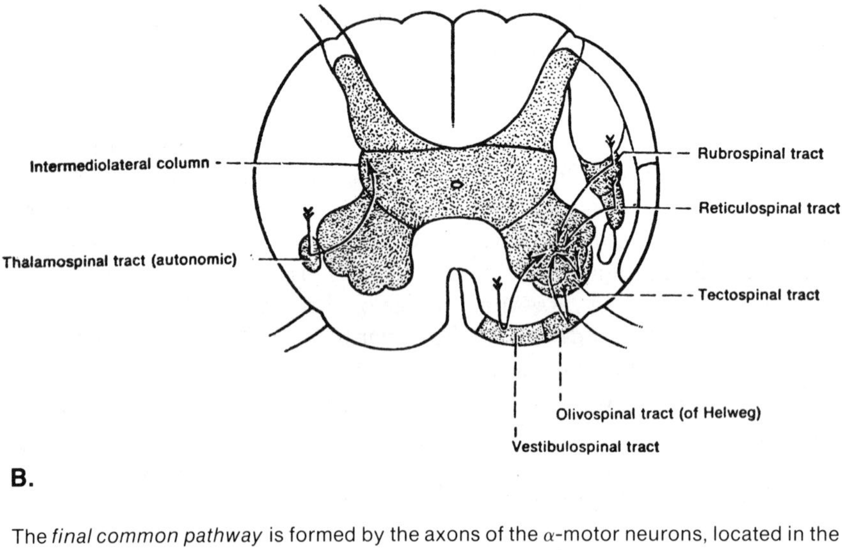

B.

The *final common pathway* is formed by the axons of the α-motor neurons, located in the ventral horn and receiving all the impulses of the descending tracts.

Figure 2.13. The pathways and synaptic junctions of the (**A**) pyramidal and (**B**) extrapyramidal systems. *(Bossy, J. Atlas of neuroanatomy and special sense organs. Philadelphia: W.B. Saunders, 1970, p. 115.)*

tion arise from the anterior horn cells of the spinal cord. The upper motorneuron refers to all of the descending tracts of the spinal cord and certain sensory impulses. Because of the importance of the corticospinal or pyramidal tracts they are sometimes referred to as the upper motorneuron. Many of the extrapyramidal descending fibers act in a collaborative fashion with those of the pyramidal descending motor tracts.

The rubrospinal tract is located and emanates from the red nucleus located in the mesencephalic tegmentum. The corticorubral tract is comprised of fibers from the cerebellum and the cerebral cortex and pass to the red nucleus. The functions of these tracts is believed to be the transmission of motor impulses necessary for muscle tone and synergistic contractions of skeletal muscles, especially some of the flexor groups.

The vestibulospinal tract originates in the nucleus of the pons and medulla (pontine–medullary) junction. It receives fibers from the vestibular portion of the ear (VIII) and some specific cerebellar fibers. Its major function is to mediate equilibrium and posture in a synergistic manner.

The reticulospinal tract primarily emanates from the reticular formation in the pons and medulla. The actions of this tract are not clear but it is believed that they include both somatic and visceral autonomics.

The tectospinal and tectobulbar tracts arise primarily from the superior colliculus, an optic center. It is believed that the function of the tectospinal tract is to mediate reflex posture through auditory and visual stimuli.

The medial longitudinal fasciculus is responsible for corrective eye movements. That is, it allows the eyes to remain fixed on the object they are visualizing when the head is moved.

The autonomic pathways in the spinal cord originate in the autonomic centers of the hypothalamus, tegmentum of the midbrain, pons, and medulla. These preganglionic cells are ultimately responsible for innervation of visceral structures.

The fasciculi proprii are mixed tracts having both ascending and descending fibers. Their functions include the unconscious coordination of spinal reflexes such as adjusting one's posture.

From an anatomical standpoint alone, individual differences in the overlapping and decussation of nerve fibers and the complexities of pain transmission may make assessment of a patient's pain problem a very difficult task. These same difficulties are also encountered when attempting therapeutic neurosurgical transection and ablative procedures for pain relief.

The overall function of the brain is believed to be accomplished through *activation* and *inhibition* in the cortex. This means that the brain has *centrifugal* ability through a *feedback loop* between the brain and the sensory fibers. These descending messages may either inhibit or facilitate the ascending transmission of potentially painful impulses. Not all impulses travel at the same speed nor do they follow the same route as described above. Eventually impulses reach the sensory cortex where the perception of pain is interpreted. The individual may take action immediately or may store the information for retrieval and use at a later time.

Interactional Systems—The Dimensions of Pain

We now begin to see possible mechanisms for the interaction of psychological and cognitive factors with the sensory or physical ones in the perception of pain. For example, emotions could initiate messages in the brain that travel antidromically (in the opposite direction) to the spinal cord and in turn affect the transmission of pain impulses upward to the brain. Most of our attention up until now has focused primarily on transmission and processing of sensory signals to produce the perception of pain. We will now turn our attention and focus on a model of pain that considers reciprocal neurophysiological, cognitive, and psychological relationships which culminate in the pain experience: perception and response. Such a model is illustrated in Figure 2.14. The material in this section is adapted from the work of Melzack (1973, pp. 93–124) and serves as a basis of the gate control theory discussed later in this chapter. For other related works to the dimensions of pain, the reader is referred to the works of Casey & Melzack, 1967; Melzack, 1965; 1969; Melzack & Bridges, 1971; Melzack & Casey, 1968; Melzack & Torgerson, 1971; and Melzack & Wall, 1965; 1970. There will be some redundancy of neurophysiology in an attempt to present the model in a logical and understandable manner.

Examples in the literature of *hyperalgesia*, congenital insensitivity to painful stimuli, and pain asymbolia, the inability to appreciate pain in a normal way or to comprehend its significance, have led to the conclusion that there are *three interactional systems* necessary to account for the perception and response to pain. The three systems elucidated are the sensory-discriminative, motivational-affective, and the cognitive-evaluative. In the literature these systems sometimes are simply referred to as the sensory, motivational, and cognitive systems. Each of these systems has a specialized physiological system subserving it. How patients and physicians describe these three components of the pain experience is referred to as the *language of pain*. This is illustrated in Figure 2.15. The language both quantifies and qualifies the pain experience.

As we have seen, the *sensory-discriminative system* processes information about the strength or intensity of nociception and the temporal and spatial aspects. The *neospinalthalamic tract* communicates this information through projections to the ventrobasal thalamus and somatosensory cortex.

The *motivational-affective system*, unlike the highly specific sensory-discriminative system, is subserved by fibers that have very wide receptive fields in the brain and receive input from other converging somatosensory fibers such as those of hearing and vision. The areas in the nervous system that are of particular importance to the motivational-affective system are the reticular formation and the limbic system in the brainstem. These areas receive input from the anterolateral somatosensory pathways, particularly projections from the spinoreticular and paleospinothalamic components. The role of the reticular formation in the pain experience is to produce an aversive drive and concommitant responsive behaviors such as attempting to interrupt the painful stimuli. Within the reticular formation there are areas with considerable variation in their specialization of function. Thus damage to the reticular formation may result in either increasing or decreasing one's responsiveness to pain and one's ability to cope with it. In animals it has been found that stimulation of these areas may even result in pleasure instead of pain. In addition to the described functions above, the reticular formation is involved in mediating light touch and pressure.

The reticular formation is the gateway to another system intimately involved with the motivational-affective dimension of the pain experience, the limbic system. The reticular formation projects onto the medial thalamus and the hypothalamus which in turn project onto the frontal lobe. Stimulation of some areas of the limbic system, the hippocampus and the amygdala may evoke escape or other attempts to stop the pain. Surgical section and ablative procedures have been used to decrease the responsiveness to noxious stimuli, the *negative affect*, associated with intractable pain.

In addition to the aversive drive, the limbic and the hypothalmic structures are involved in other behaviors that comprise the motivational-affective dimension of pain, namely, approach responses and other behaviors aimed at maintaining and prolonging stimulation. Therefore, there may be an overlapping of the structures involved in aversion and reward. For example, intense stimulation usually evokes avoidance to noxious stimuli, whereas light or mild stimulation such as touch evokes approach. The reward areas are in the lateral hypothalamus.

The *cognitive-evaluative* activities have roots in such things as culture, past experience with pain, and anxiety. These functions are based on activities in the higher cortical centers. They may significantly affect both the sensory-discriminative and the motivational-affective components of the pain experience. Some functions of the cognitive-evaluative system appear to block pain (sensory-discriminative), whereas others appear to modulate pain (motivational-affective). These functions include the identification, evaluation, and selection of input to be processed. The processing must be done by rapidly ascending and descending transmission in the frontal cortex which receives input via the intracortical fiber system from virtually all sensory and associational cortical areas and projects strongly to reticular and limbic structures. Furthermore, these cognitive functions must be performed *before* information in the more slowly conducting pathways is transmitted so that they can influence that information. It is believed that the dorsal column and the dorsolateral projection pathways function as a forward-feeding limb of this circuitry. To give precedence to cognitive-evaluative information, the dorsal column pathway must adapt quickly and conduct rapidly to the cortex so that central processes can be activated. The descending control fibers from the central system and the pyramidal fibers transmit information of a sensory-discriminative nature via the ventrobasal thalamus to the dorsal horn cells in the spinal cord. These cells modulate the information before it is transmitted to the motivational-affective and cognitive-evaluative systems. These rapidly transmitting systems account for the powerful role of the psychological processes in determining the intensity and quality of pain.

Melzack says that the neural mechanisms underlying the motor as-

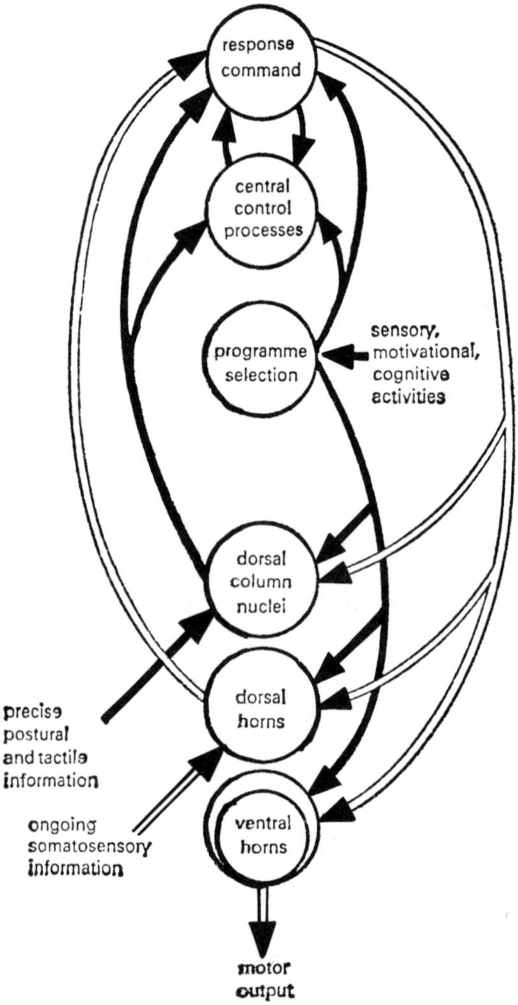

pects of pain are at least as complicated as those of the sensory aspects. Melzack & Wall (1965, p. 979) have described these and are quoted by Melzack (1973, p. 119).

> Sudden, unexpected damage to the skin is followed by (1) a startle response; (2) a flexion reflex; (3) postural readjustment; (4) vocalization; (5) orientation of the head and eyes to examine the damaged area; (6) autonomic responses; (7) evocation of past experience in similar situations and prediction of the consequences of the stimulation; (8) many other patterns of behavior aimed at diminishing the sensory and affective components of the whole experience, such as rubbing the damaged area, avoidance behavior, and so forth.

Melzack (1973, p. 119) goes on to say "This total complex sequence is hidden in the simple phrase 'pain response'." How one responds to such a pain experience is referred to as the *"response program"* and is determined by activities of the moment in the sensory-discriminative, motivational-affective, and affective-evaluative systems. The complex interactional neural circuitry simultaneously interacting with each other in several parallel systems produces a myriad of patterns that are a part of the total perception of intensity and quality of the pain experience and response.

Figure 2.14. Schematic model of the neural mechanisms that underlie purposive motor behavior in the pain experience. Sensory, motivational, and cognitive activities at a given moment selectively activate neural circuits (Program Selection) that represent a small number of alternative behavior programs to attain a goal. The output of the programs is projected to areas at several levels of the nervous system. Neuron pools in the dorsal column nuclei are selectively facilitated, and project precise postural and tactile information to (a) areas (Central Control Processes) that evaluate the selected programs in terms of prior experience, and (b) areas that activate the final response command. Motorneuron pools in the ventral horns, which have been facilitated by the earlier program selection to produce several possible behavior patterns, are selectively activated by the large and small efferent fibers, and produce the final pattern to muscles. The efferent activity to the dorsal column nuclei and the dorsal horn cells may continue to modulate the input during the ensuing motor behaviour. Open lines represent the traditional S-R circuit. Solid lines represent the circuits involved in program selection prior to the central response command that produces overt behavior. (*Melzack, R. & Bridges, J.A. Dorsal column contributions to the motor behaviour. Exp Neurol, 33: 53, 1971. As applied in Melzack, R. The Puzzle of Pain. New York: Basic Books, 1973 p. 120–121, with permission.*)

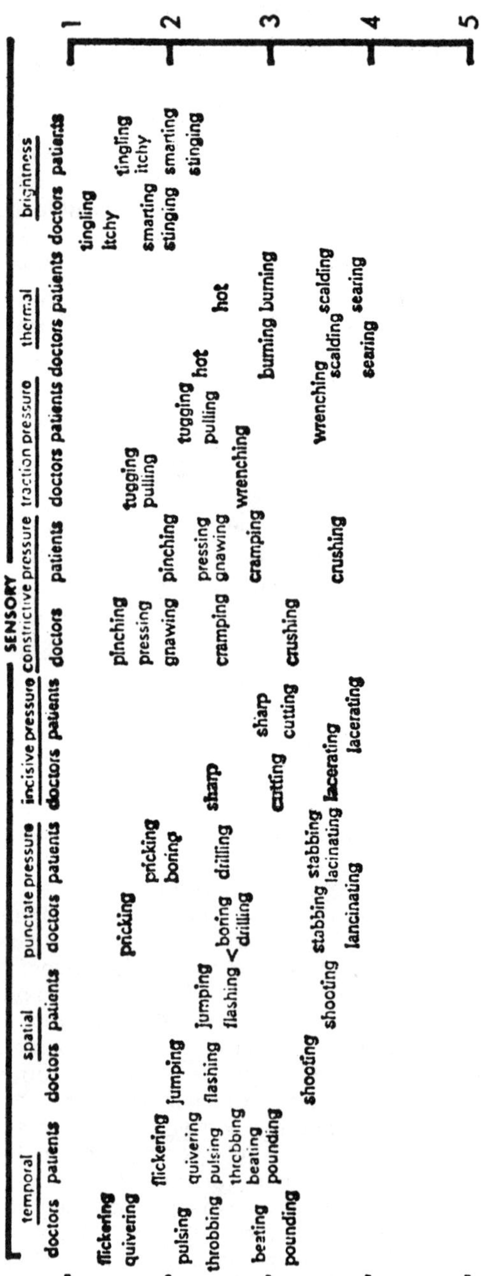
SENSORY
temporal
spatial
punctate pressure
incisive pressure
constrictive pressure
traction pressure
thermal
brightness
doctors
patients
1
2
3
4
5
flickering
quivering
pulsing
throbbing
beating
pounding
jumping
flashing
shooting
pricking
boring
drilling
stabbing
lancinating
sharp
cutting
lacerating
pinching
pressing
gnawing
cramping
crushing
tugging
pulling
wrenching
hot
burning
scalding
searing
tingling
itchy
smarting
stinging

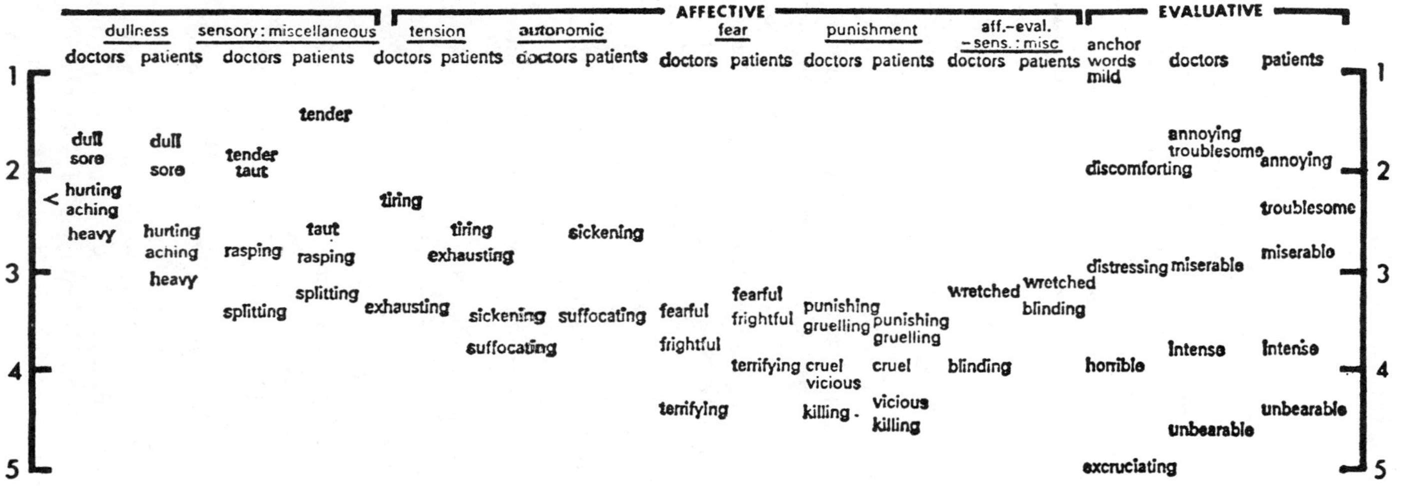

Figure 2.15. Language of pain illustrating the three interactional dimensions. Spatial display of pain descriptors which have the same rank order, on an intensity scale, for doctors and patients. The scale values range from 1 (mild) to 5 (excruciating). Two words connected by an arrowhead have the same mean scale value. (*Melzack, R. & Torgerson, W.S. On the language of pain. Anesthesiology, 34: 50, 1971, with permission.*)

Transmission and Processing of Information in the Nervous System

The Synapse Transmission of information in the nervous system requires that *all* information be converted into electrical impulses. For example to experience pain the nervous system must convert the sensory stimulus and thoughts and memories about the stimulus into impulses that ultimately become nociception. To accomplish this, the nervous system functions like a complicated electrical computer. It has electrical input circuits, output circuits and a mechanism, the *synapse*, where the transmission of impulses from neuron to neuron occurs. The synapse, the computer mechanism illustrated in Figure 2.16, is a specialized junction or contact point where the fine branches of one axon of one neuron, the *presynaptic neuron*, terminate and are in contact with the dendrite, soma, or sometimes another axon of another neuron, the *postsynaptic* neuron. There is no actual structural union, rather the membranes of the presynaptic and postsynaptic neurons are separated by a space called the *synaptic cleft*. There are hundreds of swellings on the surface of the neuron, primarily on the dendrite but some are on the soma, called *synaptic knobs, terminal buttons, presynaptic terminals,* or *end-feet*. These synaptic knobs contain synaptic vesicles and mitochondria. *Synaptic vesicles* of excitatory knobs contain an excitatory neurotransmitter and synaptic vesicles of inhibitory knobs contain an inhibitory neurotransmitter. The mitochondria provides adenosine triphosphate (ATP), a substance required to synthesize new transmitter substance.

When an impulse reaches a *presynaptic terminal*, the action potential spreads over the surface of the presynaptic knob causing it to depolarize and empty one or more of the synaptic vesicles into the synaptic cleft. The *postsynaptic membrane* of the neuron contains a receptor that the transmitter substance binds to. Excitation and inhibition are determined by the response of the receptor in the postjunctional membrane. The postsynaptic neuron integrates the excitatory or inhibitory information and responds accordingly. The postsynaptic potential is significantly influenced by both electrolytes in the extracellular fluid and the number of vesicles emptied. Usually many synaptic knobs must empty at the same time or in rapid succession to evoke a response. Thus, fluid and electrolyte balance may be of marked significance especially in the perception of acute pain where fluid and electrolyte imbalance are coexisting problems.

Synapses may occur vertically, horizontally, or obliquely. Axons of motor neurons synapse with skeletal muscle fibers and produce motion. Visceral efferent neurons synapse with smooth muscle, cardiac muscle, and glands evoking their respective function. In different parts of the nervous system, neurons vary in the number and types of synapses they possess, which at least in part accounts for the differing functions of neurons.

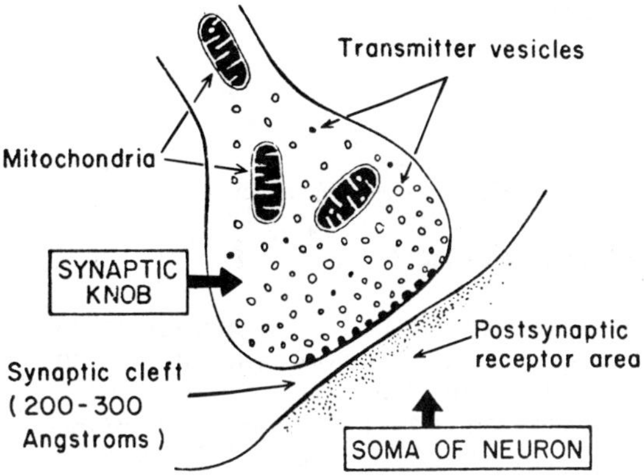

Figure 2.16. Physiologic anatomy of the synapse. *(Guyton, A.C. Textbook of medical physiology (6th ed.). Philadelphia: W.B. Saunders, 1981, Figure 46.6, p. 565.)*

Chemical Transmission of Signals

Neuroregulators Pain is *usually* experienced while tissue damage is being done. As we have seen, before impulses reach the level of awareness in the cortex, considerable regulation takes place. Rather than passing through the spinal cord without interruption, impulses undergo various types of ascending and descending neural-hormonal processing. Neuroregulators may be divided functionally into two groups—neurotransmitters and neuromodulators. Neurotransmitters are also referred to as neurohumoral agents or neurohormones. Neuromodulators are known as the endorphins. By virtue of their specific function, and through hyper- or hyposecretion, neuroregulators may significantly alter pain experience. For example, it is believed that the cause of pain in patients with chronic pain may be due to a depletion of endorphin. We will now consider the possible implications for the role of the neuroregulators in the pain experience.

Neurotransmitters *Neurotransmitters* are responsible for transmission of impulses across the synaptic cleft. If the neurotransmitter released is an *excitatory transmitter* then it excites the postsynaptic membrane to additional presynaptic excitatory impulses called an *excitatory postsynaptic potential (EPSP).* If the neurotransmitter released is an *inhibitory transmitter,* it actively reduces irritability of the motorneuron and minimizes the firing level, referred to as an *inhibitory postsynaptic potential (IPSP).* Evidence indicates that the IPSP are produced by terminals of special interneurons called Golgi bottle neurons. These interneurons lie between afferent and motorneurons. Golgi bottle neurons are of special importance in pain because they have the ability to transform excitatory input into inhibitory output in the spinal cord. Conversion of signals is illustrated in Figure 2.17.

There are specific criteria that chemical substances must meet to be

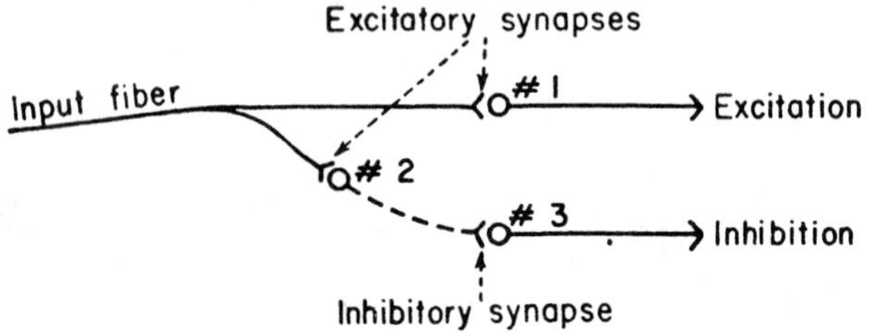

Figure 2.17. Conversion of an excitatory signal into an inhibitory signal. In this figure the input fiber divides and secretes excitatory transmitter at both its endings causing excitation of both neurons 1 and 2. Because neuron 2 is an inhibitory neuron, which secretes inhibitory transmitter, excitation of this neuron will result in inhibition of neuron 3. *(Guyton, A.C. Textbook of Medical Physiology, 6th ed. Philadelphia: W.B. Saunders, 1981, Figure 47.7, p. 580, with permission.)*

classified as a neurotransmitter. At this time, there are only four substances which are *proven* neurotransmitters. However, there are many other substances which have been strongly implicated as neurotransmitters because they meet some of the criteria. These substances are referred to as *putative neurotransmitters*. Proven neurotransmitters include acetylcholine, norepinephrine, epinephrine, and dopamine. Putative neurotransmitters include glycine, aspartic acid, glutamic acid, γ-aminobutyric acid (GABA), serotonin (5-hydroxytryptamine), and histamine.

We will now consider the relevance of neurotransmitters to the experience of pain. Pain may be produced by mechanical, chemical, or thermal stimuli irritating and/or injuring tissues and initiating a process at the cellular level, which leads to the perception of pain. The most frequent nociceptive stimuli to skin, muscles, tendons, ligaments, and viscera are chemical.

The *pH* in the tissues in pain states is highly acidic. The acid metabolites seem to heighten the sensitivity in pain fibers. For example, when inflammation occurs, it is difficult to anesthetize the tissues. The exact basis for this response is unknown (Linderoth, 1981). A common example of pH tissue change occurs in muscle spasm. Both blood flow to and the rate of metabolism of the tissues are factors. The contracting muscle compresses the intramuscular blood vessels and increases the metabolic rate of the muscle. Both of these factors result in ischemic pain.

Although many toxins and other naturally occurring substances do produce pain, there is controversy over whether or not one substance has unequivocally been proven to be the *only pain-producing substance (PPS)* activated or released by cellular injury. Mountcastle (1980) believes the identity of a transmitter PPS is still uncertain, and that the origin, mechanism of release, and mode of action are equally obscure. Benedetti (1979), on the other hand, describes it and its role as fact. As such, he says that *Substance P* (PPS) is an excitatory neurotransmitter peptide necessary for the transmission of pain impulses from the periphery to the higher cortical centers in the brain. When enkephalin or morphine bind to the receptor sites, they inhibit the release of substance P, thereby preventing the transmission of pain impulses. Descending substance P pathways have been identified in the ventrocaudal area surrounding the *aqueductus cerebri* and they synapse with neurons in the nucleus raphe magnus.

Lewis (1942) describes the *triple response,* the reaction which occurs when the skin has been injured. In the injured tissue, initially there is an area of intense vasodilatation. Soon this is followed by edema which results in a wheal formation surrounded by a wider area of less intense redness. The erythema is caused by vasodilatory flushing of the skin. The areas of injury and that area immediately surrounding it exhibit an increased response to pinprick and there occurs a lessening of the pain threshold. In the wider area of erythema there may also be an increased sensitivity to pinprick, however, there is no lowering of the pain threshold. After transection of peripheral nerves, the full triple response still occurs. The vasodilatation is believed to be caused by impulses which travel antidromically to the small C nociceptive afferents which ellicit vasomotor changes. It is proposed that the antidromic effect on the C fibers releases or causes the formation of a substance which both activates the nerve endings of nociceptive afferents and releases the smooth muscles of the arterioles (Mountcastle, 1980, pp. 400–401).

It is strongly suspected that inflammatory processes are somewhat related to both acute and chronic pain. The possible series of events is described here according to Weissman's (1977a, b) theory.

When there is an acute insult to the cell, *mediators* are launched within a few minutes. These *acid metabolites* are algogenic, capable of provoking pain. They include *histamine, kinins* (e.g., *bradykinin*), *prostaglandins,* and *serotonin.* For example, when platelets encounter an abraded surface, prostaglandins and serotonin are released.

Following the mediators within minutes or hours is another set of substances called *intermediators.* Up to this point there has been no irreversible cell damage, but the intermediators are very damaging to cell membranes and connective tissue. They may break down intracellular compounds and attack the cell membranes. During this time, phagocytic cells are activated by the injurious stimuli and by the mediators. During activation the phagocyte undergoes metabolic stimulation. The resulting end products are toxic and capable of injuring cell membranes of previously involved cells, causing further injury.

In the next and final stage, inflammatory mediators called *leukokines* are released from lymphocytes. Many leukokines are seen days after injury and also are found in chronic lesions. They mimic many of the actions of the first two sets of mediators, including the production of pain.

The body has mechanisms for reducing and eliminating the pain mediators. Otherwise, we would suffer pain for a very long time after even minor injury. Certain drugs also are used to interfere with the mediators. A common example is aspirin, which blocks the production of prostaglandins, known to block the action of the enkephalins.

The action of aspirin and other nonnarcotic analgesics can be used to illustrate the complexity of interactions at the cellular level with respect to pain. Prostaglandins, one of the initial pain mediators, induce only moderate pain by themselves but they seem to increase sensitivity to bradykinin. Thus, if aspirin interferes with the production of prostaglandins, it may decrease pain by decreasing the ability of bradykinin to produce pain. The action of aspirin and other nonnarcotic analgesics is illustrated in Figure 2.18.

In addition to the description of the role of leukokines, prostaglandins, and bradykinin, other putative neurotransmitters are involved in nociception. *Serotonin (5-Hydroxytryptamine)*, one of the cell mediators mentioned above, is found in the raphe nuclei of the medulla which is part of the pain receptor system. Serotonin depletion antagonizes both *stimulation-produced analgesia* (SPA) and opiate analgesia (Akil & Mayer, 1972; Bausbaum & Fields, 1978; Hayes et al., 1977; Tenen, 1968; and Vogt, 1974). Depleted serotonin levels are found in patients with chronic pain, peripheral nerve lesions, endogenous depression, and prior to the onset of migraine headaches (Almay et al., 1978, 1980; Asberg et al., 1976; Sicuteri, 1976, Sicuteri et al., 1973; and Terenius, 1981). It is believed that serotonin inhibits the transmission of nociceptive impulses in the dorsal horn or increases the pain tolerance. Injection of serotonin in the subarachnoid lumbar space produces profound analgesia in rats (Wang, 1977).

L-tryptophan is a precursor of serotonin. When inhibited or depleted, it decreases serotonin synthesis. Studying all three together, norepinephrine, dopamine, and serotonin, Akil & Liebskind (1975) noted depletion inhibited opiate analgesia and SPA. The original level of analgesia could be restored by injection of the precursors of serotonin or dopamine (L-tryptophan and *L-dopa*). It is believed that dopamine and norepinephrine exist in the hypothalamus, hippocampus, corpus striatum, septum, and cortex although their action is not known. In order to have a functional descending *antinoceptive* system, all three must be present. *Adrenocorticotropic hormone* (ACTH) and *b-Melanocyte Stimulating Hormone* (b-MSH), endogenic antagonists (antagonize endorphins), decrease the analgesic effects of morphine (Winter & Flataker, 1951; and Zimmerman & Krivoy, 1973). This antagonist effect of ACTH is dose-related (Paroli, 1967). ACTH is

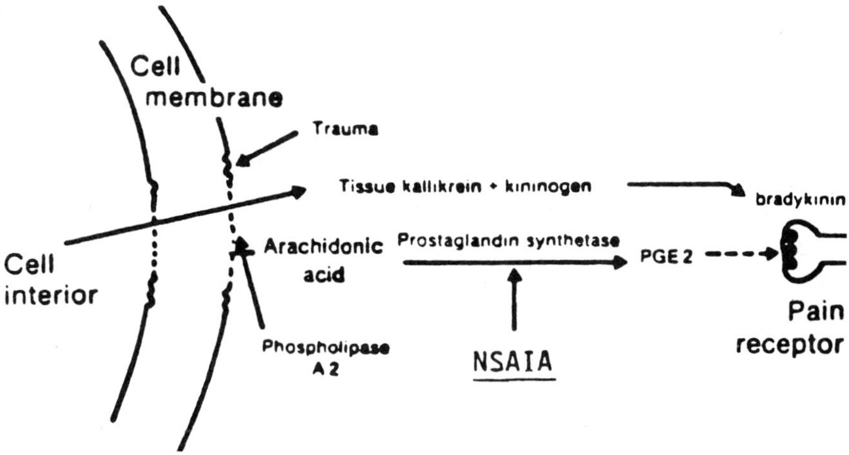

Mild Analgesics

Generic Name	Trade Name	Normal Analgesic Dose (mg)	Site of Action
Acetylsalicylic acid (Aspirin)	Generic, Bufferin Bayer's aspirin	325–650	Peripheral
Acetaminophen	Tylenol, Datril, Bayer's non-aspirin	325–650	Peripheral
Codeine	—	30–60	Central
Propoxyphene hydrochloride	Darvon, Dolene, SK-65	65	Central
Propoxyphene napsylate	Darvon-N	100	Central

Figure 2.18. Mechanism of action of nonnarcotic analgesics. (*Pittman, A.W. & Rudd, G.D. Analgesic Therapy, Part 2: Analgesia for Severe Pain. Indianapolis, MD: Eli Lilly and Company, 1980, p. 7, Pharmaceutical Division, with permission.*)

believed to be stored in the same cells as *b-lipotropin*. Pain usually produces high physical and emotional stress levels which increase ACTH and norepinephrine, both analgesic antagonists which lead to hyperactivity and increased pain perception. Patients with chronic pain usually experience a reactive depression. Depleted serotonin levels may be at least partially the cause of or aggravate the chronic pain patient's depression.

Bonica (1953) reported improvement in patients with chronic pain who were treated with *amphetamines*. Forrest et al., (1977) reported that 10 mg of dextroamphetamine almost doubled the analgesic effect of 12 mg of morphine. It also decreased the side effects of respiratory depression and lethargy. How the amphetamines actually effect their response is controversial. Some believe that amphetamines probably act on the serotonin receptors in the brain or by releasing dopamine or norepinephrine. Norepinephrine is connected with either increased pain or increase pleasure (Oleson, 1981).

Neuromodulators—The Endorphins The most promising scientific finding in relation to potential pain relief in recent years is the identification of the neuromodulators, the endorphins. These neuromodulators modulate or modify neuronal activity. It is believed that they act indirectly by increasing and decreasing the effects of particular neurotransmitters. The mechanism of the action of narcotic analgesics including enkephalin is illustrated in Figure 2.19.

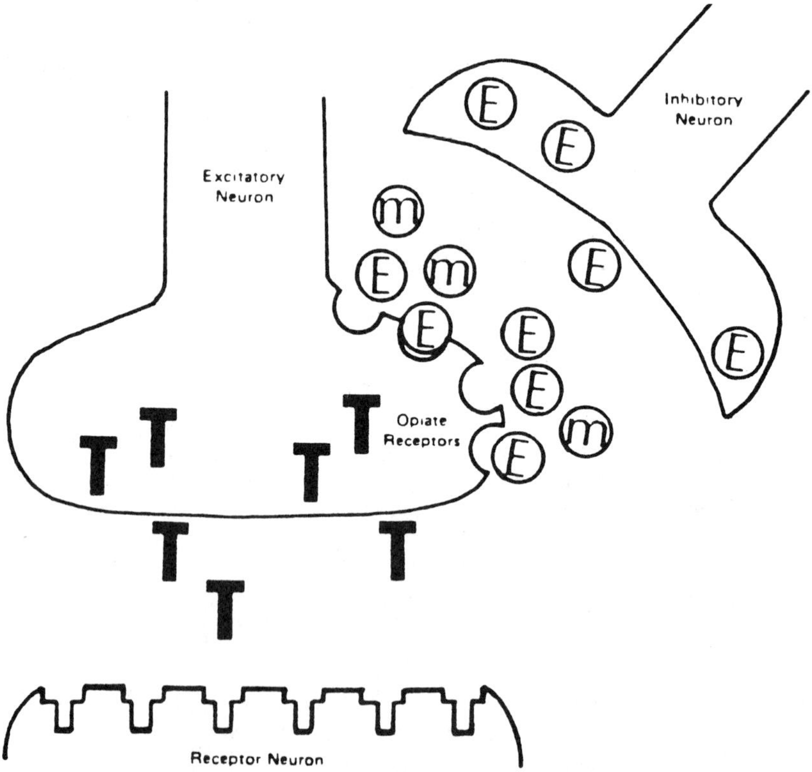

Figure 2.19. Mechanism of action of narcotic analgesics. The opiate receptor is thought to be located on the endings of excitatory neurons. Binding of enkephalin (E) or morphine (m) may inhibit release of transmitter **T**, and thereby lead to alteration in pain perception. *(Pittman, A.W. & Rudd, G.D. Analgesic Therapy, Part 2: Analgesia for Severe Pain. Indianapolis, M.D.: Eli Lilly and Company, Pharmaceutical Division, with permission.)*

Endorphin is a combination of two words, endogenous and morphine, meaning "morphine within," morphine being a potent narcotic analgesic. Endorphins are endogenous opiod peptides which are morphine-like in their pharmacologic action. Peptides contain two or more amino acids and are the building blocks of proteins. The endorphin chain is illustrated in Figure 2.20. It is believed that the exact natural equivalent of morphine has not been isolated and therefore there may be other endorphin systems not yet identified. Some endorphins are more potent analgesics than others. Some may have more to do with emotions and learning than with pain.

Over a decade ago, Reynolds (1968) demonstrated that electrical stimulation of the periaqueductal gray matter in the midbrain produced analgesia. Pert and Snyder (1976) identified stereospecific opiate receptors in the brain. Through the use of SPA and microinjections of opiates these receptors have been mapped. They are found to occur in varying concentrations in the brain, spinal cord and gastrointestinal tract.

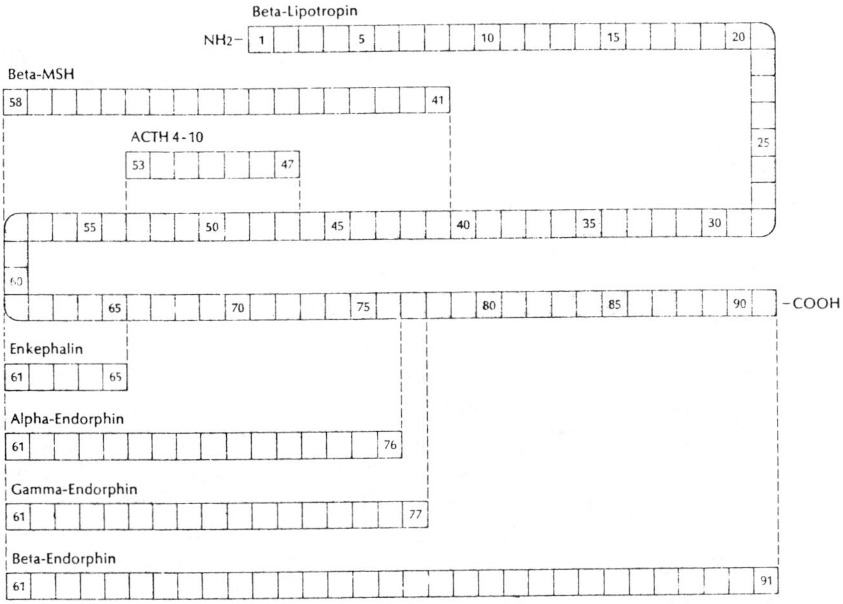

Figure 2.20. The large 91-amino-acid beta-lipotropin molecule, first isolated from the pituitary gland, contains the amino-acid sequences of several smaller biologically active peptide molecules, as illustrated in the schematic above. These include beta-melanocyte-stimulating hormone (beta-MSH), the ACTH fragment 4–10, the enkephalins, and alpha-, gamma-, and beta-endorphin. (*Krieger, D.T. & Hughes, J.C. Neuroendocrinology. Sunderland, MA.: A Hospital Practice Book, Sinauer Assoc., Inc., 1981, p. 69, with permission.*)

The brain has the highest concentration of opiate receptors. At the brainstem, receptors are found in the periaqueductal gray matter and in the periventricular gray matter of the mesencephalon, particularly the nucleus raphe magnus. In the forebrain, receptors are in the hypothalamus and the limbic system, especially the amygdaloid nuclear complex, the area believed to control emotions and inner feelings. This anatomical finding helps explain the involvement of emotions with pain. The next highest concentration of receptors is found in the substantia gelatinosa of the dorsal horn of the spinal cord and the fewest are found in the gastrointestinal tract (gut). The finding of these receptors led to the search for substances which would bind with them. The discovery of this substance, *enkephalin*, arrived in 1975 when Terenius & Hughes, working independently, identified an opiod-like peptide from the brain. Soon after other molecularly similar peptides were identified and this total classification was given the generic name "endorphins."

Since that time literally thousands of articles have been published on endorphins. Reviews of the current status of relevant neuroanatomy and neurophysiology of endorphins in pain modulation occurs in Bausbaum and Fields (1978), Benedetti (1979), Mountcastle (1981), Sherman & Liebeskind (1980) and Terenius (1981). The reader is referred to these well-documented sources.

To date, the endorphins which have been identified are:

1. *Beta-lipotropin.* This peptide is a 91-amino-acid hormone from the pituitary gland. It contains the following:
   a. *Beta-endorphin.* This is 61–91 on the amino acid chain. It may be a "biochemical switch" and may be degraded into compounds that can either enhance or inhibit pain. Beta-endorphins are larger molecules than the enkephalins and have an increased affinity for opiate receptors in the hypothalamus and the pituitary gland. They produce analgesia which is many times more powerful than morphine when injected intracerebrally. This has been confirmed in the treatment of terminal cancer patients (Oyama, 1980). Beta-endorphins are less resistant to proteolytic enzymes. When they are administered intravenously they can produce analgesia lasting for 2–3 hours.
   b. *Gamma-endorphin.* This is 61–77 on the amino acid chain. It provides some analgesia and may have to do with violent behavior.
   c. *Alpha-endorphin.* This is 61–76 on the amino acid chain. It is less analgesic than beta-endorphin.
2. *Enkephalin.* Enkephalins are peptides found in both the brain and in the spinal cord. They are localized to nerve fibers and their endings. They may be cleaved from beta-lipotropin. They are considered weakly

analgesic. Proteolytic enzymes rapidly destroy enkephalins when they are injected intravenously or intracerebrally. However, enkephalins have been synthesized and can be administered intravenously and orally. They have been found to be more potent and longer acting than morphine and resist degradation. It is believed that enkephalins act locally as neurotransmitters or neuromodulators and centrally on pain. This neuroregulator contains:

a. *Met-enkephalin*
b. *Leu-enkephalin*

3. *Dynorphin.* This is another compound word, "dynamite endorphin." It is a peptide with an analgesic potency 50 times greater than beta-endorphin. One end of its structure incorporates leucine (leu) enkephalin. It is either a hormone or a neurotransmitter.

Snyder (1977) has proposed that the mechanism of enkephalin inhibition may be indirect. Instead of acting directly on the receiving nerve cell, enkephalin may block the release of excitatory neurotransmitters. This would reduce the receiving cell's excitatory input. Mudge et al. (1979) have suggested that enkephalins may be released in response to a noxious stimulus or some central inhibitory mechanism. It has been noted that enkephalins inhibit the release of Substance P, preventing transmission of noxious impulses.

How does one test the action of the endorphins? At the present time, the relevance of blood plasma and urine studies is considered doubtful. However, endorphins can be measured in other ways. Endorphins are found in the central nervous system, therefore direct brain tissue analysis and the concentration of endorphins in the cerebral spinal fluid (CSF) can be measured. Because of the complexities involved in obtaining endorphin samples with these approaches, such as the problems of access and the danger of possible complications to the patient, it is difficult to justify repeated studies in human subjects. The endorphin levels are known to fluctuate under some circumstances such as depression. Therefore, repeated studies are highly desirable to establish a baseline. Pharmacologic approaches have less risk. The potency of the endorphins can be studied by direct injection to their receptor sites, which prevents proteolytic degradation. Again, this procedure makes repeated studies difficult to justify. Injection of an opiate antagonist has less risk. Opiate antagonists have the ability to reverse the analgesic effects of the endorphins. Naloxone is such a substance and it is used with frequency for this purpose.

Both stress and pain are known to activate the endorphin system. Also, it is believed that pain modulation is one of the normal functions of the central nervous system. Because naloxone only partially reverses SPA it is believed that other systems also inhibit pain. It now has been clearly demonstrated that SPA and opiate analgesia activate a descending pathway that inhibits pain by stimulating neurons in the base of the brain in the periaqueductal-periventricular gray matter. This activation comes through the limbic system and in turn stimulates the raphe nuclei which activates a descending pathway down to the interneurons of the dorsal horn of the spinal cord where pain inhibition occurs in the segmental levels (Sherman & Liebskind, 1980). Therefore, activation of the endorphin system actually controls pain at the primary afferent neurons. Some lesions of the dorsal spinal column decrease or abolish the analgesic effect of SPA and opiate drugs by inhibiting their effect in the brainstem. Another possible method of action of the endorphin system is to block excitatory neurotransmitters by decreasing excitatory output.

Placebos are also known to activate the descending system leading to release of endorphins in some patients. It is not clear why some persons are able to activate their own endorphin system and others are not. Halpern (1980) believes that, on psychological grounds, at least 40 percent of the population should be able to mobilize their own endorphins. He reported a study at the University of Washington on two groups of postoperative renal transplant patients. One group of patients received analgesics for postoperative pain and the other group did not. The patients who received no analgesics postoperatively had a "miserable" first postoperative day for about 8 hours after surgery. Thereafter, it is believed autogenic release of enkephalins resulted in sedation and analgesia. During the next four days, these patients showed better pain control and better sedation than if opiates had been used. Patients who did receive opiate analgesics postoperatively had some of their discomfort eased during the first postoperative day, but they never achieved elevations of their pain threshold or levels of comfort as high as those patients who were not given analgesics.

It is not known to what extent pain intensity triggers endorphin release (Terenius, 1981). There is a limited amount of data correlating endorphin release in modulation of acute pain. However, it has been shown that individuals with a decreased preoperative CSF endorphin level require more analgesia than individuals with a high endorphin level (Tamsen, et al. 1980). In Sweden, on a serial study of 45 patients with chronic pain, three investigators independently rated factors related to pain perception (Almay, et al. 1978). One conducted a neurological assessment, one a psychiatric assessment, and the other measured endorphin and serotonin levels. The final evaluation, a composite of each patient, was not made until data from each of the three categories were completed. The findings for these patients with chronic pain were that the endorphin levels were frequently low. This was particularly true for patients with peripheral nerve lesions whose pain was neurogenic. A corresponding portion of these patients also had very low serotonin levels. Another correlation from this study is one that had been noted before (Asberg et al., 1976). That is, the correlation between low serotonin levels and endogenous depression (Almay et al., 1980). Sicuteri et al. (1978), found that patients with migraine headaches have lower endorphin and serotonin levels during their attack and the vascular receptors are extremely sensitive to serotonin.

The knowledge about the endorphins already has been applied therapeutically. In addition to the report of Oyama (1980) it has been demonstrated that low frequency *transcutaneous electrical stimulation (TENS)* seems to release endorphins, as does *acupuncture*. Salar et al. (1981), studied endorphin levels in patients without pain problems using TENS. They found that all subjects during and after 20–25-minute treatments had an increase in their endorphin levels, regardless of their basal level. They also found that the use of TENS triggers therapeutic endorphin levels within the first hour. After that period, stimulation may not relieve pain. Based on their findings they recommended the use of TENS in 1-hour cycles several times a day. They theorized that after the initial stimulation of endorphins for therapeutic pain relief, the endorphins were depleted. Suspension of TENS is necessary to allow the endorphin level to recover. It has been found that one may become addicted to one's own endorphins, and the endorphins have the same side-effects as classic opiates (Terenius, 1981).

The clinical application of the endorphin and enkephalin knowledge at this time is still tentative and exploratory. It has been suggest that because of its rapid onset of action and short-lived effect the enkephalins will be useful in the treatment of acute pain. Because of the modulatory effect of beta-endorphin and its longer lasting effect it has been speculated that its greatest use may be in chronic pain. One possible goal could be to isolate and administer these substances as a natural morphine. The theories about endorphins explain some of the differences in sensitivity to pain. For example, in some people anxiety about their pain may release their endorphins. In chronic pain, endorphin systems apparently cease to function in some individuals. It is possible, as described previously, to stimulate the central nervous system to release endorphins by surgically implanting electrodes in the periaqueductal gray, by acupuncture, TENS, and placebos. It is now possible to identify chemicals which inhibit enzymes that inhibit endorphins; D-phenylalamine is one such chemical.

Terenius (1981, pp. 173–174) points out what he believes are two of the major contributions endorphin research has made to pain therapy from a practical therapeutic point of view. First, "there is now less conservatism in the use of opiates when they are really needed. Since the body makes its own opiates it should not be unethical to use such drugs." Second, endorphin research has provided "the rational basis for various stimulation techniques."

Unfortunately, *Science News* (1979) says, about the complexities of the endorphins, that "things are going to get more confusing before they are fully understood."

Other Factors Influencing Transmission Transmission of information in the nervous system is contingent upon the characteristic properties of neurons, namely irritability and conductivity. *Irritability* means that the neuron is capable of being stimulated and *conductivity* means that the neuron is capable of conducting or propagating impulses.

Nerve fibers are almost never singly stimulated. Rather impulses are transmitted in groups of parallel fibers known as a signal. A *signal* refers to the overall pattern of impulses in a nerve fiber or tract. It is more accurate and descriptive of how the information is actually transmitted. For example, nociceptive signals transmit information about pain.

The area in the neuronal pool in which incoming nerve fibers spread is called the *stimulatory* or *excitory field* of the neuron. Incoming stimuli to the neuronal pool may be either *excitory*, capable of causing the neuron to *discharge*, or *subthreshold*. Areas in the neuronal pool in which all of the neurons discharge are called the *discharge zone*. Areas peripheral to the discharge zone are called the *facilitated, subthreshold,* or *subliminal zone*. These areas are illustrated in Figure 2.21.

As signals pass through neuronal pools they may converge or diverge. *Convergence*, illustrated in Figure 2.22, means that a single neuron may be controlled by the input from two or more separate nerve fibers from the same nerve or from several nerve sources, such as a nerve tract. An example of this is seen in the brain where several nerve tracts converge. *Divergence*, illustrated in Figure 2.23, is when a single input nerve stimulates multiple output fibers. This may occur in either the same tract which is referred to as *amplifying divergence* or in more than one tract which is referred to as *divergence in multiple tracts*. These concepts are important in the transmission of nociceptive impulses because they have the ability to inhibit or excite multiple neurons thus influencing one's pain experience.

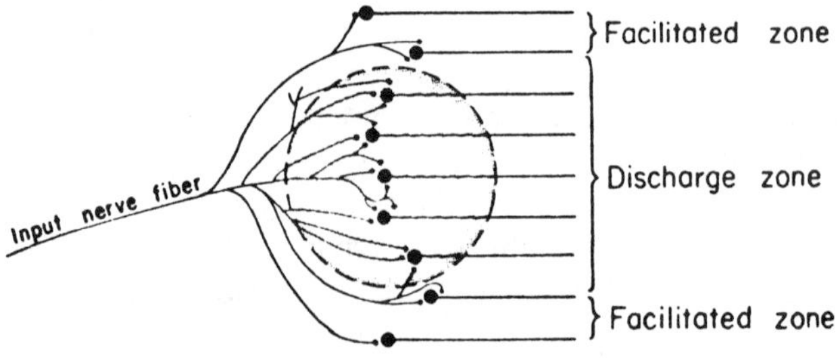

Figure 2.21. Discharge and facilitated zones of a neuronal pool. Note that the largest number of synaptic knobs lies in the center of the discharge zone whereas fewer knobs lie in the facilitated areas. (*Guyton, A.C. Textbook of Medical Physiology, 6th ed. Philadelphia: W.B. Saunders, 1981, Figure 47.5, p. 580, with permission.*)

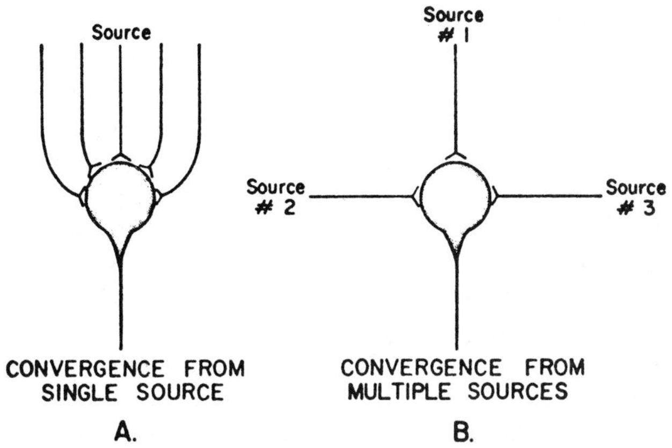

Figure 2.22. Convergence of multiple input fibers on a single neuron. In A, input fibers converge from a single source. In B, input fibers converge from multiple sources. For example, interneurons in the spinal cord may be processing information about the sensory, emotional, and cognitive components of pain all at the same time. (*Guyton, A.C. Textbook of Medical Physiology, 6th ed. Philadelphia: W.B. Saunders, 1981, Figure 47.8, p. 581, with permission.*)

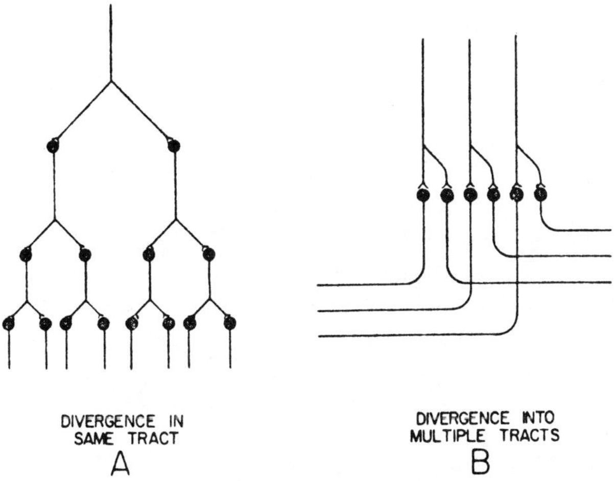

Figure 2.23. Divergence in neuronal pathways. In A, the divergence within a pathway causes amplification by the input signal spreading to an increasing number of neurons as it passes through successive pools of a nervous pathway. In B, divergence into multiple tracts, the signal is transmitted into separate directions from the pool to different parts of the nervous system. (*Guyton, A.C. Textbook of Medical Physiology, 6th ed. Philadelphia: W.B. Saunders, 1981, Figure 47.9, p. 581, with permission.*)

Summation quantifies the intensity of the pain sensation. It is determined both by the amplitude and frequency modulation of signals. *Spatial summation (multiple fiber summation)* or *amplitude* modulation is illustrated in Figure 2.24. It refers to the number of nociceptive receptors stimulated. The greater the number of nerve fibers stimulated the greater the strength of the pain signal. Spatial summation implies that if a pain stimulus which is subthreshold over a small area is applied to a larger area, the central additive effect of *the recruitment of additional fibers* will evoke pain sensations. Also, a *supraliminal stimulus* to a small area may elicit more intense pain sensations when applied to larger areas (Mountcastle, 1980, p. 395).

In general, however, pain intensity is not increased by the summation of impulses from noxious stimulation at *different sites* (Hardy, 1956). Therefore, multiple minor injuries *do not* result in excruciating pain. For example, in a hypothetical situation, a patient has five abrasions, each causing a pain intensity equal to an arbitrary value of two. The patient will tend to perceive pain at the value of two rather than ten. The intensities of the lacerations are not added together to cause overwhelming pain. However, because of the emotional component of the pain experience, it is not unlikely that some individuals will include the diameter of spatial involvement when evaluating their pain. That is, the total experience of pain, in contrast to the pain sensation may be influenced by spatial summation. For example, total body involvement in a burn patient may influence the total pain experience associated with the burn.

Temporal summation illustrated in Figure 2.25, refers to the number of impulses that are transmitted along the nerve fiber. Pain stimuli must travel at a given *frequency* or intensity (*threshold speed*) to be perceived as painful. With continued speed or a higher speed the pain sensation will escalate rapidly to an unbearable level. A common example of temporal summation occurs when a nurse is administering intravenous medications which may be irritating to the blood vessels. If the medications are administered rapidly, the patient may complain of severe pain. If the medications are administered more slowly, the patient may experience no pain.

There does not appear to be *neurological adaptation* or *habituation* to stimuli felt as painful. Nociceptors adapt not all or almost not all. A person may adapt to thermo- and mechanoreceptors. For example, with continued application of cold or pressure the sensation may decrease in intensity or disappear. Unfortunately, this does not seem to happen with pain. When the pain stimulus continues for a period of time, the excitation threshold may become progressively lower. It may then take less of a stimulus to activate the receptor sites. Therefore, the patient may experience increasing sensitivity to pain, a condition referred to as *primary hyperalgesia*. A common example of hyperalgesia occurs in patients with neurological

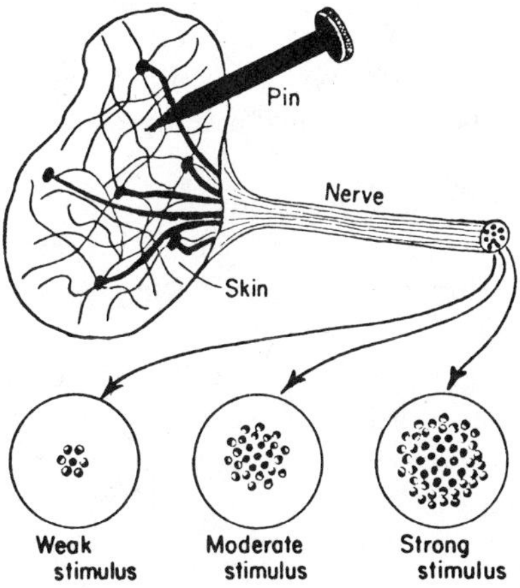

Figure 2.24. Spatial summation is illustrated in a sensory nerve. Each nerve fiber divides and spreads (arborizes) extensively over an area of skin. In the very center of the receptive field, the number of nerve endings from each fiber is large and becomes less and less toward the periphery. Thus, a pin pricking the skin stimulates the nerve fiber strongly if the point of simulation is in the center of its field of reception, but if the point of the stimulus is in the periphery of the field it stimulates the fiber only weakly. The lower part of the figure illustrates three separate views of the cross-section of the nerve bundle leading from the skin. On the left is shown the effect of a weak stimulus, with only a single nerve fiber in the middle of the bundle stimulated very strongly (represented by the solid black fiber) while several adjacent fibers are stimulated weakly (half-solid black fibers). The other two views of the nerve cross-section show the effect respectively of a moderate stimulus and a strong stimulus, with progressively more fibers being stimulated. (*Guyton, A.C. Textbook of Medical Physiology, 6th ed. Philadelphia: W.B. Saunders, 1981, Figure 47.1, p. 578, with permission.)*

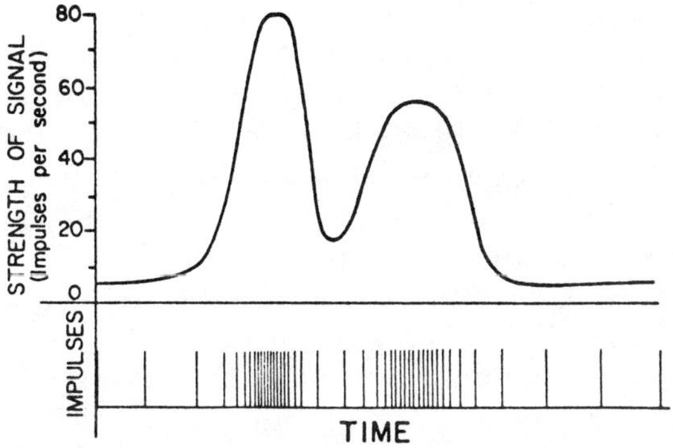

Figure 2.25. Temporal summation illustrating that the frequency increases and decreases with the strength of the signal. In the upper part of the figure the changing strength of the signal is illustrated and in the lower part the actual impulses transmitted by the nerve fiber are shown. (*Guyton, A.C. Textbook of Medical Physiology. Philadelphia: W.B. Saunders, 6th ed. 1981 Figure 47.2, p. 578, with permission.*)

disorders, such as Trigeminal Neuralgia (Tic Doloreaux). These patients experience increased activation of their pain receptors with time. Their receptors become so hypersensitive that normal activities, such as talking or chewing and environmental factors such as mildly cold or windy weather, may trigger intense pain. Intense *secondary hyperalgesia* refers to facilitation of sensory transmission in the CNS. It is believed that secondary hyperalgesia may be the mechanism underlying central pathological pain syndromes such as the thalamic syndrome. Hypoalgesia is decreased sensitivity to pain. Individuals sometimes are congenitally hypoalgesic.

Perceptual dominance of the most painful sensations tends to occur. When a patient is experiencing pain and another source of pain is imposed on him, one of the pain sensations may become dominant and alter the perceived intensity of the other pain sensation. When the patient experiences intense pain in one area of the body, the threshold of sensory perception in other areas is raised (Berlin et al., 1958). In other words, intense pain in one area of the body causes the patient to be less sensitive to a milder pain in another area of the body. In fact, he may not feel the milder sensation. The presence of pain may also raise the thresholds of perception for other sensory inputs, such as hearing, vibration, and temperature.

One patient, for example, experienced a severe migraine headache during her hospitalization for the management of intractable cancer pain. During this period of time, she demonstrated increased thresholds for her nerve root compression pain and for auditory stimulation. When the nurse entered the room to administer an injection of ergotamine, she asked this patient to turn to her side. The nurse's tone of voice was the one she ordinarily used in conversing with this patient. However, this patient did not respond until the request was repeated in a louder voice. After the injection the nurse told this patient that she could turn onto her back again. This patient asked, "But aren't you going to give me something?" When the nurse said she had already given the injection, the patient said she had not felt it. The perceptual dominance of her headache made her less sensitive than usual to even the usually rated severe cancer pain sensation and to the milder pain sensation of the injection and to auditory input. However, if one pain sensation is not sufficiently intense to gain dominance over another, the patient may be aware of both pain sensations at the level of intensity he would perceive them if they occurred separately.

Perceptual dominance is an important concept when working with patients with pain. It is not uncommon for a patient with multiple pain sites to report only the pain site that is most dominant or distressing. The health team initiates strategies to decrease this reported pain and, indeed, the patient evaluates their strategies as successful. However, the patient then reports pain in another site. When this sequence recurrs, the staff may give less credence to the patient's pain reports, label him or her a malingerer, and fail to thoroughly assess the patient's pain complaints.

Melzack (1973, pp. 110–119) applies the concepts of summation, adaptation and perceptual dominance to normal and pathological nociception. He says that the effect of the input signals is determined by the types of patterns involved. For example, in normal individuals vibration modifies the amount of pain perceived, whereas in individuals with causalgia or neuralgia the pain is enhanced by mild stimulation. In these individuals, strong stimuli such as vigorous massage, heavy pressure, and pinching may not only not evoke pain but they may produce pain relief. Other findings that he reports relating to pain patterns involve the timing of stimuli and the size of the pain stimuli (spatial and temporal summation). For example, an electric shock may be minimized by a slap on the skin either preceeding or following it. This theory has been applied by some nurses in administering injections to patients who have anticipatory fear. Melzack also reports that a shock delivered to one arm raises the pain perception threshold in the other arm, known as *metacontrast* which is explained later as perceptual dominance. This theory has also been used in pain relief. When an involved area is too painful to touch, TENS applied contralaterally has been found to provide pain relief. This latter approach has also been found to be true for sites distant to the painful site.

In individuals with causalgia, neuralgia, and other pathological pain syndromes, when the area stimulated is increased so is the intensity of the pain. Because this does not occur in normal skin, Melzack suggests that when the larger area of normal skin is stimulated, the inhibitory area surrounding it may be able to cancel out the additional excitatory impulses.

Light touch may result in an *afterglow*, a tingling that not only may persist for several minutes but occassionally presents a *mirror area* on the other side of the body. Another point that Melzack makes about patterning of pain signals is that a warm probe used to stimulate the skin may produce a sharp stinging pain that far outlasts the stimulation. Other patients report a *zone of awareness* instead of, or after, afterglow. This zone has been described as an area of heightened awareness or pulsations that the individuals believe reflect their own blood vessels in the skin or their own breathing rate. Later, after the zone of awareness has subsided, these individuals can sometimes evoke the zone by intense concentration. Melzack believes that these sensations suggest the involvement of one's cognitive processes facilitating the transmission of impulses and is in part due to input from blood vessels or surrounding tissue. That is nociceptive input may produce long-lasting memories just as those produced by other somatosensory input such as those from vision and hearing. This input results in changes in the central neural activity. He says that these concepts are supported by experimental evidence in both man and animals.

THEORIES OF THE PAIN MECHANISM

Many attempts have been made to use the current data about pain to formulate a model or theory that could explain how the pain mechanism all works together. Considering that there is a vast amount of information that nevertheless contains enormous gaps, any such attempt is admirable. Here are some theories that grew out of the information available when they were formulated. As more knowledge accumulates, the theories are criticized and revised. Each theory contains some useful and, so far, accurate aspects. The theories discussed here are illustrated in Figure 2.26.

Specificity Theory

The specificity theory is the oldest, over 200 years old, and most orthodox view of pain. Pain is explained as a primary sensation like hearing and smell. This model suggests that there is a specific pain modality that can be stimulated only by painful stimuli and, therefore, these impulses are always felt specifically as pain and only pain. The theory assumes that there is a direct and invariant relationship between stimulus intensity and perceived pain. It proposes that undifferentiated free nerve endings located in various organs and substructures are the major, if not the specific, pain receptors that generate pain impulses. These impulses are carried from the specific receptors by specific sensory pain fibers, A-delta and C, in peripheral nerves through the dorsal horn. They synapse in the substantia gelatinosa and travel via the lateral spinothalamic tract to a "pain center" in the thalamus where they are perceived as pain (Sweet, 1959; Sternbach, 1968; Melzack & Wall, 1970).

There seems to be little question that peripheral system pathways have specialized functions related to pain, but there is doubt that any of them comprise an exclusive pain modality in which there is a fixed stimulus–response relationship. Some opponents of the specificity theory feel that one of its major weaknesses is its psychological assumption. To say that certain receptors and/or fibers respond only to noxious stimulation is a physiological statement. But to say that this stimulation will always be *felt* as pain is a psychological statement. Stimulation of pain-specific receptors and fibers does not always produce pain, and pain is not the only sensation that may be produced. Many variables affect the transduction properties of receptor–fiber units, such as rate of adaptation and thresholds to mechanical distortion or chemical change. Opponents of this theory suggest that the physiological specialization of nervous system pathways in the pain mechanism can be accepted as fact without also accepting that stimulation of these pathways will invariably result in feeling pain (Melzack & Wall, 1970).

The specificity theory is helpful in explaining how a person with an

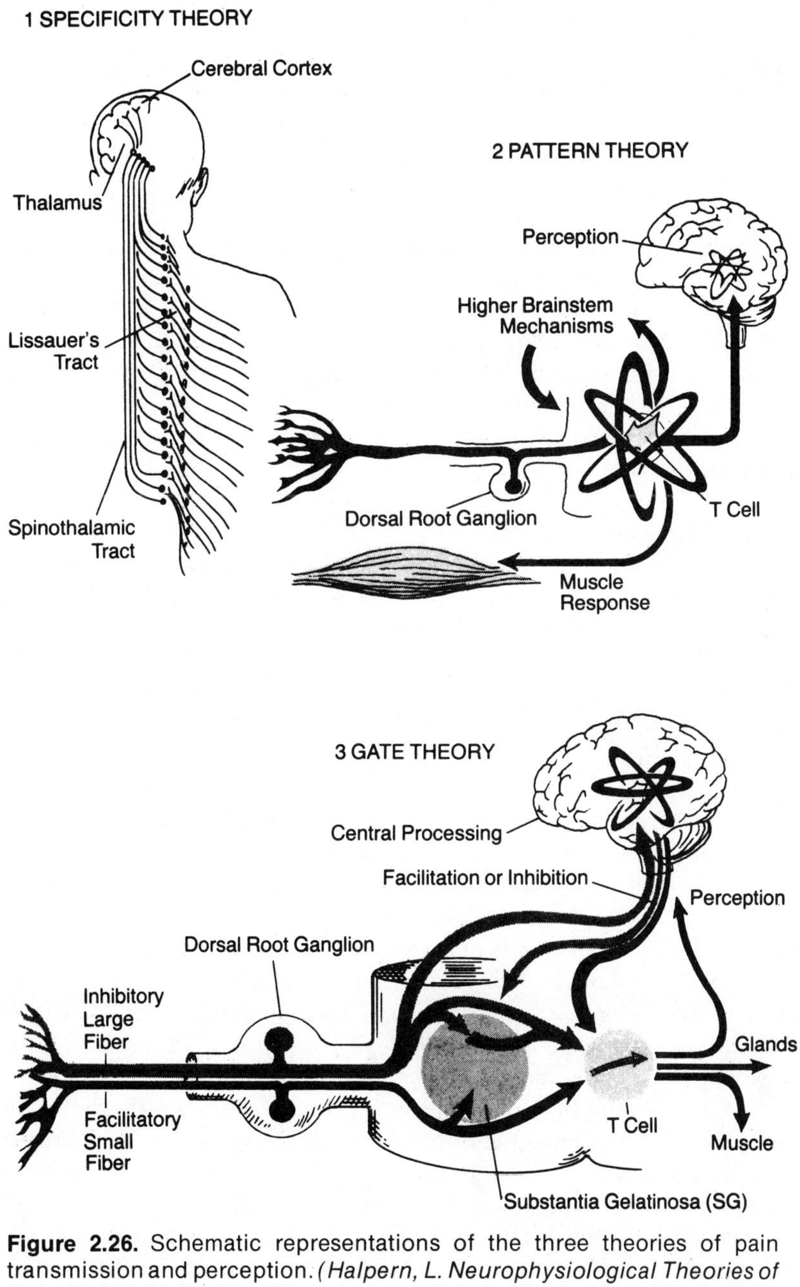

Figure 2.26. Schematic representations of the three theories of pain transmission and perception. *(Halpern, L. Neurophysiological Theories of Pain. Plainfield, NJ: The Management of Pain in Surgical Practice. Symposium: The Management of Pain in Surgical Practice, Boston, MA, Sept. 22–23, 1978. Copyright © New York: Pfizer, Inc., 1979. Adapted from Pearson, H.P. Pain Pathways—An overview. In Recent Studies on the Nature and Management of Acute Pain: HP Publishing Inc. Jan. 1976, p. 15, with permission.)*

intact neurophysiological system perceives and responds to pain when impending or actual tissue damage triggers impulses that travel over the nervous system pathways. In other words, he feels pain because pain pathways have been stimulated. However, when comparable stimuli are applied to several people, it does not explain why one person will perceive intense pain, another moderate pain, and still another no pain at all. There is not a fixed stimulus–response relationship if tissue damage does not always result in pain. Further, the specificity theory explains why pain may be alleviated after alterations in the pain pathways, such as chordotomy or thalamotomy, but it does not explain why pain may continue or return. An example of another still unanswered question is why does warmth, which is perceived as comfortable, when carried to the extreme of heat, is perceived as painful.

Pattern Theories

Because of some of the problems encountered in the specificity theory, a pattern theory of the pain mechanism was proposed. The pattern theory actually includes several slightly different theories. All of these theories generally have in common the concept that patterning of the nerve impulses generated by receptors forms the basis of a code that provides the information that there is pain. It is widely accepted that the basis of sensory perception is provided by the temporal and spatial summation of nerve impulses, that is, the patterns associated with the length of time a stimulus lasts and the area it covers. One of the pattern theories stresses a *reverberating circuit mechanism* (Livingston, 1943). Another pattern theory is a *specialized input-controlling system* (Noordenbos, 1959). Still another suggests that the pattern for pain is produced by intense stimulation of *nonspecific receptors* (Weddell, 1962). The latter proposes that all fiber endings are alike, except for those that innervate hair cells. It ignores the evidence that indicates that nervous system pathways have specialized functions related to pain.

The *input-control theory* suggests that two fiber systems are involved in pain: (1) a rapidly conducting system, and (2) a more slowly conducting system that transmits pain impulses. Normally, the rapidly conducting fiber system inhibits synaptic transmission in the more slowly conducting system that carries the signal for pain. Under pathological conditions, the slow system conducting pain establishes dominance over the fast system. The fast system is then unable to inhibit the transmission of pain impulses. This theory explains that pathological pain states result from the central summation of impulses in the slowly conducting fiber system. It also explains that failure to relieve pain by sectioning pain pathways in the spinal cord is due to a "leak" of impulses past the point of sectioning by way of the diffuse connections of the anterolateral pathways. But sectioning of the latter may fail as well, which is often the problem for patients who have received such surgical treatment for chronic pain.

The *reverberating circuit mechanism* also relies on central summation and proposes that pathological stimulation sets up *reverberating circuits* in spinal inernuncial neurons. These circuits are believed to be closed loops of nerve fibers that stimulate one another in a circular fashion. Once established these circuits can then be triggered by normally nonnoxious inputs. This generates the abnormal volleys of nerve impulses up the spinal cord to the brain where they are interpreted as pain. For example, a trigger point may develop in a limb that has been previously injured. The initial injury sets up the reverberating circuit. Then merely touching the limb can stimulate the circuit to generate more impulses that would be felt as pain. Even in the absence of touch, the abnormal activity may continue in the circuit. Therefore, pain may continue in the absence of peripheral stimuli. Since at this point the source of pain is actually in the spinal cord itself, it is understandable why some procedures such as neurectomy and sympathectomy do not always alleviate pain. This does not explain, however, why severing pathways in the cord or thalamus may not relieve pain, nor why brain stimulation may also fail.

Gate-Control Theory

In 1965, Melzack & Wall proposed the gate-control theory, the most comprehensive model of pain formulated to that date. It was expanded by Casey & Melzack in 1967 and in 1975 Melzack and Wall emphasized the importance of the central mechanisms of modulating nociception. This theory has been a major force in renewing interest in the study of pain and in generating new ideas in pain therapy. In the years since the theory was proposed, virtually every article on pain at least mentions the contribution made by these men. On the other hand, the theory is also criticized on many levels. However, ideas need not be entirely accurate to be fruitful.

The gate-control theory retains concepts from both the specificity and pattern theories, including ideas about spatial and temporal summation and specificity of pain receptors. In addition, as its name implies, the theory suggests that the transmission of pain impulses can be modulated by a gating mechanism all along the central nervous system and that impulses can flow in both ascending and descending directions. In other words, the entire nervous system is involved in the perception of and response to pain. Conceptually, when the gate is open, pain impulses flow through easily; when the gate is closed, no pain impulses flow through; when the gate is partially open, only some of the pain impulses flow through. Moreover, the gate-control theory established that pain is not just a physiological function of tissue damage, but that psychological variables interact to influence the perception of pain in intensity and quality. Prior beliefs were that pain was a primary sensation and that psychological and cognitive variables were secondary to the perception of pain. The gate-control theory rather demonstrated that this relationship of variables involved a complex balance between the peripheral and central nervous systems. Because some information such as location and type of stimuli reach the brain before other kinds of information, the gate can actually intervene *before* pain impulses evoke the perception of, and response to, pain stimuli.

The gate-control theory relies upon fairly complex neurophysiological processes, and this is one of the most questionable aspects of the theory. It has been suggested that the processes involved are far more complicated than the theory originally stipulated, and it is now thought that the actual mechanisms and location of the gate are erroneous. The notion of gating mechanisms may be accurate, however, since it is known that there are places in the central nervous system where pain impulses can be inhibited (Nathan, 1976). Others, too, have disagreed with some of the basic neurophysiological assumptions of the gate-control theory. They have pointed out that additional and more complicated mechanisms probably are involved such as presynaptic inhibition by the dorsal root reflex and certain postsynaptic activity (Crue et al., 1976). Thus, with increasing information, some parts of the gate-control theory were restated in 1976 (Wall).

In clinical practice, one of the most useful portions of the gate-control theory is the conceptualization of what may influence the transmission of impulses eventually felt as painful (see Table 2.2). It has been duly noted that "lacking hard physiological facts or not, the theoretical base of the gate theory is being applied clinically and with a great deal of success" (Whidden & Fidler, 1977, p. 51).

The proposed location of the gating mechanism is in the substantia gelatinosa in the dorsal horn of the spinal cord (see Figure 2.8). The substantia gelatinosa normally modulates nociceptive impulses by keeping the gate partially closed. The gating mechanism is presynaptic. Activation of the substantia gelatinosa closes the gate further and inhibition opens it more. Activity in both the peripheral nervous system and the central nervous system could potentially alter the opening and closing of the gate. Hence, the transmission of pain impulses from the spinal cord to the level of awareness could be inhibited or facilitated.

It has also been theorized that there are ascending neurons in the spinal cord called *T (trigger) cells* which are activated by the A-delta and C fiber impulses after they have synapsed in the cord. The longer and wider the gate is open, the more impulses reach the T cells. At a given level of activity in the T cells, they in turn trigger the brain's pain reaction system. Thus, if all other neurophysiological processes are intact and functioning the individual will experience pain. T cell activity is usually limited by the normally partially closed gate in the substantia gelatinosa. At this time, no specific T cell has been identified. Three categories of activity appear to influence the opening and closing of the gate, thereby affecting the transmission of pain impulses from the spinal cord to the cortex (Melzack, 1973):

TABLE 2.2. Nursing Practice Aspects of the Gate Control Theory of Pain

Major Contributions

(1) An integrated conceptual model for appreciating the many factors that contribute to individual differences in the experience of pain.
(2) Conceptualization of categories of activity that may form a theoretical base for developing various pain relief measures.

Nature of the Gate

The transmission of potentially painful impulses to the level of conscious awareness may be affected by a gating mechanism, possibly located at the spinal cord level of the CNS.

Structures Involved	*No Pain or Decreased Intensity of Pain Results From Closing the Gate by:*	*Pain Results From Opening the Gate by:*
nerve fibers	(1) activity in the *large diameter nerve fibers*, e.g. caused by skin stimulation	(1) activity in the *small diameter nerve fibers,* e.g. caused by tissue damage,
brainstem	(2) inhibitory impulses from the *brainstem*, e.g. caused by sufficient or maximum sensory input arriving through distraction or guided imagery, or	(2) facilitory impulses from the *brainstem*, e.g. caused by insufficient input from a monotonous environment, or
cerebral cortex and thalamus	(3) inhibitory impulses from the *cerebral cortex* and *thalamus*, e.g. caused by anxiety reduction based on learning when the pain will end and how to relieve it.	(3) facilitory impulses from the *cerebral cortex* and thalamus, e.g. caused by fear that the intensity of pain will escalate and will be associated with death.

1. *Activity in the Large, A-delta and Small, C, Nerve Fibers.* The C-fiber system is excitory and carries the largest percentage of potentially painful impulses. When the gate is open, impulses travel from the periphery through the dorsal column fibers to the cortical level of awareness. Excitation of C fibers inhibit the activity in the substantia gelatinosa. This results in opening the gate even more and, thus, allowing more nociceptive impulses through. However, the gate may be closed and the nociceptive impulses blocked by stimulation of large-diameter A-delta afferent fibers. These fibers are known to exert an activating effect on the substantia ge-

latinosa, an inhibitory action at some places in the central nervous system. Pain impulses from A-delta fibers originating in the peripheral nervous system would be stopped at the spinal cord level and would not reach the brain or level of awareness. Since many cutaneous fibers are large-diameter fibers, stimulation of the skin by rubbing or other means may result in pain relief.

The concept of a gating mechanism resulted in the 1960s in the use of *dorsal column stimulation* (DCS) for the relief of chronic pain, e.g., low back pain. This required a laminectomy for the implantation of electrodes next to the dorsal column of the spinal cord. The electrodes were anchored to a stimulation plate. Connecting wires passed subcutaneously from the electrodes to a receiver implanted beneath the skin some distance away, usually in the chest or back. Externally, a battery-operated antenna was placed over the receiver. When this was activated by the patient, electrical stimulation of the dorsal column resulted, leading to feelings of buzzing or paresthesia in the painful area of the body. This was effective pain relief for many patients, but not all. Also, complications were fairly common (McCaffery, 1975).

Fortunately, it was discovered that electrical stimulation could be applied externally without any surgical procedure. Electrodes simply could be placed over the skin and activated by a battery-operated device to provide tingling or vibrating sensations in the area of pain. This resulted in pain relief with far fewer problems. This method is referred to by many terms, such as Transcutaneous Electrical Nerve Stimulation (TENS).

Nurses are familiar with many other methods of externally stimulating the large-diameter cutaneous fibers, such as heat, cold, and massage. The theory underlying the use of cutaneous stimulation techniques for pain relief is this portion of the gate control theory—closing the gate to the transmission of pain impulses by increasing activity in large-diameter nerve fibers.

2. Projections from the Brainstem Reticular Formation. The reticular activating system regulates or adjusts incoming and outgoing signals, including the amount of sensory input referred to as the *central biasing mechanism*. For each person, there seems to be an optimum amount of sensory input. If a person receives sufficient or excess sensory input, it appears that the reticular system may project inhibitory signals to the spinal cord. That is, if there is no need for additional sensory input, the reticular formation may cause the gate to be closed decreasing the summation of nociceptive impulses. Hence, pain signals would not reach the level of cortical awareness—no pain. Or, few pain signals would reach the brain—less intense pain.

Most people are aware of similar sensory-discriminative processes occurring in daily life. It is said that the price of perceiving anything at all is that not all can be perceived. Thus, most of us realize that under certain circumstances we "tune out" stimuli in favor of perceiving other stimuli. For example, if you are engrossed in reading an interesting book, you may not hear a very loud siren. Very young children often accomplish "tuning out" when watching television, a fact most parents can attest to.

Pain-relief measures based somewhat on this part of the gate-control theory include distraction strategies. Some patients may be distracted from their pain by providing them with certain auditory, visual, and tactile-kinesthetic stimuli. However, it appears that in actuality this does not always close the gate to the transmission of pain impulses, i.e., usually it does not cause a decreased intensity of pain. Rather, it appears that pain simply is made more tolerable by placing the sensation on the edge of awareness rather than at the center of attention. On the other hand, guided imagery and hypnosis, the intense use of one's imagination, may markedly decrease or eliminate pain.

Opening the gate to the transmission of pain impulses theoretically can be achieved by reducing sensory input available for processing in the reticular formation. In other words, pain can be caused or increased in the patient who is exposed to a reduction in the amount, variety, or quality of sensory input. This is called sensory restriction and is discussed in Chapter 8.

3. *Projections from the Cerebral Cortex and Thalamus.* Processes related to thoughts, emotions, and past experiences are subserved at least in part by neural activity in the cortex and thalamus. By way of the descending fibers, these structures can send messages to open or close the gate to the transmission of pain impulses. Therefore, the individual's own unique thoughts, feelings, and memories can influence whether or not pain impulses reach the level of awareness. These potentially painful impulses can be evaluated in terms of their meaning to the individual *before* they are felt as a sensation as well as afterwards.

This portion of the gate-control theory dealing with projections from the cerebral cortex and thalamus clearly has a wide range of application in clinical practice. It suggests how many pre-existing factors influence the individual's pain experience. For example, the patient is taught the expectations of those in his or her culture and has previous experiences of pain. These memories are stored in the brain, and for the rest of his or her life they are capable of influencing the transmission of potentially painful stimuli. This is helpful in understanding some of the relatively stable ways that a person may respond to both acute and chronic pain.

This concept is particularly relevant to chronic pain syndromes in which there is little or no identifiable organic pathology for the pain. Some types of chronic pain may be at least in part a "bad memory." At the spinal level or at the higher centers there may be memory storage laid down as a learned experience. That is, memories of pain are learned, stored, and later reactivated. Activation of the pain memory that results in the current sensation of pain may be accomplished by peripheral stimuli that usually are felt as nonpainful or by descending influences from the cortex or thalamus. This process would be almost entirely subconscious or unconscious (Crue et al., 1976).

Thoughts and feelings are also generated by the circumstances surrounding a current episode of pain. These, too, can influence the gating mechanisms by projections from the cerebral cortex and thalamus. Many pain-relief activities are aimed in part at reducing anxiety about pain and, thus, can attenuate pain. The nature of the relationship the nurse has with the patient with pain can result in considerable anxiety reduction if, for example, she conveys that she believes the patient has pain and wants to help him. Patient teaching about when pain may occur, how long it will last, and other aspects obviously contribute to reducing anxiety. Anxiety may also be diminished chemically with medication such as tranquilizers. Almost everything that is done to relieve a patient's pain potentially affects the patient's thoughts and feelings, thereby contributing to pain relief by way of inhibitory signals from the cerebral cortex and thalamus that will close the gate to pain.

The gate-control theory has made numerous major contributions to the study and relief of pain. In particular, examination of the gate-control theory is a very helpful way of gaining an appreciation of the individuality of the pain experience. Considering all the possible signals that could, at any given moment, be coming from the skin, brainstem, cortex, and thalamus, it is little wonder that people perceive and respond to pain differently. Not only are there differences between individuals but there will be variations in the individual from one time to another. For many reasons, comparable stimuli or lesions in different people will not produce comparable sensations of pain.

Even though the current information available on the neuroanatomy and physiology of nociception and its relation to pain perception is far from complete, one thing becomes increasingly clear, and that is the uniqueness of the pain experience. Sir Thomas Lewis (1942) succinctly states that pain is "known to us by experience and described by illustration." Much of the dilemma of diagnosing the patient's pain and/or attempting to second guess him about his pain can be eliminated if we just believe the patient.

In the next chapter, cultural factors which may influence pain perception are considered.

REFERENCES

Akil, H., & Liebskind, J.C. Monoaminergic mechanisms of stimulation-produced analgesia. Brain Res 94: 279–296, 1975.

Akil, H., & Mayer, D.J. Antagonism of stimulation-produced analgesia by p-CPA, a serotonin synthesis inhibitor. Brain Res 44: 692–697, 1972.

Almay, B.G.L., Johansson, F., Von Knorring, L., et al.: Relationships between CSF levels of endorphins and monoamine metabolites in chronic pain patients. Psychopharmacology 67: 139–142, 1980.

Almay, B.G.L., Johansson, F., Von Knorring, L., et al.: Endorphins in chronic pain. I. Differences in CSF endorphin levels between organic and psychogenic pain syndromes. Pain 5: 153–162, 1978.

Asberg, M., Thoren, P., Tränskman, L., et al.: "Serotonin depression"—A biochemical subgroup within the affective disorders? Science 191: 478–480, 1976.

Bausbaum, A.I., & Fields, H.L. Endogenous pain control mechanisms: Review and hypothesis. Ann Neurol 4: 451–462, 1978.

Benedetti, C. Neuroanatomy and biochemistry of antinociception. In J.J. Bonica & V. Ventafridda (Eds.), Advances in Pain Research and Therapy (Vol. 2), New York: Raven Press, 1979.

Berlin, L., Goodell, H., & Wolff, H.G. Relation of pain perception and central inhibitory effects of noxious stimulation to phenomenon of extinction of pain. Arch Neurol 80: 533–543, 1958.

Bonica, J.J. The Management of Pain, Philadelphia: Lea & Feiber, 1953, p. 32.

Bonica, J.J. Pathophysiology of pain. In: Current concepts in postoperative pain. New York: HP Publishing Inc., 1978, p. 6.

Bonica, J.J. Management of Acute and Chronic Pain—An Introduction. In Proceedings: Recent Advances in the Management of Acute and Chronic Pain, a symposium held in conjunction with the Second World Congress on Pain, Montreal, Canada, August 26, 1978. New York: HP Publishing Co., 1979.

Bossy, J. Atlas of neuroanatomy and special sense organs. Philadelphia: W.B. Saunders, 1970, p. 5. Modified from Ham, A.W. Histology (5th ed.). Philadelphia: J.B. Lippincott, 1965, pp. 115, 554.

Casey, K.L. & Melzack, R. Neural mechanisms of pain: A conceptual model. In E.L. Way, Ed. New Concepts of Pain and Its Clinical Management. Philadelphia: F.A. Davis, 1967.

Chusid, J.G. Correlative neuroanatomy and functional neurology, (17th ed.) Los Altos, CA: Lange Medical Publishers, 1976, pp. 66-67.

Crue, B.L., Kenton, B., & Carregal, E.J.A. Neurophysiology of pain—peripheral aspects. Bull LA Neurol Soc 41: 13–42, 1976.

Forrest, W.H., Brown, B.W., Brown, C.R., et al.: Dextroamphetamine with morphine for the treatment of postoperative pain. N Eng J Med 296(13): 712–715, 1977.

Guyton, A. Textbook of Medical Physiology (6th ed.). Philadelphia: W.B. Saunders, 1981.

Halpern, L. Neurophysiological Theories of Pain. Plainfield, New Jersey: The Management of Pain in Surgical Practice. Symposium proceedings—The Management of Pain in Surgical Practice, Boston, MA, Sept. 22-23, 1978. Copyright New York: Pfizer, Inc. 1979.

Hardy, J.D. The nature of pain. J Chron Dis 4: 22–51, 1956.

Hayes, R.L., Newlon, P.G., & Rosecrans, J.A., et al. Reduction of stimulation produced analgesia by lysergic acid diethylamide, a depressor of serotonergic neural activity. Brain Res 122: 367–372, 1977.

Hughes, J. Isolation of an endogenous compound from the brain with pharmacological properties similar to morphine. Brain Res 88: 295–308, 1975.

Jensen, D. The Human Nervous System. New York: Appleton-Century-Crofts, 1980.

Kreiger, D.T., Hughes, J.C. Neuroendocrinology. Funderland, MA: A Hospital Practice Book, Sinauer Assoc., Inc., 1981, p. 69.

Lewis, T. Pain. New York: Macmillan, 1942.

Linderoth, B. Personal communication, August 30, 1981.

Livingston, W.K. Pain Mechanisms. New York: Macmillan, 1943.

McCaffery, M. Dorsal column stimulation. Nurs 75 5: 54–55, 1975.

Melzack, R. The Puzzle of Pain. New York: Basic Books, 1973.

Melzack R: The role of early experience in emotional arousal. Ann NY Acad Sci 159: 721, 1969.

Melzack, R. Effects of early experience on behavior: Experimental and conceptual considerations, In P.H. Hoch, & J. Zubin (Eds.), Psychopathology of Perception, New York: Grune and Stratton, 1965.

Melzack, R., & Bridges, J.A. Dorsal column contributions to motor behaviour. Exp Neurol 33: 53, 1971.

Melzack, R., & Casey, K.L. Sensory, motivational, and central control determinants of pain: A new conceptual model. In D. Kenshalo (Ed), The Skin Senses, Springfield, IL: Charles C. Thomas, 1968, pp. 423–443.

Melzack, R. & Torgerson, W.S. On the language of pain. Anesthesiology 34: 50, 1971.

Melzack, R., & Wall, P.D. Pain mechanisms: A new theory. Science 150 (Nov. 19): 971–979, 1965.

Melzack, R., & Wall, P.D. Psychophysiology of pain. In H. Yamamura (Ed.), Anesthesia and Neurophysiology. International Anesthesiology Clinics, Boston: Little, Brown and Co., 1970, pp. 3–34.

Mountcastle, V.B. Medical Physiology (Vol. 1), (14th ed.). St. Louis: C.V. Mosby, 1980.

Mudge, A.W., Leeman, S.E., & Fischbach, G.D. Enkephalin inhibits release of substance p from sensory neuron in culture and decreases action potential duration. Proc Nat Acad Sci 193: 1227–1229, 1976.

Nathan, P.W. The gate-control theory of pain: A critical review. Brain 99: 123–158, 1976.

Nathan, P.W., & Wall, P.D. Treatment of post-herpetic neuralgia by prologed electrical stimulation. Brit Med J, 3 (Sept.): 645–649, 1974.

Noordenbos, W. Pain. Amsterdam: Elsevier, 1959.

Oleson, T. Personal communication, November 30, 1981.

Oyama, T., Jin, T., Yamaya, R., et al.: Profound analgesic effects of b-endorphin in man. Lancet i: 122–126, 1980.

Paroli, E. Indagini sull effetto antimorfinico dell' ACTH, Relazioni con il corticosurrene ed i livelli ematici degli 11-OH steroidi. Arch Ital. Sci Farmacol 13: 236–237, 1967.

Pearson, H.P. Pain pathways—An overview. In Recent Studies on the Nature and Management of Acute Pain. New York: HP Publishing Inc. 1976, p. 15.

Pert, C., & Snyder, S. Opiate receptor: Demonstration in nervous tissue. Science 179: 1001–1014, 1973.

Pittman, A.W., & Rudd, G.D. Analgesic Therapy, Part 2: Analgesia for Severe Pain. Indianapolis, MD.: Eli Lilly and Company, Pharmaceutical Division, 1980.

Reynolds, D.V. Surgery in the rat during electrical analgesia induced by focal brain stimulation. Science 164: 444–445, 1969.

Ruch, T. & Patton, H.D. Howell-Fulton Physiology and Biophysics, The Brain and Neural Function. Philadelphia: W.B. Saunders, 1979.

Salar, G., Job, I., Mingrino, S., et al.: Effect of transcutaneous electrotherapy on CSF b-endorphin content in patients without pain problems. Pain 10: 169–172, 1981.

Schultz, D.P. Sensory Restrictions. New York: Academic Press, 1965.

Science News: Vol. 116, Aug. 11, 1979.

Sherman, J.E., & Liebeskind, J.C. An endorphinergic, centrifugal substrate of pain modulation: Recent findings, current concepts, and complexities. Research Publications—Association for Research in Nervous and Mental Disease, New York: Raven Press, Vol. 58, 1980, (126 ref.), pp. 191–204.

Sicuteri, F. Headache: disruption of pain modulation. In J.J. Bonica, & D. Albe-Fessard (Eds.), Advances in Pain Research and Therapy (Vol. 1). New York: Raven Press, 1976, pp. 871–880.

Sicuteri, F., Anselmi, B., & Del Bianco, P.L., 5-Hydroxtryptamine supersensitivity as a new theory of headache and central pain: A clinical pharmacological approach with p-chlorophenylalanine. Psychopharmacologia 29: 347–356, 1973.

Sicuteri, F., Anselmi, B., & Del Bianco, P.L. Systemic non-organic central pain: A new syndrome with decentralization supersensitivity. Headache 18: 133–136, 1978.

Snyder, S.H. Opiates receptors and internal opiates. Sci Amer 236 (March): 44–56. 1977.

Sternbach, R.A. Pain: A Psychophysiological Analysis. New York: Academic Press, 1968.

Sweet, W.H. Pain. In J. Field, H.W. Magoun, & V.E. Hall (Eds.), Handbook of Physiology, Vol. 1, Sect. 1, Chap. XIX. Washington, D.C.: Amer Physiol Soc, 1959, pp. 459–506.

Tamsen, A., Hartvig, P., Dahlstrom, A., et al.: Endorphins on-demand pain relief. Lancet i: 769–770, 1980.

Tenen, S.S. Antagonism of the analgesic effect of morphine and other drugs by p-chlorophenylalanine, a serotonin depletor, Psychopharmacologia 12: 278–285, 1968.

Terenius, L. Endorphins and pain. In L.H. Rees, & T.B. von Wimersma Greidanus (Eds.), Frontiers of Hormone Research, Vol. 8. Sweden: In Press, 1981. pp. 162–172.

Terenius, L., & Wahlstrom, A. Search for an endogenous ligand for the opiate receptor. ACTA Physiol Scand 94: 74–81, 1975.

Vogt, M. The effect of lowering the 5-hydroxtryptamine content of the rat spinal cord on analgesia produced by morphine. J Physiol (Lond) 236: 483–498, 1974.

Wall, P.D. Modulation of pain by nonpainful events. In J.J. Bonica, & D. Albe-Fessard (Eds.), Advances in Pain Research and Therapy (Vol. 1), New York: Raven Press, 1976, pp. 1–16.

Wang, J.K. Antinociceptive effect of intrathecally administered serotonin. Anesthesiology 47: 269–271, 1977.

Way, L. Abdominal Pain. In M.H. Sleisinger, & J.S. Fordtran (Eds.), Gastrointestinal Disease—Pathophysiology, Diagnosis and Management. Philadelphia: W.B. Saunders, 1973, p. 327.

Weddell, A.G.M. "Activity Pattern" hypothesis for sensation of pain. In R.G. Grenell (Eds.), Progress in Neurobiology, Neural physiology (Vol. v.). New York: Hoeber, 1962, pp. 134–177.

Weissman, G. The pain mediator. Considerations in Management of Acute Pain. Symposium held in conjunction with the annual meeting of the American Society of Anesthesiologists, San Francisco, Oct. 11, 1976. New York: H.P. Co., 1977, pp. 17–21. (a)

Weissman, G. Pain mediators and pain receptors. Considerations in Management of Acute Pain. Symposium held in conjunction with the annual meeting of the American Society of Anesthesiologists, San Francisco, Oct. 11, 1976. New York: H.P. Co., 1977, pp. 28–30. (b)

Whidden, A., & Fidler, Sister M.R. Pathophysiology of pain. In A.K. Jacox (Ed.), Pain: A Source Book for Nurses and Other Health Professionals. Boston: Little, Brown and Co., pp. 27–56, 1977.

Winter, C.A., & Flataker, L. The effect of corticosterone, desoxycorticosterone and adenocorticotrophic hormone upon the responses of animals to analgesic drugs. J Pharmacol Exp Therapeut 103: 93–105, 1951.

Zimmerman, E., & Krivoy, W. Antagonism between morphine and the polypeptides ACTH, $ACTH_{1-24}$ and B-MSH in the nervous system. Prog Brain Res 31: 383–394, 1973.

SUGGESTED READINGS

Akil, H., Mayer, D.J., & Liebeskind, J.C. Antagonism of stimulation-produced analgesia by naloxone, a narcotic antagonist. Science 191: 961–962, 1976.

Alexander, G. Pain-killer in brain may explain "placebo" effect. Los Angeles Times, Part I, Aug. 28, 1978, p. 3, 14.

Andersson, S.A. Pain control by sensory stimulation. In J.J. Bonica, J.C. Liebeskind, & D. Albe-Fessard (Eds.), Advances in pain research and therapy (Vol. 3). New York: Raven Press, 1979, pp. 569–586.

Barchas, J.D., Akil, H., Elliott, G.R. et al.: Behavioral neurochemistry: Neuroregulators and behavioral states. Science 200: 964–973, 1978.

Barber, T.X. Toward a theory of pain: Relief of chronic pain by prefrontal leucotomy, opiates, placebos, and hypnosis. Psychol Bull 56: 430–460, 1959.

Cannon, J.T., Liebeskind, J.C., & Frenk, H. Neural and neurochemical mechanisms of pain inhibition. In R.A. Sternbach (Ed.), The Psychology of Pain, New York: Raven Press, 1978, pp. 27–47.

Chance, W.T., Krynock, G.M., & Rosecrans, J.A. Antinociception following lesion-induced hyperemotionality and conditioned fear. Pain 4: 243–252, 1978.

Current Concepts on Pain and Analgesia: Endorphin update. 5: 3–4, 12, 1978.

Fincher, J. Natural opiates in the brain. Human Behav 5: (Jan.) 28–32, 1979.

Jessell, T.M., & Iversen, L.L. Opiate analgesics inhibit substance p release from rat trigeminal nucleus. Nature 268: 549–551, 1977.

Konishi, S., & Otsaka, M. The effect of substance P and other peptides on spinal neurons of the frog. Brain Res 65: 397–410, 1974.

Levine, J.D., Gordon, N.C., & Fields, H.L. Evidence that the analgesic effect of placebo is mediated by endorphins. In Pain Abstracts, 1978, (Vol. 1) Seattle: International Association for the Study of Pain, p. 18.

Levine, J.D., Gordon, N.C., & Fields, H.L. The role of endorphins in placebo analgesia. In J.J. Bonica, J.C. Liebeskind & D. Albe-Fessard (Eds.), Advances in Pain Research and Therapy (Vol. 3). New York: Raven Press, 1979, pp. 547–552.

Liebeskind, J.C., Mayer, D.J., & Akil, H. Central mechanisms of pain inhibition: Studies of analgesia from focal brain stimulation. In J.J. Bonica (Ed.), Advances in Neurology: Pain, (Vol. 4). New York: Raven Press, 1974, pp. 261–268.

Lindblom, V., & Tegner, R. Are the endorphins active in clinical pain states? Narcotic antagonism in chronic pain patients. Pain 7: 65–68, 1979.

Mannheimer, J.S. Neurophysiology of Pain. Papers presented at the conference on pain management, Des Plaines, IL. May 14–15, 1977.

Mayer, D.J., & Hayes, R.L. Stimulation-produced analgesia: Development of tolerance and cross-tolerance to morphine. Science 188: 941–943, 1975.

Mayer, D.J., Price, D.D., Barber, J., et al.: Acupuncture analgesia: Evidence for activation of a pain inhibitory system as a mechanism of action. In J.J. Bonica & D. Albe-Fessard (Eds.), Advances in Pain Research and Therapy, (Vol. 1). New York: Raven Press, 1976, 751–754.

Messing, R.B., & Lytle, L.D. Serotonin-containing neurons: their possible role in pain and analgesia. Pain 4: 1–21, 1977.

Nathan, P.W. The gate control theory of pain: A critical review. Brain 99: 123–158, 1976.

Sjolund, B., Terenius, L., & Eriksson, M. Increased cerebrospinal fluid levels of endorphins after electroacupuncture, Acta Physiol Scand 100: 382–384.

Sternbach, R.A., Janowsky, D.S., Huey, L.Y. et al.: Effects of altering brain serotonin activity on human chronic pain. In J.J. Bonica & D. Albe-Fessard (Eds.), Advances in Pain Research and Therapy. New York: Raven Press, 1976, Vol. 1, pp. 601–606.

Wall, P.D. Modulation of pain by nonpainful events. In J.J. Bonica, & D. Albe-Fessard (Eds.), Advances in Pain Research and Therapy, (Vol. 1). New York: Raven Press, 1976, pp. 1–16.

Villet, B. Opiates of the mind. Atlantic Monthly (June) pp. 82–89, 1978.

3

Cultural Influences

Culture constrains and regulates our daily behavior, attitudes, and values in many latent and manifest ways. It circumscribes the ways in which societies and ethnic groups solve their problems and derive meaning from their lives. Because people rely on learned behavior, or culture, for survival, it is the prime source of our adaptability (Freidman, 1981, p. 271). Richards et al. (1980, p. 355) found, in some patients, specific psychocultural factors such as older, more intelligent individuals living in difficult psychosocial situations experience higher levels of subjective pain. Pain occurs in a total integrated human being who has had a variety of physical, emotional, and intellectual life experiences. It is not surprising, then, that different people respond to pain in different ways.

Some of the fairly stable and sometimes unalterable personal attributes that affect the individual's response to pain will be examined in this chapter. The purpose is to foster an understanding and acceptance of the possibility that the person with pain may respond in a variety of ways. Some of the reasons for these variations among patients cannot necessarily be changed by the nurse, but they should be considered.

The influencing factors discussed here cannot be viewed as having a predictable or specific relationship to the patient's response to pain. As yet, there is no agreement about cause and effect. However, these factors often seem to be *associated* with similarities and differences in reactions to the pain experience and acceptance of pain treatments.

In discussing the relationship of culture to pain, Lewis (1978, p. 122) makes two important points about viewing another person in pain. First, our ability to sympathize with another person depends on our ability to identify imaginatively with him. And, second, we are less concerned by hurt to individuals that we do not know. The individual's pain experience definitely affects us as participants and observers in his care. Research indicates that it may significantly color our response to the patient, which would also influence our objectivity in pain assessment. Craig & Neidermayer (1974) and Craig & Prkachin (1978) found that, if the patient has relatively good control over her or his pain behaviors, it has a calming effect on the individual who observes her or him. Krebs (1975) found that those who were sympathetic to the individual suffering were likely to attempt to assist him with his pain. Whereas Baron (1974) found that, if an observer was initially angry with a suffering individual, it affected his relationship with the individual negatively. The observer then tended to intensify his efforts to *increase the suffering individual's distress.*

Winsberg & Greenlick (1967, p. 227) found that the nurse's assessment of the patient's pain was in close agreement with that of the medical staff. More importantly they found that patients tend to see their pain as more severe than the medical staff did. Thus staff may agree with each other that the patient's pain is not as bad as he finds it.

Another factor that may effect the patient is how the staff believe he should express his pain. Zborowski (1952) found that the staff tended to uphold "Old American" values which strongly condone stoicism during pain. He found that the individual was expected to report his pain but not the emotional reaction to it. Further, he found that when the reaction was expressed the staff tended to label it negatively. This was evidenced in his finding that the staff believed that the Italians and Jews overreacted to their pain, were too emotional about it, and complained excessively about it.

Katz (1979) studied conditioned anxiety and pain in children with leukemia undergoing repeated diagnostic and treatment procedures often perceived as painful, such as bone marrow aspirations, lumbar punctures, and intravenous and intramuscular injections. Following the painful procedures, independent ratings of the children's anxiety were done by the child and the nurse-observer. On self-report, children in the 6-10 year age range did not indicate that they experienced decreased anxiety and/or pain during their repeated procedures. The nurse observers recording behavioral responses during the same procedures did not record behaviors consistent with any decreased anxiety and/or pain. Yet, when the nurses personally evaluated the child's anxiety they indicated that it decreased with repeated procedures. Katz says that "This suggests that the nurse may not be as attentive to all behavioral variables, or that they may be biased due to their personal knowledge and experience with some children" (p. 5). One of the common misconceptions is that repeated experience with pain leads to increased ability to handle it and/or less sensitivity to it. In fact, it may be only that the observer becomes less sensitive to the patient's pain experience, as we shall see later.

Adherence to ethnic health beliefs and practices will be related to the degree of acculturation. Harwood (1981a, p. 483) identified eight determinants which are often intercorrelated and that are helpful in assessing acculturation:

1. A relatively high level of formal education (probably a minimum of several years of secondary school).
2. Greater generational removal from immigrant status.

3. A lesser degree of encapsulation within an ethnic and family social network.
4. Experience with medical services that incorporate patient education and personalized care into treatment.
5. Previous experience with particular diseases in the immediate family.
6. For immigrants, immigration to this country at an early age.
7. Urban, as opposed to rural, origin.
8. Limited migration back and forth to the mother country.

APPLICATION TO NURSING

Knowledge of different cultural beliefs and traditions can be used by the nurse on behalf of the patient in two major ways. First of all, the nurse learns that there are ways of responding to pain other than her own. Although some of these may be frowned upon in her personal and professional cultural groups, they may be not only accepted but very desirable in the patient's culture. This knowledge helps the nurse understand and appreciate the many different behaviors she may see, and it assists her in discounting her own cultural traditions as a basis for assessing the patient's pain experience. Hopefully, this will prevent the nurse from avoiding and punishing the patient who behaves in a manner that is unacceptable in her own culture. In addition, she will know that the presence or absence of expressions such as crying and moaning do not necessarily indicate the same pain experience in people of different cultural backgrounds. For example, mild pain may elicit crying in one patient. Another may never cry regardless of the intensity or implications of the pain, and a third may cry only with intense pain.

Secondly, knowledge of the various cultural attitudes toward pain assists the nurse in determining the significance of pain to the patient. Her intervention will be more effective when she seeks such clues as those that indicate whether the pain is viewed as punishment or identification with God, whether the patient seeks immediate relief or a cure for pain, and whether the patient both expects and accepts pain or merely expects but cannot accept pain.

The following discussion will focus on variations in attitudes toward pain and responses to pain which are due to the different cultural expectations resulting from the patient's sociocultural background, his sex, age and religion, the body part involved in the pain, and the roles ascribed to members of the health team. The significance of some of these cultural influences in clinical nursing practice is summarized in Table 3.1.

In an attempt to foster greater understanding and acceptance of cultural differences we will now consider determinants which may influence the patient's pain experience. First, we will consider general factors such as

TABLE 3.1. Significance of the Cultural Influences on Pain for Nursing Practice

Avoid stereotyping: Do not assume that the characteristics commonly associated with a particular sociocultural group will occur in all patients who are members of that group.

Studying the wide variety of cultural expectations with respect to pain assists the nurse in appreciating that:

1. The way she learned to respond to pain may not only be different from but quite the opposite from what someone else has learned.
2. Each person usually considers that the ways he has learned to regard and to respond to pain are both natural and correct. His behavioral responses are effective methods of communicating about pain with members of his culture.
3. The patient's attitude and behavioral responses to pain may be influenced more by his cultural background than by the intensity of his pain.
4. Similar responses to pain do not necessarily reflect similar attitudes toward pain.
5. Cultural expectations may be very detailed and varied regarding
   a. appropriate, acceptable, and effective behavioral responses to pain;
   b. when, how, and by whom pain should be treated; and
   c. the meaning or significance of the pain.

age and sex, followed by information on the most predominant ethnic subgroups in the United States, then research in relation to pain differences in ethnic groups, and lastly the application of all of this information to the patient with pain.

CULTURAL DIFFERENCES

As a person becomes acculturated he learns what the members of his culture expect and accept with regard to painful experiences. The cultural expectations may be very detailed, specifying such things as: different reaction patterns according to sex, age and occupation; whether curative or palliative treatment should be sought; the intensity and duration of pain that should be tolerated; what responses should be made; to whom the pain should be reported; and what types of pain require attention. It is this latter aspect of cultural prescription that may influence the pain sensation itself. For example, a cut or bruise obtained under conditions such as participation in a sport may be an expected and accepted consequence, and the victim may perceive the pain as being of lesser intensity than he would if a comparable injury occurred in a situation where it was not expected.

THE FAMILY

In spite of the fact that the family is usually more influenced by society than the society is influenced by the family, the family remains the basic unit of our society and the primary group for the individual. Beliefs, values, and customs of a culture are transmitted from one generation to another through the process of modeling in the family. In fact, the family "so influences the development of an individual that it may determine the success or failure of that person's life" (Freidman, 1981, p. 3). For the purposes of our discussion of pain we will use Freidman's definition of the family as "two or more people emotionally involved with each other and who live in close geographical proximity" (p. 8). This broad definition allows for all "significant other" relationships in the individual's life from the traditional nuclear and extended families to all variant family forms such as single individuals living alone, in communes, or nursing homes to group marriages and homosexual unions. Some support for this broader definition of family is seen in the observation of Kalish & Reynolds (1976) that the Japanese-Americans and Mexican-Americans have large family support systems in contrast to the narrower ones for Anglo-Americans and blacks. The later groups, however, are more likely to have larger support groups in friends and the community.

As a buffer between society and the individual, the family must meet the needs of both. At times the needs of one may predominate over the other's. For example, when an individual is in pain, as the family rallies around the suffering individual, all other family functions are likely to be suspended. On the other hand, during a societal crisis such as a war or natural disaster, even an individual's pain experience can be expected to be superseded. Because families tend to be involved in some way in the patient's decisions regarding health and illness, the nurse must consider the potential influence the family has on the individual's pain experience. Studying the white family in the United States, Litman (1974) found that the mother was the major determiner of the family health behavior 67.7 percent of the time, and the father, 15.7 percent of the time (p. 502).

Acculturation of the desired behaviors in relation to pain begins in early childhood or infancy when certain behavioral responses to pain are rewarded and others are punished or ignored. In one culture, the child's crying response to pain may be followed by cuddling and sympathy from the parent. In another, the crying may be ignored and the parent may matter-of-factly care for the injury, praising the child when he stops crying. With each painful experience the child learns more of the nuances of acceptable attitudes toward pain and responses to pain. By the time he or she reaches adulthood, these may be very firmly established reactions. If they are not and the belief or attitude is highly valued, the significant others very often persist in inculcating it in their offspring into adulthood. One mother with a painful terminal illness refused to take narcotics for pain relief. Both of her children, now in their twenties, had been convicted of using "street drugs" during their teenage years and were continuing to use them. This patient stated that her greatest desire before she died was to be able to convince her children that under no circumstances were narcotics safe to use. Until her death she continued to model this belief and refuse narcotic analgesics.

AGE AND SEX

The patient's age and sex often determine the acceptability of certain deviations from the norm of his cultural group. In most cultures, the female child is allowed greater freedom in the expression of pain than are any other members. In the United States, where the Old American cultural traditions are dominant, young boys are taught at an early age to be brave and not to cry when they hurt themselves. One example of this effect occurred with Bob, 20 months old, a white child from a rural area in the mountains of Tennessee. During his hospitalization a cut-down for intravenous fluid was performed. At the beginning of the procedure, as the local anesthetic was being injected, he looked up at his mother standing beside his crib. He was clenching his teeth and tears were forming in his squinted eyes. After a few seconds, his mother told him it would be all right to cry, and he did so, loudly (McCaffery, 1969).

By middle childhood, the ages of 10 and 11 years, boys in the United States are expected to suppress fear and control emotions in times of stress, but girls are allowed to express fear and hurt feelings. In the face of pain, boys tend to say that they do not want to cry, but they also express simultaneously feelings of bravery and fear. Girls, on the other hand, tend to admit to feeling afraid without also needing to say they feel brave. Girls also are more likely to admit that they want to cry but will not (Schultz, 1971).

There are divergent findings in relation to pain and age. It is often assumed that neonates and young children are less sensitive to pain than adults. This may be true for neonates. Terenius (1981, p. 166) reports that neonates do respond to pain, but the sensitivity increases significantly even after a few days. The full behavioral response to pain occurs between 3 and 12 months, leading Terenius to speculate that this time period may be when interindividual differences in response to pain are established. Haslam (1969) studied children 5–18 years of age and demonstrated that the younger the child the more sensitive he was to pain (lower pain perception threshold). Kaiko (1980) reports a study correlating pain relief and age in cancer patients. He also found the younger the patient the greater pain sensitivity. He found 8 mg of morphine for patients 30–69 was equianalgesic to 16 mg in patients 18–29, and 16 mg in the 30–69 age group was equianalgesic to 8 mg for patients over 69 years of age. Woodrow et al. (1972) found that pain tolerance decreased with age and that men tolerated pain better than women. They also found that cutaneous pain tolerance increased with age, whereas tolerance to deep pain decreased (p. 553). Winsberg & Greenlick (1967) did not differentiate between age and parity but they found that older patients and higher parity patients seemed more cooperative and stoical. Schluderman & Zubek (1962) found that pain thresholds remained constant until the early 50s; after that they increased. Clark & Mehl (1971) think that the difference in pain perception in the elderly may be due to a tendency of the elderly to endure more pain before reporting it. Whereas Harkins & Chapman (1977) explain the difference in pain thresholds in the elderly as being due to the elderly being less accurate in discriminating pain and being less willing to call stimuli painful.

Butler & Gastell (1980) report that diagnosis and treatment of pain in the elderly may present special problems. They cite several reasons for this. Conditions which are normally painful in younger individuals such as myocardial infarction and appendicitis may present little or no pain in the elderly patient. Also such conditions may present with only behavioral changes such as confusion and restlessness. The elderly frequently have multiple diseases all of which may produce pain. He cites an example of an "80-year-old woman with leg pain due to three separate conditions—trochanteric bursitis, lumbar stenosis, and intermittent claudication" (p. 302). On the other hand, psychological and social factors such as loneliness, boredom, depression, and the desire to conceal an unacceptable problem such as memory loss may be presented as a complaint of pain. In emphasizing that pain is not an inevitable irremediable part of aging, Butler reports an anecdote about a patient who went to his doctor and complained of left leg pain. His physician asked him, "Morris, what do you expect at age 101?" To which Morris retorted: "But my right leg is also 101, and it doesn't hurt a bit. Now explain that" (p. 302).

Evidence relating to sexual differences in pain perception is controversial. Notermans & Tophoff (1967) cite five publications that conclude that pain sensitivity was greater in women than men and five publications which reported no pain sensitivity differences between the sexes. "Pain differences, similarities found," a report in *Science* (1980, p. 183), includes a report of a study by Goolkasian who found that pain perception in women in the nonovulatory stage of their menstrual cycle and men and women on oral contraceptives were identical. Women not on the oral contraceptives reported the stimuli more painful.

In addition to pain behaviors which are generally considered more acceptable for women than for men, there are expectations regarding sexual differences for pain perception and pain tolerance. Armitage et al. (1979) conducted a chart audit study of symptoms, commonly complained about by men and women, to evaluate the degree of sexism which might affect general medical care. They evaluated the medical records of 52 married couples–104 men and women who came from the same socioeconomic and geographic areas, who had nearly an identical number of visits for medical care and who all had male physicians. The findings for all five symptoms were that physical workups were significantly more extensive for men than women. Male physicians tended to take medical illnesses in men more seriously than they did in women. Armitage et al. concluded that the findings "bear out what many critics already claim: namely, that the [male] physicians . . . tend to take illness more seriously in men than in women" (p. 2187). They speculate that this may be due to the physicians "responding to current stereotypes [mentioned by Nathanson, 1975] that regard the male as typically more stoic and females are typically hypochondriacal" (p. 2187).

In an article in *Science News* (1980, pp. 182–183) a study was reported by Lack who produced data supporting the complaint that many women are victims of sex-role stereotyping by the medical profession and end up searching wider and longer for proper medical care. Eighty percent of the 166 sequential chronic pain patients who visited a facial pain clinic were women. Her findings were that "women had their pain longer before being referred, and their treatment had differed from that of men with similar complaints. [Women] received more prescriptions for minor tranquilizers, antidepressants, and analgesics, and fewer prescriptions for narcotics. [Women] also had fewer pain-related surgical procedures" (p. 183).

Nolen (1979, pp. 201–204) addresses the issue of sexual discrimination in medical care. He believes that discrimination against women does occur and that many physicians do take a flagrant chauvinistic attitude toward female patients exemplified by such practices (resulting in pain), as inducing labor for their own convenience and performing unnecessary surgeries or more radical procedures when simpler procedures would be adequate, extended anesthesia time in itself being an added risk to the patient. In fact, he says that he knows the expression "if ovaries were testicles, there'd be a lot fewer of them removed," to be true (p. 202). He attributes the chauvinism in part to the doctor's cavalier protectionism, a "sin" that is so widely committed by medical men that most doctors aren't even aware that they are guilty (p. 203). In acknowledging that it is unfair and physicians must stop this practice, he also tells women they must not allow it to continue. If they are treated in a demeaning manner, Nolen says women must take the initiative and discuss it with their physician (p. 204).

The almost exclusively female nursing profession also does its share of discriminating in the care of pain patients. In one study, nurses demonstrated more concern for reports of pain from female patients than from male patients. In spite of the fact that the male patients reported their pain as more severe and required pain relief more frequently, they actually received less medication. Further, at no time did nurses give men medication unless the patient requested it. On the other hand, women were given medications several times without requesting it (Pilowsky & Bond, 1969). This seems consistent with Lewis's (1978) report that we are more sympathetic with those with whom we more closely identify. In contrast, more recently, Cohen (1980, pp. 265–274) reported that nurses selectively gave less analgesics in the postoperative period to women than they did to men.

In general, the adult woman is allowed more emotional expression of pain than the man. The man is allowed more freedom as he grows older. For example, Zborowski (1969) told of an Irishman, who considered himself old, readily admitting to moaning and groaning, which would be unacceptable in a younger man. Any older man not only is more prone to show his pain, but delays longer in consulting a physician and tends to value the physician's personality more than his skill (Zborowski, 1969). Although social norms are associated with being young, old, male, or female, some investigators have considered the possibility that age and sex act as *biological* determinants of variations in response to pain. However, the consensus seems to be that pain sensitivity does not vary between men and women, but that pain is better tolerated by men than women (Jacox, 1977). At the other end of the age spectrum, the theory that the neonate does not perceive pain by one week of age is open to question (Swafford & Allan, 1968). "It has been suggested that even embryos seem to respond aversely to noxious stimuli" (Wolff & Langley, 1979, p. 313). There are no firm data upon which to base the assumption that infants are either insensitive to pain or less sensitive than older children (Poznanski, 1976).

LANGUAGE

The actual words used to report emotional or bodily feeling may be influenced by the ethnic group and/or the language spoken by the group. Diller (1980, pp. 24–25) reports that

> Language-specific differences in pain reporting may be partly an effect, but partly also a cause, of culturally modulated differences in pain perception. Language can exert a powerful influence on conscious attention, but probably also on semiconscious and unconscious aspects of our species' cognitive abilities to deal with meaning.

Diller (p. 9) also proposes "that varying types and degrees of looseness in semantic contrast cannot be ignored if revealing cross-cultural comparisons are to be made."

The Chinese, Japanese and English languages illustrate how ethnic differences may influence one's verbalization about his pain. The Chinese language has words equivalent to most Western diagnoses. However, it is deficient in an equivalent psychological vocabulary. In the Japanese language there are no special terms which easily describe the qualities or presumed sources of pain, and pain terms suggest a psychological experience. In English, the pain terms emphasize a physical process for pain, especially the notion of harm (Fabrega & Tyma, 1976). Sternbach (1974) suggests that many patients express psychological distress through a physical language partly because their vocabulary lacks the words for the psychological concept. An interesting example of this is cited by Mersky and Spear (1967). One woman who complained of pain required months of intensive psychotherapy to learn to talk about her intolerable "tension" rather than her intolerable pain.

RELIGION

Webster (1963, p. 724) defines religion as the "belief in a divine or superhuman power or powers to be obeyed and worshipped as the creator(s) of the universe." In most cultural groups one religion is dominant, such as the Protestant faith of the Old American. But there are many variations of each religion characterized, for example, as orthodox, reformed, liberal, or fundamental. The individuals practicing within the variations selectively accept ethical principles and philosophic views. Within each cultural group a member's response to pain may differ slightly or significantly because of his particular religious affiliation. Further, concepts of folk medicine frequently are predicated on religious beliefs.

Lambert et al. (1960) conducted two studies on the effects of religious affiliation on pain tolerance in 80 female students—40 Jewish and 40 Protestants. In the baseline studies it was found that although the Jewish women's pain tolerance scores were slightly higher than the Protestants, they were not considered significantly so. Superiority based on one's religious affiliation was tested using one's ability to tolerate pain. In reviewing these studies Wolff & Langley (1968, p. 497) concluded that although

> . . . there are no basic ethnic differences in terms of pain response between groups, cultural factors, such as those relating to religious affiliation, if made explicit, can impose a differential pain response pattern between Jewish and Protestant groups of the same sex, education, and socioeconomic status.

Poser (1963) conducted a similar study using native and immigrant Canadian Jews and Roman Catholics. His conclusions were that ethnic origin is much more significant for immigrants than for native Canadians. The native Canadians were better able to identify and follow the behavior patterns of the majority group whether they were made aware of the ethnic differences explicitly or implicitly. Citizenship and interactions were not found to be significant. Also found to be significant though was the ethnic origin of the experimenter.

In reviewing cultural studies, Wolff & Langley (1968, p. 500) speculate that because religious attitudes influence the perception of the physical self, they may also color the pain response. The patient's religious faith may serve as a source of either strength or despair. One patient may effectively use prayer and religious ritual to help tolerate pain; another may feel that pain is a punishment for sins and may pray for forgiveness. Miss Berry, 73 years old and a Southern Baptist, experienced pain from pathological fractures and prayed loudly for forgiveness when the pain became intense. In her prayers, she frequently asked God what she had done to deserve such pain.

On the other hand, when pain is viewed as punishment, it may relieve the patient's guilt feelings. He or she may therefore endure the pain with a patience and tranquility not present during health. Still another patient may see pain as a means of identifying with God, or may feel that God has a reason for providing an experience of pain.

It is important to note that the association of pain with punishment may occur for reasons other than the patient's religion. The infliction of pain is one of the oldest forms of punishment; therefore, it is not surprising that pain and punishment may be closely related in the patient's mind. A child may consciously associate the pain of illness and treatment with punishment. In the adult, this association is likely to be on a more unconscious level.

Another interesting example of the relationship of religion during the pain experience was provided by Gitelson (1981) about a 35-year-old Jewish man who had been raised in the Jewish Orthodox faith. When he was dying he felt victimized by his pain. He reported that he now found comfort by identifying with Christ, since Christ was a Jew who also had experienced extreme suffering; he had a cross to bear.

NONMAINSTREAM MEDICAL PRACTICES AND HEALERS

Although we often attribute folk and primitive medical practices to "other" cultures, Klein (1979a, pp. 205–208) and Spector (1979, pp. 31–54) point out that these practices exist in all cultures. The unifying thread in all folk medicine is the prevention of "evil" believed to be the basis for illness and the maintenance of "good" health. The basis for many folk medicine practices have medical analogies. Practices of good nutrition, adequate rest, exercise, and psychological support are components of all health care systems. Currently, these practices in the United States have become million-dollar industries; such as the health food stores, health spas and gyms, "Pop Psychiatry" and "How to" books. Many cultures use the same remedies but vary the ingredients. One example of a folk preventative measure is the wearing of a garlic on a string around one's neck to prevent colds. People are likely to avoid the wearer of the garlic, thus accomplishing the biomedical equivalent of isolation for prevention of disease. Even seemingly less scientific practices are carried out currently in the United States. Examples can be found in The Merck Manual. Lyght (1961, p. 1445) recommends the use of "Psychotherapy (Hexing)" to remove warts in children. Specific techniques included are warming it with a heat lamp and touching it with unusual objects. In a later edition Berkow (1977 p. 1587) continues to make such recommendations saying that "suggestion accompanied by an impressive manipulation such as shining a Wood's light on the wart after painting it with a fluorescent dye" may be a successful treatment. Spindler (1979, p. 229) points out that when Americans frequently go to their physician for an antibiotic for a cold, this may be a form of magical thinking.

Certain symptoms such as blood loss may be almost universally considered serious. However, all ethnic groups prioritize and interpret symptoms based on what they personally perceive as serious, and this varies with different groups. All ethnic groups tend to prefer to treat symptoms at home with their own remedies, thus delaying seeking medical care from a physician. When we are blaming patients for "not coming sooner to the doctor," it may facilitate empathy with the patient if the nurse takes an honest look at her own health care practices.

Folk healers are primarily psychosocial ethnic specialists. This inherent quality provides a distinct "in" with treating different cultural groups. In explaining the effectiveness of the witch doctor, Dr. Albert Schweitzer was quoted by Dunn (1982, p. 2) as telling Norman Cousins that

> The witch doctor succeeds for the same reason all the rest of us succeed. Each patient carries his own doctor inside of him. They come to us knowing the truth. We are at our best when we give the doctor who resides within each patient a chance of going to work.

For the most part, folk healers can be used in a complementary rather than conflictual manner with biomedicine. The most important consideration in working with folk and magical medical beliefs is to acknowledge the individual's right to and a preference for a folk healer, and to work with and around the healer in providing the best care possible.

BODY PART INVOLVED IN PAIN

In almost every culture, members are taught that certain parts of the body are socially unacceptable for viewing and as topics of conversation. Consequently, when pain strikes these areas of the body, the patient's response will differ from his response to pain in an acceptable and acknowledged part of the body. For example, in the United States pain occurring in the genitalia, rectum, or anus does not evoke much sympathy from others and is rarely discussed, so the patient may hesitate to complain of the pain. For example, the unmentionability and lack of sympathy were reported recently in relation to Herpes Genitalis (Leo, 1982). Further, the patient may find it difficult to describe because he has not been allowed to use such terminology. He may also avoid any protective or rubbing body movements that could indicate the site of the pain. For example, Mr. Call, 40 years old, was admitted for urological examination because of persistent cystitis. The physician ordered Pyridium orally q^{6}h prn for burning on urination, but Mr. Call rarely requested the medication. Most of the time he received it only when the physician, following his visit with the patient, asked the nurse to give it. Often Mr. Call would turn his head away when a nurse asked him if he had any burning. Apparently this patient was somewhat uncomfortable in making any reference to pain in his genitalia.

SOCIAL CLASS AND STATUS

Social class refers to the interplay of one's membership in a group primarily determined by socioeconomic factors such as one's level of education, occupation, and income. Status refers to one's rank or relative position in a class. Although Americans tend to downplay social class differences and ethnocentric tendencies, they are very important both in the United States and in other countries where there are explicit status differences (Simmons, 1979, pp. 102–103). This is important because of the ongoing immigration to the United States.

Class differences go beyond ethnic differences. That is, an upper-class individual in one country will hold many values similar to those of an upper-class individual in another country. Social class is considered as the major variable that molds one's value system. Freidman (1981, p. 180) says that "persons with different levels of social order, by virtue of their varied experience and exposure, come to see the world differently, to develop different conceptions of social reality, as well as different aspirations, fears, and values."

Studies by Grey (1949) and Redlich et al. (1955) have shown that the closer the patient and physician are in status, the better the treatment and the most sympathy that are afforded the patient. Further, Freidman points out that the more similar an individual's values are to that of the relevant societal value, the less they are stigmatized and the easier it is for them to adjust. When attempts are made to change a patient's perceptions of medical treatment "they are likely to collide with the individual's investment with his group affiliations," (Simmons, 1979, p. 107). This may further entrench the patient into the very value that may be counterproductive in getting pain assessment and relief.

The implications of one's socioeconomic status for obtaining pain relief relate significantly to the individual's willingness to pursue medical care. Harwood (1981b, p. 12) says, "the more educated, more affluent, and occupationally advantaged members of ethnic categories tend to differ in their health beliefs and behaviors from the less [advantaged individuals]." The more advantaged show greater similarity in relation to matters of health and illness regardless of ethnic identity. Koos (1954) found that individuals of lower socioeconomic status were slower to respond to initial symptoms; were more tolerant of high stress and even disabling diseases; may fail to recognize the significance of symptoms as needing medical care or as a part of disease; and were more susceptible to disease. Koos also found that the middle- and upper-classes seek medical care for problems that the lower socioeconomic status individuals would not. A recent example of this was cited in relation to the very painful condition Herpes Genitalis (Leo, 1982, p. 66). Ninety-five percent of the sufferers are "nice, healthy, educated, clean-cut Caucasians of the middle and upper classes." These individuals are of the self-help culture and are quick to seek medical care. Also the middle-class hygienic practices include keeping children "squeaky clean" which may prevent them from developing immunity. The poor and the black "may have more crushing problems to deal with . . . In lower income brackets almost all children develop the antibodies by age 5."

More specific to pain, Schludermann & Zubek (1962) reported that the higher socioeconomic status individual had a higher pain tolerance. One possibility for this for the patients with acute pain may be that it is less threatening to their life style in that their affluence affords them "great freedom with relatively little discipline" (Henry & DiGiacomo-Geffers, 1980, p. 1426). Other possibilities include that more affluent individuals, who are more likely to expect more attention, have better verbal skills, and greater confidence in expecting what they do express about their pain, will be taken more seriously by the equal status physicians. With chronic pain, the converse may be true because the patient may have so much at stake, not being able to control his pain through delegation to servants and through purchased luxuries and having to spend considerable time in activities related to minimizing or controlling pain. Obviously, these factors become significant when assessing the patient's pain because of the potential that they have for methods of acceptable pain relief. Even keeping a pain diary to aid in assessment may seem like a burden for some individuals.

Social class and the "system" may complicate the pain and suffering for individuals in the lower socioeconomic class. Merskey (1978) reports that individuals of the working class are more likely to complain of pain, to have had painful experiences in the past, and to have had more relatives with pain experiences. Sternbach (1978, p. 246) says being poor and engaging in physical labor predispose an individual to pain. Two other factors may further influence how the poor express their pain. First, generally they are less well-educated and such individuals are usually not familiar with psychological concepts. Second, they are usually less psychologically minded. Compounding these factors may be those which specifically relate to the economics of the situation because lower-class individuals are often financially deprived. Health care plans often pay for physical treatment but not psychological or psychiatric treatment. Also, if the individual is eligible for disability, it will more closely approximate his income than that for the more affluent patient. Thus, there may be little incentive to return to work. Unfortunately this may necessitate that the individual perpetuate pain behaviors and suffering to become eligible for disability programs, not because he masochistically enjoys pain and suffering.

MEMBERSHIP IN A PARTICULAR SOCIOCULTURAL GROUP

Although stereotyping can and does exist in relation to all of the previously mentioned information on cultural orientation, perhaps the most damaging practice occurs in relation to ethnic groups and race. A very dramatic example of stereotyping is provided by Teish (1979, pp. 185–187). According to Teish, in 1851 a physician named Cartwright defined a new illness occurring only in blacks, drapetomania. *Drapetes* means flight or running away from; and *mania*, craziness. This mental illness occurred when black slaves attempted to escape from their white masters. To perpetuate the white masters' domination and control and to force submission, the treatment devised for drapetomania was to rub down the captured slave with oil and beat him into submission.

Akin to this for the pain patient, but more subtle, perhaps is the practice of the different cultural groups, and the health care professionals, discrediting what the pain patient reports about his pain and failing to provide adequate assessment and treatment. This may be done if the patient's beliefs and wishes for pain management conflict with the unilateral biomedical model, or if the patient fails to respond to the treatments being used for his pain. In the instance of the pain patient, he is also rendered powerless and forced into submission and robbed of all dignity. Instead of being deprived of food and water, he is deprived of adequate pain relief.

Considering the effectiveness of current mass communications media and the ease with which a person can travel or change his place of residence, it is not surprising that there is an increasing number of variations within each culture. Even in adulthood this exposure to the expectations of other cultures and subcultures may result in some change in the person's behavioral responses to the pain experience, although the underlying attitudes may change more slowly. Therefore, it is wise for the nurse to avoid stereotyping a patient's behavioral response to pain on the basis of her knowledge of the expectations of his culture.

MAJOR CULTURAL GROUPS

We will not consider various attitudes and behaviors of the major ethnic and racial groups in the United States which may influence the individual's pain experience. It would be impossible to cover all of the expectations of the various cultural groups the nurse may encounter. The information presented on the cultural groups should demonstrate some of the differences in cultural traditions. The terms used to differentiate between ethnic groups are likely to be quite misleading. These terms suggest that a person can be placed in one specific group or another. This is not true and would be counterproductive because it would amount to stereotyping or generalizing about an individual. Some terms may sound racist and prejudicial, but this is not the intent. Further, as one becomes acculturated and assimilates other values, many of the characteristics presented will decrease. Generally the more anglicized an individual becomes, the more likely he will espouse and seek more biomedical care for pain problems. Therefore, it will become apparent that many of the behaviors and values cited often represent the least acculturated and lower-class patients. It is with the greatest dissimilarity that we are likely to have the least understanding and acceptance and the greatest conflicts. It is important to remember in a stratified society such as ours, that individuals are often confined to the lower class because of barriers imposed by the more advantaged. The person may not have had a choice, due to a lack of money and education, to behave differently. Thus, his or her health care values are limited by access.

Asian-Americans

The largest numbers of Asian-Americans have their roots in China, Japan, Korea, the Philippines and, more recently, Vietnam, Laos, and Cambodia. As with other ethnic immigrants, the Asians frequently live in close proximity, not only to the port of entry but also to each other to facilitate understanding and communication and, perhaps to preserve some of their values and traditions. Common examples of these include the "Chinatowns" and "Little Tokyos" in the large cities. Of the Asian groups we will consider only two, Chinese-Americans and Japanese-Americans.

Before we proceed, one comment about Asians needs to be made relative to stoicism. Klein (1979b, p. 40) points out that labeling the Oriental "stoic" is unfortunate because it has "blatantly reinforced the erroneous notion that Orientals have no feelings and are incapable of emotion and [the label] has become one used as a perjorative."

Chinese-Americans Information in this section was primarily developed from the well-documented work of Gould-Martin & Ngin (1981) and Spector (1979). Concepts of health care for the Chinese-American are based on the philosophy and teachings of Tao (604 B.C.), on the relationship of the harmony between man and nature. Accordingly, nature provides laws which guide and govern the universe and man. To live a healthy life, one must adapt and adhere to these laws (Spector, 1979, p. 213). Health and illness are based on the concept of dynamic equilibrium between two opposing yet complementary forces, Yin and Yang. Yin, the negative or female force, stores the vital strength of life, helps conserve energy, and restores physical vitality. Yin represents darkness, cold, and emptiness. Yang, the male force, represents positive energy that protects the body from outside forces such as organisms. It produces light, warmth and fullness. The body is conceptualized in relation to these two forces. The inside of the body and the front are Yin. The outside or surfaces of the body and the back are Yang. Diseases are also categorized by Yin and Yang. Diseases of winter and spring are Yin, while those of summer and fall are Yang.

When Yin and Yang are in balance, a person is considered to be "living in peaceful interaction with his mind and body in proper order" (Wallnöfer & von Rottausher, 1972, pp. 12–13). Disruptions in this balance or harmony are considered to be the sole cause of diseases (Spector, 1979, p. 215).

Chaitow (1977, p. 11) feels that the Yin–Yang theory is a colorful, although, archaic explanation for disease. Rather, he suggests discussing "the body's homeostatic tendency [to maintain] a stable internal environment . . . through the interaction of the various body processes and systems." Wolff et al. (1980, p. 81) believe that it is important to make "the distinction . . . between the mind–body and good–evil dualism in Western philosophical and religious thought and the Eastern concept of dynamic interaction . . . of the Yin–Yang model." We, too, feel this distinction is important because the Yin–Yang philosophy is likely to be held by the more traditional and/or older Asian-American patients. It is also likely to be less familiar to the more traditional Western nurse, and the information presented here is for the purpose of assisting the nurse to assess cultural differences which may influence the patient's pain experience.

Both internal and external influences may alter the balance of Yin and Yang. Internal forces include such things as age and personality. External forces include influences of other individuals which may cause stress and environmental factors such as the weather and organisms.

Blood and ch'i, "the breath of life which flows through the meredians" (specific acupuncture points or patterns on the body surface which correspond to various organs), are two other vital forces governed by Yin and Yang (Chaitow, 1977, p. 20; Gould-Martin & Ngin, p. 147). At certain points in the body, blood, and ch'i interact. To maintain health these forces must flow smoothly through the body. If blood or ch'i are lost from the body, so is energy which is difficult to replace (Gould-Martin & Ngin, p. 137).

The pulse is considered as the storehouse of the blood. A strong regular pulse is a sign of good health. There are six different pulses, each having a specific characteristic and relationship to various organs. The balance of the body is influenced by several other

> conceptual devices. These include "wind"; "hot" and "cold" polarity; "poison"; and "fright" . . . [Each has] physical manifestations and symbolic aspects that fit together into a relatively coherent system (Gould-Martin & Ngin, p. 146).

The following are examples of the application of these devices to illness. Wind may enter the body during vulnerable periods and is also present in certain foods. Warming foods stimulate health and tend to be nutritious. Poison refers to conditions that are allergic or irritating such as a wound that enlarges rather than heals, infections, allergies, and skin diseases. Fright is a condition occurring in children, similar to that described by the Mexican-Americans, in which a child's soul is believed to become scattered from the body (pp. 147–148).

As with other ethnic groups, the Chinese-American may ignore or handle minor symptoms initially himself or herself. Sometimes symptoms will be allowed to persist in order to obtain sympathy and affection from the family. However, the Chinese-American sees his or her body as a gift from his or her parents rather than a personal possession. Therefore, it must be treated with much respect and good care. Another reason that the Chinese-American usually maintains his or her body and health is that it is considered a social obligation to prevent others from having to assume one's work. With migrant workers especially, there is also the concern of jeopardizing their chances for employment. For these reasons preventative measures may be carried out, including good nutrition and seeking medical care early, in spite of a tendency to handle minor symptoms himself or herself.

Initially, symptoms are diagnosed in the family, primarily by the parents, oldest brother, and the mother-in-law. Spouses consult each other first regarding their own symptoms. Chinese-Americans usually express more concern about symptoms in their sons than daughters. In fact, sons may not be concerned about their own symptoms, but will seek medical consultation for the sake of their parents (Koo, 1976). Symptoms which are likely to receive immediate attention include such things as "fright," blood loss, and those which have special significance such as threats to a male's sexual potency (Gould-Martin & Ngin, p. 151).

Chinese-American women usually assume the major health care functions for the family. During periods of illness, they provide the direct care for physical and emotional needs, brewing herbs and preparing soups. If the male is more literate he is likely to establish the diagnosis and peruse the "medical" literature for the best possible treatments. Nonmedical individuals consulted outside of the family are those considered to have a special interest in illness, those having more than the average knowledge about it, and those who are more accessible to the patient.

There are primarily two health care systems to which the Chinese-American patient may subscribe, the Chinese doctor and the Western physician. Although several factors may be involved in the decision on where to seek medical care, the major deciding factor is likely to be financial, that is, the ability to pay the fee. Chinese-Americans are very moral about paying their bills, paying most of them from their savings. They may not be willing to accumulate medical bills which they know they may not be able to pay (Gould-Martin & Ngin, p. 161). The amount of time to travel to medical facilities and the time spent in waiting for the care may be other major determinants. Chinese-Americans, even women and older individuals, work long hours. They may be unwilling to allow time to get the recommended care, especially if they perceive it as nonessential, such as preventative measures. Most Chinese-American patients who do not speak English will not go to a Western physician unless a bilingual relative or friend can accompany them. This then would involve another person's time. Limited language facility with English may cause the patient to be fearful about leaving Chinatown, using public transportation, and the possibility of getting lost (Hessler, Nolan, Ogbut & Kong-ming New, 1975; UCLA Asian Health Team, 1975).

The presenting symptoms may be determinants also. The Chinese doctor is usually consulted for minor symptoms. The Western physician is more likely to be consulted for symptoms considered more serious, those which have a rapid onset, high fever, dyspnea, and problems involving blood loss.

Acculturated middle-aged suburban patients are most likely to consult a Western physician for medical care especially during the acute phase. Treatment may involve both that prescribed by the Western physician and Chinese medicine. Follow-up, especially for chronic illnesses, is likely to be done with a Chinese doctor particularly by those less acculturated.

The Chinese doctor makes his diagnosis based on eight principles of

Chinese medicine; Yin or Yang; internal or external; cold or warm; increased or decreased function (Gould-Martin & Ngin, p. 154). In addition to the pulse, as previously mentioned, the color and appearance of the tongue and vital organs also provides important diagnostic information. All treatments by the Chinese doctor are aimed at restoring equilibrium between Yin and Yang. Treatments by the Chinese doctor include prescriptions for herbs and patent medicines, acupuncture, massage and exercise, and moxibustion, which is a treatment based on the therapeutic value of heat and is used for diseases where there is an excess of Yin. This is in contrast to acupuncture, a cold treatment for diseases caused by an excess of Yang. The Chinese doctor also offers recommendations for general good health measures such as nutrition and rest, and provides emotional support. One attractive aspect to treatment by the Chinese doctor is that his recommendations do not involve very painful diagnostic procedures and treatments (Chan & Chang, 1976, Louie, 1975). Another benefit is the relatively inexpensive cost.

Western medicine may be sought because it is considered more expedient in providing symptom relief and a complete cure. On the other hand, Western medicine may be veered away from or abandoned prematurely because medications and treatments are believed to be too drastic, with high risks and dangerous side effects.

In general, the Chinese-American patient usually respects the Western physician because he or she is considered to be a scholar. A physician must earn the respect of the Chinese-American patient, however, by demonstrating not only competence but also qualities highly valued by the Chinese-American patient such as politeness, seriousness, graciousness, and benevolence. The fee is considered an ethical matter, and high fees are incompatible with moral rectitude or humanitarian physicians (Louie, 1975).

If a Chinese-American patient needs hospitalization, he prefers to go to a hospital with a Chinese-speaking staff. However, even hospitals which are most likely to be utilized by the Chinese-Americans are severely underutilized (UCLA Asian Health Team, 1975). Perhaps this is partly because Chinese-Americans believe that the hospital is a place to die. They wait until they are almost dead before submitting to hospitalization. In Asia, when a patient is hospitalized, the family provides most of his routine care. Nurses only provide medically related procedures such as injections. This may be an expectation of the hospitalized Chinese-American.

Acupuncture is a popular treatment for many health problems including pain. In China, even children are often well-informed on the benefits and techniques of acupuncture. In some areas of China, children are instructed on the location of meredians and practice needle insertion on stuffed socks, themselves, and others (Wall, 1974, pp. 31–34; Capperauld, 1972, pp. 440–445).

Japanese–Americans In one study, Payne (1971) described the values of Japanese-Americans during health and illness and, more specifically, expectations and behaviors during the pain experience. She says that the Japanese "culture appears as the dynamic factor related to virtually every state of health or disease" (p. 17). Values modeled and reinforced by the family and community include "maintenance of correct personal relationships, harmonious coexistence, . . . conformity and obedience, respect for authority and a corresponding low degree of acting-out, overt rebellion, and independence" (p. 31). Self-control, resignation, and gratitude are also considered very important.

> Interpersonal relationships are implied in the *enryo* syndrome typical of patients even during a lengthy period of diagnosis and treatment, and a painful recovery. The *enryo* syndrome is characterized by behavioral reserve seen in the individual's restraint, reservation, and discretion in personal relationships with hospital staff and family members even under the most trying circumstances (p. 53).

Gaman, or forbearance, is another cultural value of importance during pain (Klein, 1979b, p. 40). As a cultural law, *enryo* "requires that one not intrude upon another's privacy, even when the desire is to help and [prohibits] off-loading one's troubles onto another" (Payne, pp. 4–5).

The major religion practiced by the Japanese is Buddhism. It is based on kindness and simplicity which also reinforces the cultural values as do suffering and hard work which are believed necessary for the building of character.

The Japanese are oriented toward the collective needs of the family and community. The individual's needs are of a lower priority. Manifestations of ethical behavior are so valued by the Japanese that any defiance of family or societal expectations brings shame and guilt to the family. In the family, parents are greatly respected, and there is a sense of "extreme obligation and willingness to defer to the parents" (Payne, p. 35). The highest respect is paid to the father. During illness he is expected to receive full support of all family members. The eldest son customarily assumes the responsibility for the parents. Children are treated with reverence which is believed to enhance their self-reliance.

In general, the Japanese patient likes to be taken care of when he is ill and is willing to be dependent and submissive. He may verbalize this with words such as "I'm putting myself in your hands." In Japan, for example, illness is sometimes used as an "egosyntonic impulse," minor symptoms being used to receive care and attention from loved ones (Payne, p. 30). During periods of illness, the Japanese prefer to care for the patient at home, providing both assistance with physical needs and companionship.

Traditionally a family member is present continually to do so. When this is not possible, a *tsukisoi*, a subprofessional nurse, may be employed to fulfill these functions.

The Japanese tend to communicate their feelings through behaviors rather than words. Cooperative behaviors imply approval. Dislike or displeasure are displayed by withdrawal, closing the eyes and mouth tightly, refusing to communicate, and patients may sometimes refuse to eat, drink, or take medications.

As with other ethnic groups, variation in health care practices can be expected in the Japanese-American patient. In one ethnic comparative study on death and dying, the Japanese-American displayed the greatest amount of intraethnic diversity and it correlated largely with generational identity (Klein, 1979b, p. 41). Thus, it is important to know the Japanese-American patient's place of birth and generation. There are large Japanese-American populations in Hawaii and California. *Issei* are first generation individuals who have immigrated to the United States; *Nisei* are second generation; *Sansei* are third generation; and *Yonsei* are fourth generation. Most *Issei* do not speak English, whereas *Nisei* understand and speak English and may only understand Japanese, and *Sansei* and *Yonsei* may perceive the Japanese language as a foreign tongue (Payne, pp. 31–32).

In relation to pain and illness, the *Issei* are usually the most stoic, disregarding minor symptoms as unimportant. Sometimes they ignore symptoms until a disease is out of control or even terminal. The *Issei* are loyal to their physicians. The *Nisei* tend to seek attention for minor illnesses rather rapidly. However, they lack the loyalty to their physician and, if they disagree with him, they may discharge him. The *Sansei* immediately attend to minor illnesses and are very selective in their choice of health professionals (Payne, p. 24).

Consistent with their communication style and *enryo*, the Japanese-American patient accepts pain as an integral part of illness, as does his family and physician, if his physician is Japanese. Further, patients are willing to submit completely to diagnostic procedures and treatments without complaint even though they may be extremely uncomfortable or painful (Payne, pp. 53–54).

The Japanese-American patient feels that it is extremely disgraceful to make a sound or cry out even during intense pain. One patient exemplifying this value said, "Once you let the cry of pain pass your lips, you may not bring it back" (Payne, p. 41). Another patient, a man who had extensive bowel surgery, made only one comment prior to his death: "I can't stand this any longer." Payne attributed this comment to severe pain and wondered if the health team had not perceived the "depth of this patient's suffering" (pp. 8–9). Indeed, some physicians working with Japanese women in labor "wonder if Japanese women feel pain" (Payne, p. 8).

In addition to the Japanese–American's reluctance to express pain, the Japanese patient may not expect to receive medication for pain. Further, if it is prescribed, the Japanese–American patient will not ask for it. Moreover, when it is offered he may refuse it. In fact, Japanese and Japanese–American physicians, tend to forget to prescribe analgesics even for patients expected to experience severe pain (p. 53). Because of this stoicism it is imperative that the nurse be especially attuned to nonverbal expressions of pain in the Japanese patient. "Body tension is one of the cues which Japanese–American funeral conductors observe to signal the need for a supporting hand" (Kalish & Reynolds, 1976, p. 135), one which may be helpful for the nurse to recognize in relation to the pain experience.

Black–Americans

Black, like white, is not an ethnic group but a race which is widely heterogenous, representing many ethnic groups with differing health care values. Jackson (1981, pp. 114–115), in a well-documented reference, says that because "a number of people both black and white still believe that blacks are culturally unique it is important to consider urban blacks as a group to help mainstream medicine improve their delivery of health care to them." We will first consider more general information about blacks and then consider how it may influence their pain experience.

> The etiology of disease identified by blacks is based on folk, popular, and biomedical sources, depending on the types of knowledge that are most prevalent among specific groups of urban blacks. Older blacks tend to rely more heavily on folk or popular sources, as do many rural migrants. Younger blacks, who are generally better educated, rely more heavily on biomedical sources, although many of them still retain folk and popular conceptions (Jackson, p. 75).

Most blacks initially treat themselves for symptoms. In this respect, blacks do not differ from other groups.

Differences in health care behaviors in the black culture do exist, and they are significantly determined by factors related to social class structure. Billingsley (1968, p. 123) divided black families into three classes. The upper class, 10 percent of the population, was comprised of both old and new wealth. The middle class, 40 percent of the population, was comprised of professionals, clerical workers and the skilled blue collar workers. The lower class, 50 percent of the population, was divided into the working poor, nonworking poor, and the underclass. Freidman (1981, pp. 285–287) identifies four social classes within the black culture: upper-class, middle-class, working-class, and lower-class. She did not include information on the upper-class blacks due to the lack of availability of such information. Briefly, Freidman describes features of the black middle-class family as tending to be nuclear; both parents usually work; the wife is often a professional, whereas the husband may or may not be; both spouses earn approximately the same income; they plan college education for their children; spouses have an egalitarian pattern of interaction, sharing decisions; socialization patterns are largely congruent with the dominant culture; grandparents and older siblings or extended family members usually play a more active role in the socialization process; and religion generally has a higher priority for black middle-class than for white Anglo-Saxon Protestant (WASP) middle class families (p. 285).

The black working-class family tends to be nuclear, but having more children than the middle-class family; greater likelihood that a relative or boarder may be part of the household; both parents generally hold jobs, and men usually are involved in semiskilled work; parents generally have not completed high school; parents desire more education for children; couples usually marry early and start families very soon after; although husbands and wives usually have traditionally assigned roles the relationship is usually egalitarian; women usually have more economic control in matters relating to home and children; owning one's home is highly valued; bearing and rearing children is considered to be an important function; religion plays an important function, second only to the home as the emotional center of life; parental lessons imbued to children include respectfulness, obedience; children are assigned household chores and are encouraged to seek away-from-home work for pay when old enough; and parents often have to work different shifts to cover child-care responsibilities, often sharply minimizing time for family activities (p. 285).

Distinguishing features of the black lower-class include three-fourths of members are working poor; poorer households are more likely to be single-parent; extended families are common especially in the absence of the husband; they generally have more children than other blacks and poor white families; if the husband is present he is often unemployed and the mother is on welfare; movement and instability are great in areas of jobs, residence, and relationships, which are criticized by society at large; adolescent boys and girls have sexual experiences at an early age and tend to get married earlier than other blacks because of stresses associated with family life; marriage is looked upon ambivalently and often negatively; although the husband is the titular head of the family, the wife is expected to care for the children and home and to make the husband feel welcome and comfortable when he is at home; the wife makes necessary decisions and has the greatest sense of responsibility for the family; intense loyalty exists between mothers and grandmothers and their children; grandparents often take on child-care roles and act as prime socializers; strong loyalty and reciprocity exists between siblings; family values are distinct and incongruent with wider society's value; fatalism, hoping for little and expecting less is a common value; although sexually involved, men and women are afraid to trust and commit themselves to each other; dependency rather than self-sufficiency is an orientation accepted as a reality; lack of achievement and work ethic is apparent as is the lack of the value of education and future planning; although confined to be home with small children there is no deep involvement and constant solicitousness in contrast to other blacks and other middle-class and working-classes from other ethnic backgrounds, and the loosely organized home is a reflection of the mother's sense of impotence in facing the street system (pp. 285–287).

In relation to health care, Jackson (p. 216) believes that "groups of low-income Southern blacks constitute a health culture of their own." Elesh & Schollaert (1972, p. 238) say that "formal education creates a common culture—one which places a high value on medical care and this can explain most of the differences attributed to other measures of cultural predisposition." Ring & Schein (1970) found this to be true when education and income were controlled for in one study of 388 black middle-class households. For a variety of psychiatric-related symptoms 87.4 percent of respondents were oriented toward mainstream medical care. Whereas Snow (1978) found that low-income blacks who were proponents of folk medicine made no distinction between science and religion and viewed the difference between mental and physical illnesses as irrelevant, considering the cause as the most important consideration. White (1977) maintained that because of humiliation, lack of money, and lack of trust in health workers, folk medicine has been perpetuated in the black community.

Regardless of social class structure, the black family is considered to be a matriarchial structure with a strong kinship system whether voluntary or out of a sense of obligation. Two distinguishing features of this are seen in the higher proportion of adult extended-family members living within households and the strong informal adoption network for children. For example, 90 percent of babies born out of wedlock are adopted into the family (Freidman, 1981, p. 294). Hill, as reported by Williams (1978, p. 77) believes that "the extended family is still one of the most viable institutions for the survival and advancement of black people today." In rural or urban areas, the extended family may not be available or in a position to assist with health care.

As the matriarch, the wife and mother most often assumes the primary responsibility for the family's health care including the assessment of symptoms, determining the treatment approach, providing for preventative measures and arranging for the care of the sick. If the wife or mother is not able to fulfill these responsibilities, then they are usually assumed by the eldest female child. Friends and neighbors also may help out. Single parents may be less stringent in defining illness behavior in children. Although health is usually an individual responsibility for adults, occasionally the wife may assume responsibility for her husband's health. Women tend to delay consultation for their own health problems longer than they do for their families (Jackson, pp. 82–89). Emphasis is placed on preventative health measures such as adequate nutrition, rest, and cleanliness. Rocereto (1973) points out that an individual who believes in spells believes that the use of preventative measures are helpful in avoiding folk illness.

Mechanic (1969, p. 201) says that "regardless of socioeconomic, demographic, or psychological characteristics the nature of the symptom is the most powerful factor blacks use in defining whether or not an individual is ill and will seek care for his symptoms." Also important in the decision about who should be sought out for discussion and treatment of symptoms is the previous experience the individual has had with the symptom. If the symptom is related to physical origin or produces pain or other intolerable discomfort, most urban blacks will discuss it with the person they feel is knowledgeable and seek medical care (Jackson, p. 84). Children most often discuss symptoms with those within their household or, if at school, their peers and school personnel. Ministers, pharmacists, and friends also may be consulted, especially if the friends work in health care settings. Unfortunately, such individuals are often attributed with knowledge that they may not possess.

In reporting their illnesses, James (cited in Jackson, p. 75), a black physician in private practice for almost three decades in Charlotte, North Carolina, noted that urban black patients often report their diseases in simplified terms, for example, coronary heart disease is shortened to "heart trouble" and diabetes mellitus to "sugar diabetes" or simply "sugar." No specific terms related to pain, pain perception, or pain tolerance were mentioned. Snow (1976, p. 52) believes that "every health professional who sees low-income Southern patients, black or white, soon learns the necessity of taking on another vocabulary in order to communicate effectively." Although this may not be true, the necessity for a "baseline" vocabulary understood by all those involved in the communications, obviously, is essential. Discussion of this will be considered in Chapter 9, Communication of the Pain Experience. In assessing pain with one elderly Southern white woman and attempting to establish congruent terms for pain intensity, the patient rejected words such as mild or moderate and offered "light."

The behavioral responses of blacks to pain have been reported in several studies. In some instances no differences were identified between blacks and whites with respect to reports of pain threshold in a laboratory setting. Merskey & Spear (1964) studied pain perception and reactions in male Afro-Asian and white medical students. They found no significant differences between the students. Winsberg & Greenlick (1967) studied 365 lower and middle-class black and white mothers' reports of pain intensity during labor and delivery. They found no observable differences. What they did conclude was that individual differences appear to be determined by other sets of social, psychological, and biological characteristics. In other studies, the Southern black exhibited a low pain threshold and less willingness to tolerate pain (Chapman, 1944; Chapman & Jones, 1944; Woodrow, Freidman, Siegelaub & Morris, 1972). This is especially relevant in view of McCabe's (1960) report that the Southern black hesitates to ask for pain relief, sometimes denies pain when there is sound reason for suspecting its existence, and identifies pain in general terms. Larkins's (1977) clinical experience with a black woman following bilateral total hip replacement substantiates McCabe's findings. This patient failed to verbalize pain and adamantly denied pain despite nonverbal indications to the contrary. This was accompanied, interestingly enough, by expressions of contempt for the roommate, suggesting displacement onto the roommate of her anger concerning her pain. Hence, it seems probable that in many instances of denial, black patients actually are experiencing pain. Absolutely no evidence exists to suggest that a black person is less sensitive to pain than a white person.

The concept of stress being responsible for physical illnesses is held by some blacks. It seems similar to that of Selye (1956). Accordingly, "worriation" is believed to be an etiological factor of disease. At times blacks seem to be too willing to attribute "worriation" as the cause of their diseases. "Some urban blacks who are presumably knowledgable about the causes of symptoms misinterpret them, attributing them to psychosomatic etiology" (Jackson, p. 84). This could possibly be related to a reluctance in seeking medical treatment in medical facilities. Jackson & Nixon (1970, p. 59) report several reasons both low-income and middle-income blacks may delay medical consultation. These include "the fears of a dreaded diagnosis; the fear that the treatment may make the condition worse or even be fatal; the fear that the individual may be told that he cannot work; and the fear of racial discrimination."

In spite of these fears, blacks view the physician as an individual of high prestige and authority. In turn, they expect the physician to treat them with respect. Jackson (1981, p. 99) says that whether or not a physician is white or black does not seem to be as important to the black patient as is the preference for competence. The white physician–black patient may replicate the master–slave relationship, according to Satcher (1973, p. 1499), with the master's words not to be questioned. Thus blacks who may not understand the physician's communication do not question him nor would the black patient be likely to express dissatisfaction with care. Satcher further reports that the white physician views this relationship as the "good patient" and believes that their patients are "happy." Also, the black patient has a growing suspicion and distrust of the white physicians because they call patients by first names and use them in teaching sessions according to Satcher (p. 1499). On the other hand Mayerson (1982), a white physician who obtained a considerable portion of his professional education in a large Mississippi county teaching hospital, reports that the poor black patients there preferred to be assigned to white physicians believing that they would receive better care than that provided to them by black physicians.

What seems most important is the disparity between the patient and the physician and how this may influence his ability to report and hope for adequate treatment of his pain. The use of formal versus informal communication with the black patient seems to be an individual matter and not related to being black.

Other conceivable deleterious consequences for the black patient due to fear of the predominantly white health team and a potential communication gap include the possibility that the patient will not seek medical assistance until his condition approaches an emergency state. When he does seek help, and especially if he enters the hospital, the patient may experience a quiet panic over his conflict between wanting help and distrusting it. If the patient continues with the care and hospitalization he may try to win the favor of those responsible for his care by exhibiting the responses that he knows they will approve—accepting care with unquestioning submission, not asking for information or not even requesting pain relief. The patient may fear that if he reports his pain he would be subjected to more of the care he already distrusts. As a result the patient may terminate treatment or leave the hospital against medical advice.

Because of this overriding distrust the black patient may be so dissatisfied and threatened by mainstream medical care that he seeks assistance with his health problems outside of the "system." Therefore, in treating a black patient it is important to know if he believes in folk medicine and, if he does, if he believes that his present health problems may be caused by a "hex" or someone "working roots" on him. Also important would be if he had sought assistance from a person capable of treating folk illnesses.

Snow (1979, pp. 179–184) reports on "voodoo illnesses" in the black population. She says that some patients may believe that doctors do not understand witchcraft and cannot cure its effects. Moreover, a bewitched person may believe that if he goes to the doctor his illness will become worse. In spite of this she says that, "The majority of black patients who believe their illnesses are due to sorcery go to a mainstream physician first" (p. 180). She lists terms which are often used for witchcraft as "voodoo, a fix, a hex, and working roots" (p. 180).

The hex is most often administered in food or drink by a relative or a friend close to the individual for the purpose of gaining control of his behavior. Supposedly this robs the individual of his free will. The most common reason that a person has been hexed is a triangular social relationship in which two people are fighting for control over a third person. This person usually is a lover, parent, or sibling. The goal is to remove the rival from the scene. An added danger of the hexed individual is that he may not realize that he has been hexed or that he needs help.

In one study, those interviewed about root work were unanimous in agreeing that a person could fall victim to roots and become ill, but only if he sincerely believed in root work. Pain is only one of a number of symptoms that may result from "rootin'," as it is called in Georgia (Rocereto, 1973). Because the substances used to "work roots" are administered in food and drink, gastrointestinal symptoms such as nausea, vomiting, a bad taste in the mouth, and diarrhea are common.

Although many folk healers do use folk medicine, calling in a "root doctor" may not be the treatment of choice. The patient may believe that the root doctor can kill as well as cure and be able to cast spells as well as take them away. Root doctors may offer patients dangerous substances such as mothballs to produce a dramatic physiological response, and they often charge a significant fee for their services. Even more destructive is the possibility that the patient may suspect that the physician's calling in a root doctor implies tacit approval of the root doctor (Snow, 1979, p. 184). The patient may also consider it a character evaluation by the suggesting individual and thus become distrustful of him or her.

Unless there is an atmosphere of acceptance, the patient probably will not reveal his belief that his pain is a result of root work. Questions of a general nature may be more productive in obtaining information. For example, Rocereto's (1973, p. 425) black subjects suggest that "you should teach the nurses to ask if a patient knows how he got sick or what he thinks made him sick. You just can't ask every black person outright if root work did it, because they all don't believe in it." Specific to pain questions of a general nature that may be productive in obtaining information could include "Do you know why you have this pain?" or "Do you know anything that may have caused you to have this pain?" If the nurse believes that the patient is being evasive, illiciting assistance from a black health care worker that the patient trusts and may be more willing to confide in may prove helpful in obtaining the desired information.

Snell (1967) suggests that hypnosis can be effectively used by psychiatrists in the treatment of the hexed patient without the psychiatrist believing in it or pretending to the patient that such a belief exists. White (1977) feels that humiliation, lack of money and a lack of trust in the health workers have perpetuated folk medicine in the black community.

Many blacks have a strong religiosity that may influence their acceptance of pain. Concepts such as heaven and hell may be involved in their illness behavior. A black patient with these beliefs may be willing to attribute an illness to "God's will" or fear that he or she may be doomed to hell.

Johnston (1977, p. 78) believes that "when scientific knowledge is presented so that it appears incompatible with a patient's traditional beliefs, the traditional way will probably win, and the best health information may be rejected."

Because black patients often stop treatment when symptoms abate, mainstream medicine can be most helpful to the black patient in attempting to control and work with factors which may result in termination. In general, acceptance of the medical regimen by the black patient is likely to occur when some control can be exerted over the extent to which expected roles need to be modified; when the treatment regimens are not too complex; when there are not long waiting periods for scheduled appointments; when there are not undue delays in receiving diagnostic reports (especially those related to serious illnesses); and when the patient is subjected to less racism (Jackson, 1981, p. 97). This is extremely unfortunate since so many of the lower class blacks are dependent for their health care on the city and county clinics and hospitals where *they have to wait for everything*.

It seems likely that any member of a minority group that is deprived educationally, economically, and occupationally may respond in some of the same ways. If his daily life is controlled by a dominant group and if existence is a day-to-day struggle, he can hardly be expected to trust members of the dominant group. Of necessity he has a more present-oriented attitude. He may attempt to behave in a manner approved of to gain acceptance by the dominant group since, as Zborowski (1969) found with Italian-Americans, for example, he knows expressive behavior annoys the Old American.

Mexican-Americans

In addition to the 12 million Hispanic-Americans reported by the United States Census Bureau in 1978, there are estimates of 7.4 million Hispanic-American illegal aliens in the United States. The Hispanic-American population is composed of Mexican-Americans, Cubans, Puerto Ricans, Spanish, and Carribean Island blacks (Freidman, 1981, p. 275). The only group we will consider with some depth is the largest group, Mexican-Americans.

Age, geographic area of residence, and socioeconomic factors somewhat determine what a Mexican-American prefers to be called. However, in an attempt to avoid negative stereotyping by alien "Anglos" or "gringos," some Mexican-Americans have elected to refer to themselves as "Mexicans," "Chicanos," "Latin-Americans," "Latins," "Latinos," "Spanish-Americans," or "Spaniards."

In studying Mexican-Americans, Freidman (1981, p. 276) points out that the pattern of labor utilization of the Mexican-Americans provides a key to understanding, similar to that provided by studying black slavery. She further identifies several factors which have served to isolate and which act as a wedge separating the Mexican-American from acculturation. These include continued use of their native Spanish language, close identification with the strong Roman Catholic religion, cultural and social class differences, drastic increases in population in some Southwest areas, and negative stereotyping by other Americans. Martinez & Martin (1979, p. 188) add to this that the Mexican-Americans have "on their own part separated themselves from the larger community by living in barrios, which have served to isolate them and preserve many of their folk beliefs."

The most significant characteristic of the Mexican-Americans is their strong family orientation. The family is usually a large closely knit group composed of both nuclear and extended members. Ties beyond the nuclear family are strong and extensive, linking grandparents, aunts, uncles, and cousins, and it often further extends to *compadrazgo* or "ritual coparenthood." *Compadres* and *comadres* assume the rights and obligations of relatives and are assimilated into the extended family (Clark, 1959, pp. 157–161; Schreiber & Homiak, 1981, p. 306).

The traditional roles, responsibilities, and communication patterns differ significantly in the Mexican-American culture in comparison to other American cultural groups. The Mexican-American male is the unquestionable head of the household, being "hard, unyielding, and strong" (Castro, 1978, pp. 19–32). His arbitrary powers are displayed by his machismo, aggressiveness, insensitivity, invulnerability, and superiority (Paz, 1973, p. 23). The female or wife, on the other hand, is characterized as "a soft, nurturing, self-sacrificing woman whose place is in the home, responsible for the children and to her husband. The children are socialized into absolute respect and obedience toward their father and are expected to place family duties before their personal ambition" (Freidman, p. 277). It is not surprising then that the communication pattern is authoritarian and that the male and older members of the household direct the women and children.

When Mexican-Americans become ill their family orientation and communication style often results in considerable disparity with traditional medical care practitioners. The family's decisions "often supercede the authority of both the individual patient and the health care personnel" (Schreiber & Homiak, 1981, p. 317). For the patient, however, there is a strong natural support system that helps the individual cope with serious illness and pain.

Religion may also play a dominant role during illness for the Mexican-American patient, as it provides an opportunity to do penance for one's sins. Rubel (1966, pp. 172–178) and Kiev (1968) both attribute much of what the folk healers accomplish with Mexican-Americans to the power of religious traditions and rituals. God has been evoked no matter what the outcome. Having a strong Catholic orientation, many Mexican-Americans have crucifixes, statues, and images of God and the saints, and altars to them. Spiritual works such as good deeds, personal sacrifice, masses, novenas and other prayers are done in an attempt to intercede and appeal for a return to health or the acceptance of God's will no matter what that may be. Some Mexican-Americans make pilgrimages to shrines in Mexico. The religious conviction and faith of the Mexican-American in the recovery process cannot be underestimated (Frank, 1961).

Freidman (1981, pp. 278–279, 1982) has summarized the differences in the values of the Mexican-American and the American majority cultures. She says that these values of the Mexican-American exist, irrespective of class (p. 278). This information can be seen in Table 3.2.

Although a small minority of Mexican-Americans subscribe exclusively to either folk or scientific medicine, most are heterogenous utilizers of medical care. Use is largely determined by the interaction of variables such as psychosocial or socioeconomic class and the degree of acculturation (Schreiber & Homiak, pp. 298–299). Even low-class Mexican-Americans evidence some knowledge and acceptance of biomedical concepts. However, they often maintain insular categories for medical and folk illnesses and treatments.

The Mexican-American defines health as the absence of pain and the ability to function adequately. The healthy individual is a person with a "well-fleshed" body and a high level of energy. Common signs and symptoms such as a cough or diarrhea are not interpreted as illness as long as they do not interfere with the activity of the individual (Schulman & Smith, 1963, pp. 228–229). Health is also considered a matter of "good luck." A change in luck may result in a change in health (Spector, 1979, p. 251). Because health and illness are considered a matter of chance, the Mexican-American does not hold the ill person as responsible for becoming ill. The transition from health to illness is "as much a psychological process as a biophysical process—one in which there is significant mediation of symptoms by situational and social factors" (Schulman & Smith, p. 300).

The woman has been assigned the role of the "home medical specialist" (Weaver, 1970, p. 143). As a result of this role allocation, medical knowledge is transmitted primarily from mothers to daughters (Rubel, 1966, p. 180). It is not surprising, then, that symptom assessment is first done by the wife and mother. If symptoms persist or are severe, consultation occurs in the following order—family, *compadres*, neighbors, friends, folk healer, and finally the physician. During this process many Mexican-Americans employ "dual usage" of healers even though the systems are considered insular (Schreiber & Homiak, p. 301).

Symptoms in infants and young children are quickly responded to even though the cost of treatment may impose a financial hardship on the family. If there is the slightest cause for concern, the ill child will be taken to the doctor. This concern applies to that for the unborn child, thus to ensure a healthy child, pregnant women seek medical care readily.

Mexican-Americans believe that life is full of traumas and that difficulties should be borne with dignity and courage (Schulman & Smith, p. 301). Consequently stoicism is valued. Neither men nor women usually

Area/Issue	American Central Value Orientation	Traditional Mexican–American Value Orientation
Family	Americans see themselves as individuals first and secondarily as members of families.	Chicanos see themselves as members of families first and as individuals second.
Self vs. kin obligations	American culture stresses individuality and independence from family after a certain age. Self-reliance and autonomy are emphasized.	Chicanos believe in ethic of reciprocity within family and kinship group.
Respect and authority structures	Americans value democratic ideals and egalitarianism (to a much greater extent). The elderly do not receive great respect. The authority of the masculine role is gradually diminishing as a result of feminist struggles.	Value in male dominance and respect for and obedience to the elderly predominate. Authoritarianism is valued over democratic ideals.
Progress vs. tradition	Americans value progress and change.	Mexican–Americans show more reverence and respect for tradition.
Work	Work and productivity are central, prominent values of the Anglo culture. Work often becomes a value in itself (more true in the past than today).	Work is seen as a necessity in order to live. Other life experiences—social and emotional experiences—are valued more than work.
Materialism	Materialism is another central American value. Possession of material goods is seen as a sign of success and becomes an end in itself. The cynosures of society are the businessman and financier.	Material objects are viewed as necessities and not as ends in themselves. Social status and prestige are more likely to be derived from an ability to experience things directly and/or through social and family relationships rather than through past successes and accumulation of wealth. Mexican–Americans generally have great reverence for philosophers, poets, musicians, and artists.
Time	"Time is money." Punctuality is equated with goodness and being responsible.	Time is a gift to be enjoyed. The concept of wasting time is not understood. Punctuality is not an important moral value.

Present vs. future time orientation	Making plans for the future (planning) is highly valued as a means of getting ahead. Future-oriented.	Enjoyment of the present. Less concern for always living in the future. More present-oriented.
Interpersonal relationships	Americans value openness and directness in communications. (Americans are viewed as being blunt and succinct by Mexican-Americans.) Use of kidding to get messages across more indirectly is acceptable. In interpersonal conflict situations, Americans value "leveling," open dissent, and criticizing each other. Value rational expression of thoughts and not emotional expression as much.	Mexican-Americans value diplomacy and tactfulness, and show concern and respect for other's feelings and dignity. Their manner of expression is more elaborate and indirect. Mexican-Americans value agreement and courtesy, and are very sensitive to criticism regardless of manner presented. Value being expressive and showing feelings toward another person.
Environmental responses	Americans are less sensitive to the environment and its various forms of stimulation.	Mexican-Americans value greater sensory stimulation within their environments, using the full range of senses to experience their environment (vivid colors, expressive music and art, spicy foods).
Relationship to environment	Americans see themselves as mastering the environment.	Chicanos value living in harmony with the environment.
Education	Education highly valued as means to success and way to be productive. Correlated with work and productivity ethics.	Education is not [as highly valued]* primarily because it has been so inaccessible and schools so culturally incongruent with the Mexican-American values. Also, many Chicanos are not in tune with the success and scientific values which are associated with education. They are not as competitive as Americans generally and education is not pursued with the aggressiveness needed to succeed.

(From: Friedman, M. M. Family Nursing Theory and Assessment. New York: Appleton-Century-Crofts, 1981, pp. 278–279, with permission. Adapted primarily from Murillo, N. The Mexican American family. In Hernandez, C.A., Haug, M.J., Wayner N.N.: Chicanos: Social and Psychological Perspectives. St. Louis, Mosby, 1971, pp. 97–108.)

*Friedman, M.M. Personal Communication, November 2, 1982.

respond to early signs and symptoms, because it may be considered a lack of stamina and weakness. Women can be more easily relieved of their duties; therefore it is easier for them to seek treatment. Mexican-American males have a strong need to express their masculinity, referred to as "macho." It is very difficult for them to tolerate a loss of their authority or self-esteem even in front of their family. They also consider that illness reflects moral weakness and is shameful. Thus illness results in a personal loss of *dignidad*. Consequently, assuming the sick role and curtailing activities is done with much resistance (Clark, 1959).

Both sexes consider medical care embarrassing. A "good husband" will want to protect his wife's modesty and may want to be with her during examinations and treatments. Men see medical care as another affront to their masculinity and self-esteem. To protect his own modesty the male may refuse some examinations and treatments. Two things become very apparent in caring for the Mexican-American patient. Sexual topics should not be discussed in mixed groups, and during examinations and treatments the exposure of body parts should be kept to a minimum (Schreiber & Homiak, p. 319).

To varying degrees Mexican-Americans subscribe to a variety of folk ideas, to be discussed later in this chapter, about the cause and treatment of illness and disease. Many folk conditions have a corollary in traditional scientific medicine and therefore may be fairly amenable to scientific treatment. However, folk orientation requires the presence of symptoms to diagnose illness. If an abnormality is detected on examination and the patient does not have symptoms he may refuse to comply with treatment because "no disease exists."

Most female heads of household recognize the symptoms associated with folk disorders and also symptoms and signs of more serious physical conditions. Traditional folk illnesses may be categorized as *males naturales* ("natural illnesses") and *mal puesto* ("witchcraft") (Rubel, 1966, pp. 156-157). In one study of 75 housewives living in a public housing project, ages 18 to 84, 97 percent of the women knew about all five of the major folk illnesses. Eighty-five percent possessed some specific information such as the etiology and treatment for these diseases except *mal puesto* (Martinez & Martin, 1979, pp. 189-190).

The causes that Mexican-Americans may attribute folk illnesses to include imbalances between "hot" and "cold" or "wet" and "dry." The healthy body is in a state of equilibrium in relation to these qualities. Either internal or external excesses may cause disequilibrium and precipitate illness. Accordingly, the imbalance occurs in the four "body fluids" or "humors," namely: blood (hot and wet), yellow bile (hot and dry), phlegm (cold and wet), and black bile (cold and dry) (Spector, p. 251). Body organs have a specific location and function. If there is any change in these, illness may result (Rubel, 1960, p. 808). Loss of any amount of blood is believed to weaken a person and precipitate illness. The loss of blood in males is believed to impair sexual vigor (Clark, 1959, p. 181; Scrimshaw & Burleigh, 1978, p. 36). Health entails harmonious social and spiritual relationships. Any disruption or transgression of cultural values may negatively effect one's emotional and physical health (Schulman & Smith, 1963). Anglos are believed to be immune to folk illnesses; therefore, during stressful conditions or times of social change, when illness results the Mexican–American's cultural identity is likely to be reinforced.

Several common folk maladies among Mexican–Americans include: *Caida de la mollera* ("fallen fontanelle") which occurs in a child following a blow to the head or when the nipple is removed too quickly from its mouth during breast feeding. The physician or nurse may also cause it by touching the infant's head. This condition may be emotionally laden because of the possible implication that inadequate care was provided by the mother for her child. The corresponding scientific illnesses to *caida de la mollera* are dehydration, and feeding problems. High temperature, crying and restlessness are common symptoms. There are no folk cures, but Western medicine is often accepted.

Empacho ("indigestion infection") is a condition which occurs in both children and adults. It is caused when one is unable to pass a bolus of food through the digestive tract. Certain foods such as eggs and cheese may precipitate *empacho*. Symptoms include abdominal pain, nausea, vomiting and diarrhea. In the child, fever, crying, and restlessness are common. The folk treatments are to rub or pinch the spine until a "pop" is heard indicating that the bolus of food has been dislodged. Then broth or a purgative is administered.

Mal ojo ("evil eye") is a disease believed to occur most frequently in individuals with "light" blood and "weaker beings," thus children and women. *Mal ojo* is believed to be caused by heating the blood through the electricity in a stronger person's eyes or vision. A strong, admiring, or covetous glance or stare is said to result in causing the weaker person to be robbed of their ability or to act on their own behalf. Symptoms of *mal ojo* include fever, vomiting, crying, restlessness, and abnormalities of the eyes. If the disease is not successfully treated it may progress to a fatal stage called *ojo pasado*.

Susto ("fright") or *espanto* ("soul loss") is the scientific counterpart to the reactive syndromes—a culturally meaningful type of anxiety hysteria linked to role conflicts in which the individual voluntarily elects the symptoms to express the conflict and uses it to control or impose his perception of a situation on another (Rubel, 1964, pp. 278–280; Uzzel, 1974, p. 374). *Susto* may result from even the slightest fright or scare. It is believed that the trauma immobilizes the individual, rendering him helpless to remove the fear. Early symptoms are referred to as *susto nuevo* or *susto liviano*. Later on advanced symptoms which may be fatal are known as *susto pasado*. The later is characterized by wasting away of the body. Rubel (1964) says that *susto* serves as both the explanation for and the excuse for assuming the passive sick role. Because *susto* is due to the "loss of the soul" from the body, the most effective cure is to have a folk healer coax the soul back into the body. While this is being accomplished the patient is relaxed through massage.

Mal puesto ("bewitchment") is similar to the concept held by the blacks of "root work." A hex is placed on an individual through food, a photograph, or an effigy of the individual. It involves the jealousy between lovers or discord within the family or between other individuals. In response to these a *bruya* or *bruyo* (sorcerer) places a hex on the rival. Its scientific equivalent is schizophrenia. Symptoms may be both emotional and physical including uncontrolled screaming, crying, and exhibitionism. *Mal puesto* may also be used by the Mexican-Americans as a "catchall" category for any other illness which persists or is unresponsive to treatment.

There are several types of folk specialists who may be consulted to treat illnesses. *Yerberos* (herbalists) may be either the primary or adjunctive healer. The main treatments they employ are home remedies and herbs, compounding and instructing the patient in the latter. *Espiritualists* (spiritualists) may use herb diets and massage but their major role is to treat through a trance and the use of spirit mediumship. Their effectiveness seems to be greatest with psychosomatic illness. *Parteras* (lay-midwives) serve to deliver babies and are a referral source for their patients. *Sobadoras* (masseuses) primarily treat musculoskeletal disorders. *Señoras* (wise women) are middle-aged women who seem to be most knowledgeable in popular medicine. They may function in the treatment of folk disorders, delivering babies, and in caring for the extended family. *Curanderos* are holistic healers who practice the defined medical system, *curanderismo*. The Mexican-American who believes in *curanderos* views them as religious figures. Some are specialists, others are generalists. They treat physical, psychological, and social problems. Because the *curandero* has a religious orientation, treatments include "elements of both the Catholic and Pentecostal rituals and artifacts: offerings of money, penance, confession, lighting candles, wooden or metal offerings in the shape of the afflicted anatomic parts (*milagros*), and laying on of hands" (Spector, 1979, p. 256). They are considered "good intuitive psychologists with insights into intracultural and acculturational stress" (Schreiber & Homiak, 1981, p. 311). They may be especially effective because they capitalize on "paternalistic dependence," often allowing the head of the household to make decisions about the care to be given, and they offer assurance in contrast to a physician who may primarily ask many questions. They also are intimately involved with the community and therefore are aware of common problems. Other desirable aspects about the services of *curanderos* is that they expect a donation rather than a fixed fee (p. 312).

White Anglo-Saxon Protestants (WASP)

In spite of the fact that the white Anglo-Saxons (old Yankees and English) are still considered the dominant cultural group in the United States there is little social research done on this group (Harwood, 1981, p. 14). They are descendants of the English and subscribe to the Protestant work ethic which is based on personal achievement—the male being successful in his occupation and the female being a good wife and mother (Freidman, 1981, p. 173). Desired behaviors which are modeled by both men and women include self-reliance and resourcefullness, planning and allocating resources rationally, efficiently, and with consideration for future orientation, self-denial to achieve goals, and hard work (Simmons, 1979, p. 105; Freidman, 1981, p. 175). In one study, based on a national probability sample of 1247 families, it was found that 56 percent of all Americans still subscribe to these values (Yankelovitch, Skelley, & White, 1975, p. 100). This information is illustrated in Figure 3.1. These values will become

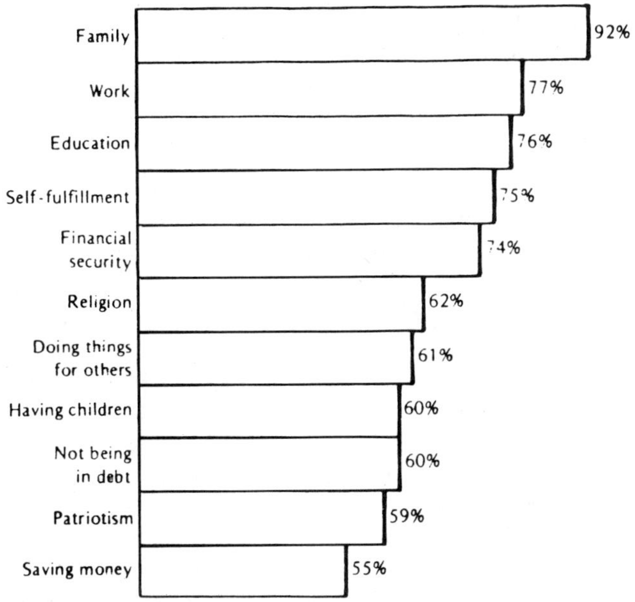

Figure 3.1. Most important personal values of the American family. (*From Yankelovitch, Skelley, and White, Inc.: The General Mills American Family Report, 1974–1975: A Study of the American Family and Money ©. General Mills, Inc. 1975, with permission.)*

evident in the following studies on Wasp culture and how it may influence their culture and pain behaviors and willingness to seek and accept relief.

Hautman & Harrison (1982) reported in their study of the health beliefs and practices of the middle-income Anglo–American that 85 percent of the individuals considered themselves in good health; 11 percent in fair health; and 4 percent in poor health. The majority of individuals reporting good health defined it as their ability to function adequately in spite of a variety of diseases. Whereas individuals with fair or poor health defined it as the absence of disease or in relation to pain, frequency of visits to the doctor, or the inability to work. Ninety-six percent of the individuals studied attributed the possible etiology of disease to viruses and bacteria, and 93 percent identified poor eating habits as a possible cause. Other possible causes identified included stress, cold air, drafts, and environmental factors. Twenty-four percent believed in hexes or witchcraft as a possible cause; 17 percent believed that punishment by God may result in ill health.

A preventative eclectic approach was identified as the best way to maintain one's health. This included diet, exercise, and use of vitamins. A good diet included foods that were considered healthy and abstinence from foods perceived as unhealthy, such as junk foods. Over 50 percent of the individuals studied had at least one book related to health or illness. Most individuals treated themselves for minor signs, symptoms, and injuries. Thirty-six percent used home remedies and 12 percent used herbs or plants. The pharmacist was consulted about the use of medications and treatments for minor conditions; however, more than 70 percent reported that they would seek consultation with a physician if they were concerned about or believed a symptom to be serious. This is in contrast to other ethnic groups previously discussed who first used a lay-referral system. The majority of patients paid for their health care through the use of private medical insurance, prepaid health plans, Medicare, military insurance, or student health plans.

In studying illness beliefs and behaviors in low-income Anglos, Bauwens (1977) found that their ideas about the etiology of illness were vague and discussed in general ways. For example, changes in the climate and impurities were frequently mentioned. Further, the pharmacist was utilized to a great degree to diagnose, recommend treatment, and give advice.

APPLICATION OF THE INFORMATION ON CULTURAL DIVERSITY TO THE PATIENT WITH PAIN

Usefulness of Research

We may be misled by research studies that attempt to evaluate pain threshold, pain tolerance, and pain relief measures. Potential danger to the patient would arise if we applied such studies in a stereotypical or cause and effect manner to him. In all pain experiences, including well-controlled studies, all the pain dimensions, sensory-discriminative, motivational-affective and cognitive-evaluative, are operative. Because pain is a highly personal subjective experience it really is impossible for us to determine at any given moment which of the interacting variables is most influential. Although the patient can be the only judge of his pain, at times even he will tell you "I'm not sure" or "I don't know." Therefore, before reviewing studies on the relation of ethnicity to the pain experience some general considerations relevant to the application of these studies in clinical practice seems important.

Because of the innumerable problems associated with designing and conducting research some of the researchers themselves point out the limitations of studies related to pain, especially their applicability to the patient with pain in the clinical setting. Some of the studies have limited validity or are completely invalid because the major relevant variables may not have been controlled for or the number of subjects studied was inadequate and thus the findings are not statistically significant. As you will see at the end of the review of the studies, in the more highly controlled studies there is remarkable similarity in the findings.

In an attempt to control important variables that can affect the outcome of studies related to pain relief, among other things, it is often necessary to control the pain-relief measure so that it is consistent. Hence, the same pain-relief measure may be used in the same way with every subject. If the research shows that the pain-relief measure is not effective or is even detrimental, the results should be viewed with caution. Such results do not always mean that the pain-relief measure should be discarded. Individualizing pain relief measures is an indispensable key to successful pain relief, and research design may prevent it.

Sometimes when research reports are cited only a limited amount of information may be provided. For example, it may not be clear whether the research was done on human subjects or animals. In animal experiments tissue damage may be inflicted, whereas in human experiments this is highly unlikely . In most human pain studies the individual is likely to know through the accompanying verbal explanation and signing of the consent that he may terminate the experiment, thus interrupting the pain at any time, though he may be strongly urged to continue his participation. In clinical practice the patient usually does not have the option of completely terminating his pain. For example, a patient with pathological pain of high intensity does not know when and if the pain will ever be relieved.

Because of the dearth of studies on the relationship of ethnicity to the pain experience, we will even include studies which seem to be dated or those that fail to control for relevant variables because they are either considered a classic or represent the only work which we were able to find on a given aspect of the pain experience. The absence of studies on some of the cultural groups in the United States reflects our inability to locate such research if indeed it has been done.

The best known study of pain in ethnic groups was done by Zborowski (1952, 1969). He selected males in four cultural groups, Old American, Italians, Jews, and Irish (as they existed in the United States), and described their pain response patterns. Following is a summary of the major characteristics of a "typical" or hypothetical member of each group as identified by Zborowski.

The Old American group as defined in Zborowski's study includes all ages of adulthood. Its members are typically born in the United States, white, Protestant, and without identification with any foreign group either nationally or socially. The cultural expectations of this group are dominant in the United States. The Old American usually attempts to give an efficient description of his pain to members of the health profession; otherwise he remains nonexpressive. He attempts to control reflexive responses of withdrawal and to avoid screaming, crying, and other manifestations of pain. He views such vocalizations as useless and indicative of a defeated condition. Only limited expressions such as an occasional jerk or "ouch" are acceptable. He takes pride in being the "good patient" who does not annoy others with his complaints. In the presence of family and friends he tries to retain his sense of humor, to minimize his pain, and not to evoke sympathy or pity. When the pain becomes severe he tends to withdraw and wants to be alone. He is optimistically future-oriented, concerned with the implications of his pain but confident that skillful health team members will effect a cure. In the meantime, however, he feels that the pain is unnecessary and expects it to be relieved by palliative measures. Before this patient seeks medical assistance, he may experience some anxiety and conflict in deciding whether his pain is insignificant or is a warning signal that something is wrong with his body. He does not want to ignore a warning signal but on the other hand he does not want to feel he is a "sissy." Pain involved in athletic performance is expected but not accepted; however, such pains as headaches, "growing pains" in the extremities, stomachaches, and sore throats are accepted as normal unless they increase in frequency and severity. With any pain, the patient may delay contacting the physician a few days to see if it goes away.

A patient of the Jewish religion tends to give rather dramatic accounts of his pain experience. He uses many adjectives such as "terrific" and "unbearable." He does not mind telling others about his more extreme responses to it. Although this behavior differs markedly from the Old American response, the Old American and the Jew share a similar attitude toward pain. Both are future-oriented and concerned with the symptomatic significance of the pain. The Jew, however, is pessimistic, especially at first, and his reactions initially tend to be more intense, apparently for the purpose of creating sufficient concern to cause others to take the best possible care of him. Unlike the Old American, he believes that crying and moaning help by mobilizing those around him to offer sympathy and assistance. He does not want to be alone with his pain. Another source of his pessimism is that he does not view the physician as an undisputable authority. He may seek the advice of several physicians, but he is not afraid of the diagnosis since it is usually less ominous than what he had imagined. Because the Jew is primarily concerned about the future implications of pain, he seeks curative measures and frequently is reluctant to take analgesics, especially if they are associated with addiction.

The Italian, like the Jew, feels that it is natural to cry, moan, complain, and use many gestures and body movements. This response apparently serves no particular purpose such as mobilization of support—it is merely natural. Unlike the Jew, he does not complain to his family for fear that he will upset them. Besides, he feels that they know of his pain without being told and that they want to help. He likes to have family and friends around (if they do not remind him of his pain by asking questions) because their presence tends to take his mind off the pain. In fact he feels he can deal better with the pain if he remains occupied to the extent of going to work. Unlike the Jew, the Italian is present-oriented. The Italian is concerned with the pain sensation itself and not the reasons for the pain. Like the Old American he wants at least palliative relief and he wants it immediately. He believes he should ask for relief as soon as pain occurs. He willingly accepts almost any pain relief measure although he tends to view drugs as unnatural. Interestingly enough, the Italian is among the very few who feel that drugs relieve pain mostly through their psychological effect. In general, he has confidence in the health team and complies with their instructions. Surgery is accepted if it relieves pain and does not reduce life's enjoyments. A chordotomy, for example, may be refused since it affects sexual functioning. To the Italian the significance of pain is related to its effect upon his state of mind. He experiences depression over the loss of energy and ability to enjoy life. His tears are not only an expression of pain but also a manifestation of grief. Relief of pain immediately relieves the depression.

The Irishman is similar to the Old American in his calm and unemotional reaction to pain. He too feels that complaining serves no purpose. He is reluctant to discuss his pain and suffering. Also like the Old American, the Irishman tends to withdraw from family and friends when he is in pain. However, underlying the Irishman's behavioral responses to pain is an attitude quite different from the Old American. The Old American wants to be alone because he does not want to be seen as weak and helpless, but the Irishman does not mind admitting to his friends that he suffers—he merely wants to suffer alone. He is not expected to share any of his troubles with anyone. It is even difficult to obtain information regarding the quality and intensity of his pain. Whereas the Old American feels pain is unnecessary and should be relieved, the Irishman seems almost proud of being able to handle pain. His two predominant methods of dealing with pain are relaxing and fighting. To use the passive technique of relaxing the patient must be undisturbed and alone to concentrate on absorbing the pain without complaint. Fighting, an active response, requires mobilizing his resources, "hanging on" and gritting his teeth, or continuing to be active by going to work. Often he goes through a long period of struggling with his pain before he consults a physician. When the Irishman finally goes to the physician, he tends to follow orders without question in spite of some skepticism. Perhaps because he has the techniques of relaxing or fighting to assist him, the Irishman is less concerned with the sensation of pain than he is with its future implications. This concern is not focused on the pathological aspects but on possible crippling and inactivity. The patient has less anxiety about this if the pain is caused by external injury such as a fall. Pains resulting from violent sport and fist fights are both expected and accepted without complaint.

Opler (1961), commenting on Zborowski's findings, suggested that the lower pain tolerance of the Italians may be due to their general preoccupation with their body. The Irish, on the other hand, pride themselves with a denial of their physical self and Opler believed that might account for their stoicism.

Sternback & Tursky (1965) studied pain in four middle-class ethnic groups of "housewives" using Zborowski's hypotheses. The groups they studied were the "Yankees" (third generation British-descent subjects mostly from New England); second-generation Orthodox and Conservative Jews; and second-generation Irish and Italian Roman Catholics. The "Yankees" had the highest pain tolerance, followed by the Jews, Irish, and lastly the Italians. The "Yankees" tended to have a matter-of-fact attitude toward pain. The Jews were future-oriented and not alarmed about their pain. The Irish were nondemonstrative about their pain. The Italians had a present orientation and focused on the immediacy of their pain. Sternbach and Tursky concluded that these four subcultural groups had attitudinal differences which accounted for their autonomic and psychophysical pain reactions.

In the article, "Pain differences, similarities found," in *Science News* (1980, p. 182) a study was reported by Lipton & Marbach at the American Pain Society meeting in New York which yielded similar results to Zborowski's. They studied the ethnic differences in 166 patients with chronic facial pain of unknown origin. The cultural groups studied included Hispanics, blacks, Italians, Irish, Jewish, other white Catholics, and other white Protestants. Conformity was found in the emotional response (tears or moans) to pain, but distinct differences were found in how patients viewed their pain and how they described it. Hispanics and blacks differed from

Italians, Jews, and other white Protestants in that they were five to seven times more likely to fear their pain was cancer-related. The Irish differed from blacks, Italians, and other white Catholics in that they were less likely to fear they were responsible for bringing on their own pain. Other white Catholics differed from all the other groups in that they more readily believed that their pain was imagined. Hispanics differed from blacks, Italians, Jews, and other white Protestants in that they were less willing to admit they lost control when describing their pain. Other white catholics differed from Italians, Irish, and Jewish participants in their description of pain. They were more willing to describe their pain as stabbing. Blacks in comparison to Hispanics were more likely to describe their pain as unbearable. Because their study was done with third- or later-generation Americans, the surprising thing to Lipton & Marbach was that the groups did not have more conformity with each other.

Differences between the Irish and Italians have also been observed by Zola (1966). The Italians tend to have more symptoms in more areas of the body along with more bodily dysfunction than do the Irish. Different attitudes also affect the extent to which people seek medical attention and what they report to the health professional. Even in patients with the same disorder, there was a tendency for the Irish, compared with the Italians, to deny the symptom of pain.

In two other studies Chapman (1944) and Chapman & Jones (1944) found that blacks were able to tolerate much less pain than Northern European subjects. They also studied Russian Jews and Italians. Their conclusions were that individuals of Mediterranean races had pain tolerance levels similar to those of the blacks. Black subjects did not complain; however, those of Mediterranean origin complained loudly. The conclusion of Chapman & Jones was that pain tolerance was due to ethnic factors.

Some comments have been made about differences between Englishmen and Americans, although no systematic studies seem to exist. Katz, who has practiced medicine in both the United States and the United Kingdom, states that patients in London will tolerate, without complaint, the passage of a large-bore intravenous needle, whereas patients in New York are much less tolerant (Katz, et al. 1974). The incidence of chronic pain, however, appears to be the same in Britain and North America (Fink, 1974).

Two of the findings of a study done on the expression of emotions and sources of support during personal loss of a significant other may be applicable to understanding and assisting these groups with a pain experience. The groups studied were blacks, Japanese-Americans, Mexican-Americans and Anglo-Americans. This study is included here because of the dearth of pain-specific research findings for two of the groups—Japanese-Americans and Mexican-Americans. Answers to the question "Would you try very hard to control the way you showed your emotions in public?" yielded the following percentages of Yes answers: blacks, 70 percent; Japanese-Americans, 82 percent; Mexican-Americans, 64 percent; and Anglo-Americans, 54 percent. Of all the groups studied, 50 to 54 percent reported that the family was who they would turn to for comfort (Kalish & Reynolds, 1976).

More recently in a tightly controlled study, Flannery, Sos, & McGovern (1981, pp. 39–50) assessed ethnicity as a factor in the pain experience of 75 women, all who had a similar episiotomy for a similar delivery and who had previous Lamaze training. The women were divided into five ethnic categories: Old Americans, blacks, Roman Catholic Irish, Roman Catholic Italians, and Conservative or Reformed Jews. The Old Americans were at least third-generation white Anglo-Saxon Protestants. This group served as the control for the four other groups. The American blacks were Protestant, of at least third-generation, whose ancestors were born in the rural South. The parents of the Irish Catholics and the Italian Catholics had to have immigrated from rural Ireland or Italy, respectively. The Jews' parents had to have immigrated from Eastern Europe.

Socioeconomic information for the 75 participants indicated that the average patient was 27 years old, married with two children, had a family income of $16,000, and had attended at least two years of college. Further, 60 percent of all subjects reported that when their mothers were in pain they were generally not expressive. Sixty-six percent reported that their fathers generally were not expressive either.

All patients were approached 12–48 hours after delivery to participate in this study. To illicit the relation of ethnicity to the pain experience, self-assessment measurements were administered to and behavioral observations were done by two of the researchers for this study. The testing included semantic pain differences, pain attitude measurements, physical awareness measurements, a manifestation of anxiety test, a urogenital anxiety test, and global episiotomy pain scale.

The findings of this study suggest that "when the experimental stimulus is held constant, when anxiety over medical procedures is minimized, and when the patient's attention span is focused, no significant differences in pain response among ethnic groups will be found" (p. 50).

These researchers offer three possible explanations to account for the significant differences both for the reported clinical experience of many health care professionals and other researchers studying the relation of ethnicity to the pain experience. First, others' findings may be valid for immigrants and first generation; however, there is an assimilation of the "Protestant ethic" including the response to pain, "silent suffering," with successive generations. Second, as health care professionals, we may mistake the effect of the patient's ethnicity on his pain experience based on *our* assumptions of how *our own* ethnic groups behave, not considering relevant demographic data such as generation and education of our patients. Our assumptions may then serve to strengthen our expectations of the ethnic behavior. Third, as health care professionals, regardless of our ethnic backgrounds, we may tend to behave in ways consistent with the Protestant ethic in some situations including our work with patients in the hospital environment; whereas, at other times, we may behave more consistently with our earlier learned ethnic patterns such as those practiced during specific ethnic rites like the Irish wake or a Bar Mitzvah.

Various values and behaviors associated with pain and general health care practice have been examined. It seems likely that any member of a minority group that is deprived educationally, economically, and occupationally may respond in similar ways. If his daily life is controlled by a dominant group and if existence is a day-to-day struggle, the person can hardly be expected to trust members of the dominant group. Of necessity he has a more present-oriented attitude. He may attempt to behave in a manner approved of by the dominant group since, as Zborowski (1969) found with the Italian, for example, he knows expressive behavior annoys the Old American. However, aside from these reasons for respecting one's ethnicity, some individuals may elect consciously to respond to pain based on their own ethnicity regardless of possible social censure of their expression. Harwood (1981, p. 5) explains this as *ideological ethnicity,* "that is, people who display ethnic markers and otherwise manifest their ethnicity in restricted social contexts, often through ethnically based interest groups" . . . in contrast to "primarily first-generation Americans for whom ethnic identity is predominantly behavioral".

Memorizing the characteristics of each ethnic group for the purpose of using them in clinical practice represents a gross misunderstanding of the relevance of this content. Hopefully the nurse will use this information to gain a greater understanding of people's needs during painful experiences.

NURSING CONSIDERATIONS FOR THE PATIENT'S CULTURE

The following three paragraphs illustrate how cultural information may be used in working with the patient in pain.

First, it becomes obvious that the pain sensation itself probably does not influence the patient's attitude and behavioral responses as much as the patient's cultural background. The nurse must realize that the patient's responses are very effective methods of communicating with members of her or his culture who may disapprove if she or he fails to respond according to their traditions.

Second, the difference between groups indicates why members of one cultural group often have difficulty understanding the attitudes and responses of members of another. Typically, the Old American is annoyed with the expressiveness of the Jew and the Italian. The Italian thinks it rather curious that the Jew and Old American are so concerned with the future. In turn, the Jew and Old American believe the Italian's behavior is childish and immature. The Italian and Jew think the Old American is rather coldblooded and selfish in not communicating his pain experience. *Each considers his own attitudes and behavior the correct ones*. The nurse must know that the patient responds in a certain way because he has been taught that this is correct and normal. If she considers that the expectations of her own culture are the only correct and normal ones, she may be prone to make the errors cited by Zborowski (1969). He found that patients with expressive and emotional responses to pain were labeled "mental cases" and sometimes were transferred to psychiatric wards. The nurse from the Old American culture should realize that if she or he were hospitalized in Italy, failure to express pain emotionally might result in being labeled masochistic.

Third, and most importantly, this survey of some cultural expectations regarding pain points out several questions the nurse must ask about her patients. Since similar responses to pain do not necessarily reflect similar attitudes toward it, and since many variations may exist between and within cultural groups, answers to these questions are very pertinent.

Is the patient concerned about the pain sensation itself or about the future implications of the pain? Is he afraid the pain indicates fatal illness, or is he afraid the pain does or will deprive him of some specific pleasures of life? Does the patient want to be asked about his pain, or would he rather not be reminded of it? Does he want to be alone for fear of showing an emotional response to pain, or does he want to be alone because he has methods of handling the pain by himself? Does he want visitors to share his pain or does he want to use them as a distraction? Does he expect to obtain pain relief immediately or does he expect he should suffer for a while? Does it matter to him whether he receives palliative or curative pain relief? Does he want to know his diagnosis or is he unconcerned or afraid of it? Does he believe drugs are unnatural pain-relief measures or does he fear the consequences of taking addictive drugs? Does he have confidence in the health care team or is he distrustful of their actions or skeptical of their skill? Does his crying mean he wants immediate pain relief, sympathy, or demonstration of technical skill? Does he view his expressions of pain as natural, serving a particular purpose, or indicative of defeat?

As you shall see as we proceed in subsequent chapters, there is such interplay of the previously mentioned sensory and cultural factors with the upcoming psychological and other factors that potentially influence communication of the pain experience that we incorporate considerations of one's culture as part of the broader topic of Communication of Pain presented in Chapter 9.

In the next chapter, we discuss preexisting psychological factors which influence the patient's pain experience.

REFERENCES

Aging and illness: It's a myth that they always go together–Growing Old: Part I. Los Angeles Times, Feb. 7, 1982, pp. 2: 18.

Armitage, K.J., Schneiderman, L.J., & Bass, R.A. Responses of physicians to medical complaints in men and women. J Amer Med Assoc 241 (20): pp. 2186–2187, 1979.

Baron, R.A. Aggression as a function of victim's pain cues, level of prior anger arousal, and exposure to an aggressive model. J Personal Soc Psychol 29: 117–124, 1974.

Bauwens, E. Medical beliefs and practices among lower-income Anglos. In E Spicer (Ed.), Ethnic Medicine in the Southwest. Tucson: Univ. Arizona Press, 1977, pp. 241–270.

Berkow, R. (Ed.) The Merck Manual of Diagnosis and Therapy, 13th ed. Rahway, New Jersey: Merck Sharp & Dohme Research Laboratories, 1977.

Billingsley, A. Black Families in White America. Englewood Cliffs, NJ: Prentice Hall, 1968.

Brink, P. (Ed.), Transcultural Nursing. Englewood Cliffs, NJ: Prentice-Hall, 1976.

Butler, R.N., & Gastell, B. Care of the aged: Perspectives on pain and discomfort. In L.K.Y. Ng, & J.J. Bonica (Eds.), Pain, Discomfort and Humanitarian Care. Proceedings of the National Conference Held at the National Institutes of Health, Bethesda, MD, Feb. 15–16, 1979. New York: Elsevier/North-Holland, 1980, pp. 297–311.

Capperauld, I. Acupuncture anesthesia and medicine in China today. Surg Gynecol Obstet 135: 440–445, 1972.

Castro, E.M. The Mexican American. How his culture effects his mental health. In R.A. Martinez (Ed.), Hispanic Culture and Health Care. St. Louis: C.V. Mosby, 1978, pp. 19–32.

Chan, C.W., & Chang, J.K. The role of Chinese medicine in New York City's Chinatown. Amer J Chin Med 4: 31–45; 129–146, 1976.

Chapman, W.P. Measurement of pain sensitivity in normal control subjects and in psychoneurotic subjects. Psychosom Med 6: 252–257, 1944.

Chapman, W.P., & Jones, C.M. Variations in cutaneous and visceral pain sensitivity in normal subjects. J Clin Invest 23: 81–91, 1944.

Chaitow, L. The Acupuncture Treatment of Pain. New York: Arco, 1977.

Clark, M. Health in the Mexican-American Culture. Berkeley: University of California Press, 1959.

Clark, W.C., & Mehl, L. Thermal pain: A sensory decision analysis of the effects of age and sex on d' various response criteria and 50 per cent pain threshold. J Abnorm Psychol 78: 202–212, 1971.

Craig, K.D., & Neidermayer, H. Autonomic correlates of pain thresholds influenced by social modeling. J Personal Soc Psychol 29: 246–252, 1974.

Craig, K.D., & Prkachin, K.M. Social modelling influences on sensory decision theory and psychophysiological indexes of pain. J Personal Soc Psychol 36(18): 805–815, 1978.

Diller, A. Cross-cultural pain semantics. Pain 9: 9–26, 1980.

Dunn, A.F. Aging and Illness: It's a Myth That They Always Go Together, Growing Old: Part I. Los Angeles: Los Angeles Times, Part VII, View 2: 18. Feb. 7, 1982.

Fabrega, H., Jr., & Tyma, S. Culture, language and the shaping of illness: An illustration based on pain. J Psychosom Res 20: 323–337, 1976.

Fink, B.R. (Moderator). Floor discussion, chronic pain behavior. In J.J. Bonica (Ed.), Advances in Neurology, Vol. 4. New York: Raven Press, 1974, pp. 431–432.

Flannery, R.B., Sos, J., & McGovern, P. Ethnicity as a factor in the expression of pain. Psychosomatics 22(1): 39–40; 45: 49–50, 1981.

Frank, J. Persuasion and Healing. Baltimore: Johns Hopkins Press, 1961.

Friedman, M. Family Nursing, Theory and Assessment. New York: Appleton-Century-Crofts, 1981.

Freidman, M.M. Personal Communication. November 1, 1982.

Gitelson, J.S. Personal Communication. February 10, 1981.

Gould-Martin, K., & Ngin, C. Chinese Americans. In A. Harwood (Ed.), Ethnicity and Medical Care. Cambridge, MA: Harvard University Press, 1981, pp. 143–171.

Grey, A. Relationship between social status and psychological characteristics of psychiatric patients. Unpublished doctoral dissertation, University of Chicago, 1949.

Harkins, S.W., & Chapman, C.R. Age and sex differences in pain perception. In D.J. Anderson & B. Matthews (Eds.), Pain in the Trigeminal Region. New York: Elsevier/North-Holland, 1977, pp. 435–441.

Harwood, A. Introduction. In A. Harwood (Ed.), Ethnicity and Medical Care. Cambridge, MA: Harvard University Press, 1981, pp. 1–36; Guidelines for culturally appropriate health care. pp. 412–507.

Haslam, D.R. Age and the perception of pain. Psychonomic Sci 15: 86, 1969.

Hautman, M.A., & Harrison, J.K. Health beliefs and practices in a middle-income Anglo-American neighborhood. In P.L. Chinn (Ed.), Advances in Nursing Science—Nursing and Culture 4(3): 49–64, 1982.

Henry, B.M., & DiGiacomo-Geffers, E. The hospitalized rich and famous. Amer J Nurs 80: 1426–1429, 1980.

Hernandez, C.A., Haug, M.J., & Wayner, D.N. Chicanos: Social and psychological perspectives. St. Louis: C.V. Mosby, 1971.

Hessler, R.M., Nolan, M.F., Ogbu, B., & Kong-Ming New, P. Intraethnic diversity: Health care of the Chinese-Americans. Human Org 34: 253–262, 1975.

Jackson, J. Urban black Americans. In A. Harwood (Ed.), *Ethnicity and Medical Care.* Cambridge, MA: Harvard University Press, 1981, pp. 73–129.

Jackson, O.J., & Nixon, W. Medicine in the black community. Calif Med, West J Med 116: 57–61, 1970.

Jacox, A.K. Sociocultural and psychological aspects of pain. In A.K. Jacox (Ed.), Pain:

A Source Book for Nurses and Other Health Professionals. Boston: Little, Brown, 1977, pp. 55–82.
Johnston, M. Folk beliefs and ethnocultural behavior in pediatrics. Nurs Clin North Amer, 1977, pp. 77–84.
Kaiko, R.F. Age and morphine analgesia in cancer patients with postoperative pain. Clin Pharmacol Rev 28: 823–826, 1980.
Kalish, R.A., & Reynolds, D.K. Death and Ethnicity: A Psycho-Cultural Study. Los Angeles: Ethel Percy Andrus Gerontology Center/University of Southern California Press, 1976.
Katz, E.R. Distress behavior in children with leukemia undergoing medical procedures. Paper presented at the Annual Meeting of the American Psychological Association Symposium: Psychological Strategies in the Management of Children with Life-threatening Illness, New York City, Sept. 1979.
Katz, R.L., Kao, C.Y., Spiegel, H., & Katz, G.J. Pain, acupuncture, hypnosis. In J.J. Bonica (Ed.), Advances in Neurology, Vol. 4. New York: Raven Press, 1974, pp. 819–825.
Kiev, A. Curanderismo. New York: Free Press, 1968.
Klein, N. Health belief systems. In N. Klein (Ed.), Wake up and die right: Death in the age of feeling. Novato, CA: Chandler & Sharp, 1979, pp. 35–42.
Klein, N. Health belief systems. In N. Klein (Ed.), Culture, curers, and contagion. Novato, CA: Chandler & Sharp, 1979, pp. 205–208.
Koo, L. C-L. Nourishment of Life—The Culture of Health in Traditional China. Unpublished doctoral dissertation, Anthropology Department, University of California, Berkeley, 1976.
Koos, E.L. The Health of Regionville. New York: Columbia University Press, 1954.
Krebs, D.L. Empathy and altruism. J Personal Soc Psychol 32(6): 1134–1146, 1975.
Lambert, W.E., Libman, E., & Poser, G. The effect of increased salience of a membership group on pain tolerance. J Personal 38: 350–357, 1960.
Larkins, F.R. The influence of one patient's culture on pain response. Nurs Clin North Amer 4(12): 663–668, 1977.
Leo, J. Coverstories, The New Scarlet Letter. Time, August 2, 1982, pp. 62–66.
Lewis, G. The place of pain in human experience. J Med Ethics 3: 122–125, 1978.
Litman, T.J. The family as a basic unit in health and medical care—A social behavior overview. Soc Sci Med 8: 502, 1974.
Louie, T. T-T. C. The Pragmatic Context: A Chinese-American Example of Defining-Managing Illness. Unpublished doctoral dissertation, School of Nursing, University of California at San Francisco, 1975.
Lyght, C.F. (Ed.) The Merck Manual of Diagnosis and Therapy, 10th ed. Rahway, New Jersey: Merck Sharp & Dohme Research Laboratories, 1961.
Martinez, C., & Martin, H.W. Folk diseases among urban Mexican Americans: Etiology, symptoms, and treatment. In N. Klein (Ed.), Culture, cures and contagion. Novato, CA: Chandler & Sharp, 1979, pp. 188–194.
Mayerson, B. Personal Communication, May 14, 1982.
McCabe, G.S. Cultural influences on patient behavior. Amer J Nurs 60: 1101–1104, 1960.
McCaffery, M. Brief episodes of pain in children. In B.S. Bergensen, E.H. Anderson,

et al. (Eds.), Current Concepts in Clinical Nursing, Vol. 2. St. Louis: C.V. Mosby, 1969, pp. 178–191.

Mechanic, D. Illness and care. In J. Kosa, A. Antonovsky, & I. Zola (Eds.), Poverty and Health: A Sociological Analysis. Cambridge, MA: Harvard University Press, 1969.

Merskey, H. Pain and personality. In R.A. Sternbach (Ed.), The Psychology of Pain. New York: Raven Press, 1978, pp. 111–127.

Merskey, H., & Spear, F.G. The reliability of the pressure algometer. Brit J Soc Clin Psychol 3: 130–136, 1964.

Merskey, H., & Spear, F.G. Pain: Psychological and Psychiatric Aspects. London: Bailliere, Tindall and Cassell, 1967.

Murillo, N. The Mexican American family. In C.A. Hernandez, M.J. Haug, & N.N. Wayner (Eds.), Chicanos: Social and Psychological Perspectives. St. Louis: C.V. Mosby, 1971, pp. 97–108.

Nathanson, C. Illness and the feminine role: A theoretical review. Soc Sci Med 9: 57–62, 1975.

Nolen, W.A. How doctors are unfair to women. In N. Klein (Ed.), Culture, Curers, and Contagion. Novato, CA: Chandler & Sharp, 1979, pp. 201–204.

Notermans, S.L.H., & Tophoff, M.M.W.A. Sex differences in pain tolerance and pain appreciation. Psych Neurol Neurochir 70: 23–29, 1967.

Opler, M.K. Ethnic differences in behavior and health practices. In I. Galdson (Ed.), The Family: A Focal Point for Health Education. New York: New York Academy of Medicine, 1961.

Pain differences, similarities found. Science News, September 20, 1980, pp. 182–183.

Payne, T.D. Behavioral Responses of Japanese Patients to Illness, Birth, Accidents, Surgery, and Death. Unpublished Master's thesis, Health and Safety Studies, California State College, Los Angeles, 1970.

Paz, O. The sons of La Malenche. In L.I. Duran & H.R. Bernard (Eds.), Introduction to Chicano Studies. New York: Macmillan, 1973, p. 24.

Pilowsky, I., & Bond, M.R. Pain and its management. Psychosom Med 31: 400–404, 1969.

Poser, E.G. Some Psychosocial Determinants of Pain Tolerance. Paper presented at the XVI International Congress of Psychology, Washington, D.C., 1963.

Pozanski, E.O. Children's reactions to pain: A psychiatrist's perspective. Clin Pediatr 15: 1114–1119, 1976.

Redlich, F.C., Hollingshead, A.B., & Bellis, E. Social class differences in attitudes toward psychiatry. Amer J Orthopsych 25: 60–70, 1955.

Richards, J.S., Meredith, R.L., Nepomuceno, C., et al.: Psycho-social aspects of chronic pain in spinal cord injury. Pain 8: 355–366, 1980.

Ring, S.I., & Schein, L. Attitudes toward mental illness and the use of caretakers in a Black community. Amer J Orthopsych 40: 710–716, 1970.

Rocereto, L.R. Root work and the root doctor. Nurs Forum 12: 415–426, 1973.

Rubel, A.J. Concepts of disease in Mexican-American culture. Amer Anthropol 62: 795–814, 1960.

Rubel, A.J. The epidemic of a folk illness: Susto in Hispanic America. Ethnol 3: 268–283, 1964.

Rubel, A.J. Across the Tracks: Mexican Americans in a Texas City. Austin: University of Texas Press, 1966.

Satcher, D. Does race interfere with the doctor-patient relationship? J Amer Med Assoc 223: 1498-1499, 1973.

Schluderman, E., & Zubek, J.P. Effect of age on pain sensitivity. Perceptual Motor Skills 14: 295-301, 1962.

Schreiber, J.M., Homiak, J.P. Mexican Americans. In A. Harwood (Ed.), Ethnicity and Medical Care, Cambridge, MA: Harvard University Press, 1981, pp. 264-336.

Schulman, S., & Smith, A.M. The concept of "health" among Spanish-speaking villagers of New Mexico and Colorado. J Health Human Behav. 4: 226-234, 1963.

Schultz, N.V. How children perceive pain. Nurs Outlook 19: 670-673, 1971.

Scrimshaw, S.C., & Burleigh, E. The potential for the integration of indigenous and Western medicines in Latin America and Hispanic populations in the United States of America. In B. Velimirovic (Ed.), Modern Medicine and Medical Anthropology in the United States—Mexican Border Population. Pan American Health Organization Scientific Publication, no. 359, 1978.

Selye, H. The Stress of Life. New York: McGraw-Hill, 1956.

Simmons, O.G. Implications of social class for public health. In N. Klein (Ed.), Culture, Curers and Contagion. Novato, CA: Chandler & Sharp, 1979, pp. 99-107.

Snell, J.E. Hypnosis in the treatment of the "hexed" patient. Amer J Psychiatr 124: 311-316, 1967.

Snow, L.F. "High Blood" is not high blood pressure. Urban Health 5: 54-55, 1976.

Snow, L.F. Sorcerers, saints and charlatans: Black folk healers in urban American. Culture, Med Psychiatr, 2: 69-106, 1978.

Snow, L.F. Voodoo illness in the black population. In N. Klein (Ed.), Culture, Cures and Contagion. Novato, CA: Chandler & Sharp, 1979, pp. 179-184.

Spector, R.E. Cultural Diversity in Health and Illness. New York: Appleton-Century-Crofts, 1979.

Spindler, G.D. Volksheilkunde. In N. Klein (Ed.), Culture, Cures and Contagion. Novato, CA: Chandler & Sharp, 1979, pp. 218-229.

Sternbach, R.A. Pain Patients: Traits and Treatments. New York: Academic Press, 1974.

Sternbach, R.A. Clinical aspects of pain. In R.A. Sternbach (Ed.), The Psychology of Pain. New York: Raven Press, 1978, pp. 241-264.

Sternbach, R.A., & Tursky, B. Ethnic differences among housewives in psychophysical and skin potential responses to electric shock. Psychophysiology 1: 241-246, 1965.

Swafford, L.I., & Allan, D. Pain relief in the pediatric patient. Med Clin North Amer 52: 131-136, 1968.

Teish, L. That nigger's crazy. In N.K. Klein (Ed.), Culture, Curers, and Contagion. Novato, CA: Chandler & Sharp, 1979.

Terenius, L. Endorphins and pain. In L.H. Rees & T.B. van Wimersma Greidanus (Eds.), Frontiers of Hormone Research 8: 162-177, 1981.

UCLA Asian Health Team (Choi, P., Kawaoka, K., Kitashima, B., Matsushima, B.). Asian Americans and Health Care in Los Angeles County. Los Angeles: UCLA School of Public Health, 1975. (Mimeographed.)

U.S. Bureau of the Census. Washington, D.C.: U.S. Government Printing Office, 1978.

Uzzel, D. Susto revisited: Illness as a strategic role. Amer Ethnol 1: 369–378, 1974.

Wall, P.D. Acupuncture revisited. New Scientist 3: 31–34, 1974.

Wallnöfer, H., & von Rottauscher, A. Chinese Folk Medicine (M. Palmedo, Trans.). New York: American Library, 1972.

Weaver, T. Use of hypothetical situations in a study of Spanish American illness referral systems. Human Org (Summer): 140–154, 1970.

Webster's Seventh New Collegiate Dictionary. Springfield, MA: G & C Merriam Co., 1963.

White, E.H. Giving health care to minority patients. Nurs Clin North Amer 12: 27–40, 1977.

Williams, L., Lord, M. Blacks: Fresh trials. Newsweek, May 15, 1978, p. 77.

Winsberg, B., & Greenlick, M. Pain responses in negro and white obstetrical patients. J Health Soc Behav 8: 222–227, 1967.

Wolff, B.C. (Rapporteur) et al. Evolution of expression of pain (acute and chronic). Group report. In H.W. Kosterlitz & L.Y. Terenius (Eds.), Pain and Society. Report of the Dahlem Workshop on Pain and Society, Berlin, Nov. 26–30, 1978. Weinheim: Verlag Chemie, 1980, pp. 81–92.

Wolff, B.B., & Langley, S. Cultural factors and the response to pain: A review. Amer Anthropol 70: 494–501, 1968.

Wolff, B.B., & Langley, S. Cultural factors and the response to pain. In D. Landy (Ed.), Culture, Disease and Healing. New York: Macmillan, 1979, pp. 313–319.

Woodrow, K.M., Freidman, G.D. & Siegelaub, M.S. Pain tolerance: Differences according to age, sex and race. Psychosom Med, 34(6): 548–556, 1972.

Yankelovitch, Skelley, & White, Inc.: The American Family Report: A Study of the American Family and Money. Minneapolis, MN.: General Mills, Corp., 1975.

Zborowski, M. Cultural components in responses to pain. J Soc Issues 8: 16–30, 1952.

Zborowski, M. People in Pain. San Francisco: Jossey-Bass, 1969.

Zola, I.K. Culture and symptoms: An analysis of patients presenting complaints. Amer Sociol Rev 31: 615–630, 1966.

SUGGESTED READINGS

Abril, I. Mexican American folk beliefs that effect health care. Arizona Nurse 28: 14–20, 1975.

Ashmore, R.D. (Ed.) Black and white in the 1970's. J Soc Issues 32: No. 2, 1976.

Bace, J.E. Some health beliefs of Spanish-speaking people. Amer J Nurs 69: 2172–2176, 1969.

Beecher, H.K. Relationship of significance of wound to pain experienced. J Amer Med Assoc 161: 1609–1613, 1956.

Berkanovic, E., & Reeder, L.G. Ethnic, economic, and social psychological factors in the source of medical care. Social Problems 21: 246–259, 1973.

Brown, E.L. Newer Dimensions of Patient Care, Part 3: Patients as People. New York: Russell Sage Foundation, 1964.

Bullough, B., & Bullough, V. Poverty, Ethnic Identity and Health Care. New York: Appleton Century Crofts, 1972.

Campbell, T., & Chang, B. Health care of the Chinese in America. Nurs Outlook 21: 245–249, 1973.

Chung, H.J. Understanding the Oriental maternity patient. Nurs Clin North Amer 12: 67–75, 1977.

Cohen, F.L. Postsurgical pain relief: Patients' status and nurses' medication choices. Pain, 1980, 9: 265–274.

Craig, K.D. Social modeling influences on pain. In R.A. Sternbach (Ed.), The Psychology of Pain. New York: Raven Press, 1978, pp. 73–109.

Craig, K.D. Ontogenetic and cultural influence on the expression of pain in man. In H.W. Kosterlitz & L.Y. Terenius (Eds.), Pain and Society. Report of the Dahlem Workshop on Pain and Society, Berlin, Nov. 26–30, 1979. Weinheim: Verlag Chemie, 1980, pp. 37–52.

Elesh, D. & Schollaert, P.T. Race and Urban Medicine: Factors Affecting the Distribution of Physicians in Chicago. Journal of Health and Social Behavior, 1972, 13, 236–249.

Fabrega, H., Jr. On the specificity of folk illness. Southwest J Anthropol 29: 305–314, 1970.

Griffin, J.H. Black Like Me. Boston: Houghton Mifflin, 1960.

Grinker, R.R. The poor, rich: The children of the superrich. Amer J Psychiatr, *135*: 913–916, 1978.

Guttmacher, S., & Elinson, J. Ethno-religious variation in perceptions of illness: The use of illness as an explanation for deviant behavior. Soc Sci Med 5: 117–125, 1971.

Haley, A. Roots. New York: Doubleday, 1976.

Hess, G. Racial tensions: Barriers in delivery of nursing care. J Nurs Admin 5: 47–49, 1972.

Hiestand, W.C. Nursing, the family, and the "new" social history. In P.L. Chinn (Ed.), Advances in Nursing Science—Nursing and Culture 8(3): Apr.: 1–12, 1982.

Hollingsworth, A.O., Brown, L.P., & Brooten, D.A. The refugees and childbearing: What to expect. RN, Nov.: 45–48, 1980.

Hoppe, S.K., & Heller, P.L. Alienation, familism and the utilization of health services by Mexican Americans. J Health Soc Behav 16: 304–314, 1975.

Houston, S. Black English. Psychol Today, March, pp. 45–48, 1973.

Hughes, L., & Bontemps, A. The Book of Negro Folklore. New York: Dodd, Mead, 1958.

Jacques, G. Cultural health traditions: A black perspective. In M. Branch & P.P. Paxton (Eds.), Providing Safe Nursing Care for Ethnic People of Color. New York: Appleton-Century Crofts, 1976.

Johnson, F., Cloyd, C., & Wer, J.A. Life satisfaction of poor urban black aged. In P.L. Chinn (Ed.), Advances in Nursing Science—Nursing and Culture 8(3) Apr.: 27–31, 1982.

Kitano, H. Japanese Americans. Englewood Cliffs, NJ: Prentice-Hall, 1969.

Knief-Hardy, M., & Burkhardt, M.A. Nursing the Navajo. Amer J Nurs 77: 95–96, 1977.

Kosterlitz, H.W., & Terenius, L.Y. (Eds.), Pain and Society. Report of the Dahlem Workshop on Pain in Society, Berlin, Nov. 26–30, 1979. Weinheim: Verlag Chemie, 1980.

Kubricht, E.W., & Clark, J.A. Foreign patients: A system for providing care. Nurs Outlook, 30: 55–57, 1982.

La Barre, W. Cultural basis of emotions and gestures. J Personal 16: 49–68, 1947.

Landy, D. (Ed.). Culture, Disease and Healing. Studies in Medical Anthropology. New York: Macmillan, 1977.

Lauranne, S. Blacks and Health Care: Spanning the Life Cycle. Presented at the New England Regional Black Nurses' Association, Inc. Meeting, Statler Hilton Hotel, Boston, MA, May 20, 1977.

Leninger, M. Nursing and Anthropology: Two Worlds to Blend. New York: John Wiley & Sons, 1970.

Leninger, M. Transcultural Nursing. New York: Masson International Nursing Publ, 1979.

Leninger, M. (Ed.). Transcultural Nursing: Concepts, Theories, and Practices. New York: John Wiley & Sons, 1978.

Li, F.P., Schlief, N.Y., Chang, C.J., & Gaw, A.G. Health care for the Chinese community in Boston. Amer J Public Health 62: 536–539, 1972.

McCaffery, M. & Hart, L.L. Undertreatment of acute pain with narcotics. American Journal of Nusing, 1976, 76: 1586–1591.

McLemore, S.D. Ethnic attitudes toward hospitalization. Southwest Soc Sci Q 43: 341, 1963.

McMahon, M.A., & Miller, P., Sr. Pain response: The influence of psycho-social-cultural factors. Nurs Forum, 17: 58–71, 1978.

Morse, J.M. Descriptive analysis of cultural coping mechanisms utilized for the reduction of parturition pain and anxiety in Fiji. (Unpublished abstract.) In P.L. Chinn (Ed.), Advances in Nursing Sciences—Nursing and Culture, *8*(3), Apr.: 65–66, 1982.

NIH: Pain in the elderly—Patterns change with age. J Amer Med Assoc 241: 2491–2492, 1979.

O'Brien, M.E. Pragmatic survivalism: Behavior patterns affecting low-level wellness among minority group members. In P.L. Chinn (Ed.), Advances in Nursing Science—Nursing and Culture, 8(3), Apr.: 13–26, 1982.

Padilla, E. Up from Puerto Rico. New York: Columbia University Press, 1958.

Palos, S. The Chinese Art of Healing. New York: Herter & Herter, 1971.

Peterson, W. Japanese Americans. New York: Random House, 1971.

Petrello, J. Your patients hear you, but do they understand? RN Feb.: 37–39, 1976.

Pilowsky, I. Abnormal illness behavior and sociocultural aspects of pain. In H.W. Kosterlitz & L.Y. Terenius (Eds.), Pain and Society, Report of the Dahlem Workshops on Pain and Society, Berlin, Nov. 26–30, 1979. Weinheim: Verlag Chemie, 1980, pp. 445–459.

Powers, B.A. The use of orthodox and black American folk medicine. In P.L. Chinn (Ed.), Advances in Nursing Science—Nursing and Culture, 8(3): Apr.: 35–47, 1982.

Rand, C. The Puerto Ricans. New York: Oxford University Press, 1958.

Santopietro, M-C.S. How to get through to a refugee patient. RN 44, Jan.: 42–48, 1981.

Scott, R. It hurts red. A preliminary study of children's perception of pain. Perceptual Motor Skills 47(3, Pt. 1): 787–791, 1978.

Shubin, S. Nursing patients from different cultures. Nurs 80, June: 79–81, 1980.

Simmen, E. (Ed.). Pain and Promise: The Chicano Today. New York: New American Library, 1972.
Skipper, J.K., & Leonard, R.C. Social Interaction and Patient Care. Philadelphia: J.B. Lippincott, 1965.
Smith, H. The Religions of Man. New York: Harper, 1958.
Snow, L.F. Folk medical beliefs and their implications for care of patients. Ann Intern Med 81: 82–96, 1974.
Spear, F.G. Cultural factors in clinical pain assessment. Int Dental J 27: 284–287, 1977.
Stringfellow, L. The Vietnamese. In A.L. Clark (Ed.), Culture, Childbearing, Health Professionals. Philadelphia: F.A. Davis, 1978.
Sue, S., & Wagner, N. Asian Americans: Psychological Perspectives. Palo Alto, CA: Science and Behavioral Books, 1973.
Szasz, T.S. The myth of mental illness. Amer Psychologist 15: 113–118, 1960.
Tao-Kim-Kim, A.M. Orientals are stoic. In J.K. Skipper, Jr., & R.C. Leonard (Eds.), Social Interaction and Patient Care. Philadelphia: J.B. Lippincott, 1965, pp. 143–153.
Tu, W. A religiophilosophical perspective on pain. In H.W. Kosterlitz & L.Y. Terenius (Eds.), Pain and Society. Report of the Dahlem Workshop on Pain and Society, Berlin, Nov. 26–30, 1979. Weinheim: Verlag Chemie, 1980, pp. 63–77.
Weaver, J.L. Mexican American health care behavior: A critical review of the literature. Soc Sci Q 54: 85–102, 1973.
Welch, S., Comer, J., & Steinman, M. Some social and attitudinal correlates of health care among Mexican Americans. J Health Soc Behav 14: 205–213, 1975.
Wintrub, R. The influence of others: Witchcraft and rootwork as explanations of behavioral disturbances. J Nerv Mental Dis 156: 318–326, 1973.

4

Preexisting Psychological Factors

A mass of literature deals with the mental processes and emotional states associated with pain (e.g., Barber, 1959; Beecher, 1959; Bonica, 1976; Craig, 1978; Crue, 1975; Jacox, 1977; Jacox & Stewart, 1973; Merskey, 1978; Merskey & Spear, 1967; Pilowsky, 1978; Sternbach, 1968; 1974. The results of both research and clinical observations are not only inconclusive, but in some cases contradictory. A review of this material is instructive and interesting, especially for the researcher. However, the emphasis here is on clinical practice.

In practice, we see that patients respond to pain differently, and what is painful for one patient may not be regarded as painful by another patient. Trying to muster a feeling of acceptance for all these different patients can be rather difficult. Knowledge is helpful. Already we have seen that some of these differences in patients can be understood by realizing that people are raised in different environments or cultures. Expectations with regard to pain may differ greatly from one cultural group to another. However, there are considerable differences among people raised in the same general culture. In this chapter, we will discuss preexisting psychological factors in relation to the pain experience, that is, certain characteristics of the person that may help explain the wide variation of responses to the pain experience.

PAIN SYNDROMES

Psychogenic Pain

Since pain often has such an obvious emotional impact on the patient, practitioners often wonder whether or not the patient's emotional state actually causes the sensation of pain. As discussed here, the significance of some of the psychological aspects of pain to nursing practice is summarized in Figure 4.1. The mind and the body cannot be separated. Efforts to do so have led to much confusion with respect to pain. Yet in clinical practice, the

All pain is real regardless of its cause

"Pure" psychogenic pain is rare

mental events alone (e.g., anxiety) → bodily change without physical change

"Pure" organic pain does not exist:

diagrammed as:

physical stimuli alone (e.g., burn, cut) → bodily pain without emotional or cognitive response

Most bodily pain is a combination of factors:

diagrammed as:

mental events + physical stimuli → bodily pain

Figure 4.1. Significance of the psychological aspects of pain for nursing practice.

application of knowledge in these areas often culminates with the question, Is the patient's pain *psychogenic* or is it *somatogenic*?

Consistent with information about the interrelationship of neurophysiological and cultural factors in previous chapters, Davis et al. (1980, p. 228) say that the dichotomy between psychogenic and somatogenic pain is an artificial one because "all perceptual experience has a physiological basis and all physiological stresses have psychological effects." Their point of view is shared and extended by Melzack & Dennis (1978, p. 1) regarding the relationship of mind and body to pain perception. First, "it is now recognized that every physiological explanation of pain contains an implicit psychological concept that has a profound impact on both the study and treatment of pain." Secondly, "it is essential to remember that stimulation of receptors does not mark the beginning of the pain process. Rather, stimulation produces neural signals that enter an active nervous system which even in the young child is already the substrate of past experience, culture, anxiety, and so forth." When the dichotomy is made, *somatogenic pain* usually is defined more in physical terms referring to physiological processes involving the somatosensory system. *Psychogenic pain*, on the other hand, usually implies that the pain originated in the mind, that is, it is a somatic delusion.

Why then does the differentiation of psychogenic versus somatogenic pain assume such importance? First and foremost, a diagnosis of psychogenic pain is often used against a patient. Associated with the diagnosis of psychogenic pain often are negative stereotypes incorporating such notions as "malingering," "hypochondriasis," and "hysteria," or even more pejorative, "demanding," "manipulative," or of the patient on medications, "clock watcher." Patients, health care professionals and significant others all get caught up in attempting to authenticate and legitimize the presence of the patient's pain. The more the patient attempts to convince others that he does have "that much pain," the more likely he may be to reinforce or increase their disbeliefs (Weiner, 1975). Proving the presence of pain is so problematic that physicians "continue to seek a procedure in laboratory tests that will differentiate between so-called organic and psychogenic pain. Some have called this the 'lie detector' approach to diagnosis" (Davis et al., 1980, p. 228).

Variations on this proposed terminology are the phrases *psychological overlay* and *functional overlay* used in conjunction with a diagnosis of organic or somatic pain. They simply mean that the patient's response to the identifiable or organic pathology involves intense mental processes such as worry or anxiety. Crue et al. (1979, p. 19), in discussing "functional overlay," say that the percentage may vary from 100 percent psychogenic to 100 percent organic in the same patient. Even in a chronic pain center where patients are often more carefully studied, they say they "may be occasionally fooled by a malingerer or sociopath, but faking is very rarely seen" (p. 20).

A second reason for clarifying the use of the terms psychogenic or somatogenic is that describing pain in psychological language, or labeling the pain psychogenic, tends to lead to many other misunderstandings. We seem to have a much better appreciation of somatogenic pain. Therefore, it is important to review those areas where Sternbach (1974) points out misconceptions frequently exist.

Psychogenic pain is not simply grief or some other unpleasant emotional experience. Neither is psychogenic pain "painless" or "imaginary." It is not necessarily experienced any differently than pain from obvious physical injury. *The location, severity and other qualities of psychogenic pain can be exactly like those of somatogenic pain.*

The idea that any pain can be *imaginary* is an interesting notion. Many patients say they have difficulty recalling the specific characteristics of pain once it is gone. To imagine what pain feels like is even more difficult. It is very easy to imagine the taste of a lemon, for example. The taste sensation exists in a few moments and salivation often occurs. But try experiencing the same degree of sensation by imagining that your finger is painfully burned. This usually is far more difficult.

Especially with respect to chronic pain, it is often presumed that the patient with psychogenic pain will differ psychologically from the patient with somatogenic pain. Of major interest is the finding that there are *no significant differences in psychological test scores* between patients with psychogenic pain and those with somatogenic pain. Anxious, complaining, and depressive mood are characteristic of both kinds of chronic pain patients (Sternbach, 1974). Thus, two seemingly different kinds of pain have remarkably similar outcomes.

A third reason that the differentiation is not helpful is that psychogenic pain usually does not represent a scientific diagnosis. Major authorities in the field of pain work are critical of the use of the diagnostic label "psychogenic pain." Davis et al. (1980, p. 228) view the diagnosis of psychogenic pain as a negative one—one based on *excluding* physical causes *rather than* one based on *positive evidence*. Crue et al. (1979, p. 18) concur. They say it is usually invoked as the explanation of a clinical pain syndrome when there is a dearth of objective physical findings to explain the situation in organic terms. In working with chronic pain patients their finding is in agreement with Freud and Breuer (1895) that even psychogenic pain processes started with a "genuine" organic process.

Even a tentative or presumed diagnosis or labeling of a patient's physiological problem often has merit because definitive diagnostic and treatment modalities can be fruitfully used in its resolution. With pain, however, labeling often scapegoats the patient and may reflect our lack of knowledge and our personal feelings of inadequacy in helping the patient with pain. This is illustrated by a woman with headaches that had begun twenty years before in childhood. They were rather clearly emotionally precipitated by increased physical activity or stress. As the years passed they became more frequent and severe. During that time her physician referred her to several specialists, including an internist and a psychiatrist. The consensus was that she worried too much. Worrying seemed to precipitate the headaches so her problem was described in psychological language and the pain was considered psychogenic. Eventually she was seen by a neurologist who discovered a rare type of highly vascular brain tumor. This tumor had grown to the point of being life threatening. After a procedure that destroyed the tumor by occluding the blood supply, the patient was pain free. Thus, after twenty years, the patient's pain was described in physical terms and considered somatogenic.

One other point on the discussion of psychogenic pain: there is no *personality type* that automatically results in psychogenic pain. "Pure" psychogenic pain is best understood as a state or condition that may occur in a variety of personalities, perhaps more frequently in some.

Characteristics associated with the patient who has received a diagnosis of psychogenic pain include an unconcerned attitude although the patient may have requested an appointment with urgency or presented at an emergency room. Also, in discussing his pain the patient may report it in an inconsistent manner, with many contradictions; the primary pain complaint and the secondary symptoms being vaguely defined in relation to location, onset, and other characteristics.

It is felt that the primary cause of these pains is due to muscle tension or an excessive preoccupation with one's body. Although the patient usually does not appear ill, he or she *does* appear to be suffering. Often pain offers a way for the individual to obtain help for a problem which may be unrelated. When these syndromes occur in adolescents, factors repeatedly identified include "the death of a parent, separation from significant others, marital discord between parents, family pathology, similar complaints of pain in parents or siblings, [and] difficulties in school (either academic or with teachers or peers)" (Caghan et al., 1978, p. 20).

Hysterical Pain

Hysterical neuroses, or *conversion hysterias*, are *states* in which there is an involuntary psychogenic loss or disturbance of body function. *Hysterical pain* may occur in relation to such a state. The state results from unconscious emotional conflicts that have their origins in the past. However, the state may be precipitated by a recent emotionally charged event. Pain is only one of the symptoms that may occur. Literally, any physiologically based symptom may present as a hysterical one including blindness or paralysis (Mastrovito, 1974; Pinsky, 1979).

A hypothetical situation illustrates how hysterical pain may occur. An event may cause a person to feel impelled to do something they have always wanted to do but felt they should not. Pain is used to repress the desires for which guilt is felt. An adult male may harbor strong but conflicting love and aggression toward his father since early childhood. He suddenly develops severe pain in his arm during an argument with his father, because he wishes to strike his father. The pain allows him to repress this conflict; it prevents him from yielding to the desire to hit his father and also punishes him for the temptation to do so. Such a mechanism is entirely unconscious and the patient is aware only of the resulting pain.

Hysterical neurosis often is confused with hysterical personality and further misunderstood because of the layman's usage of the word "hysterical." The *hysterical personality* is a lifelong character structure, a particular pattern of personality organization. It is not a state, as is hysterical neurosis, and it may not result in hysterical neurosis. When the layman describes a person as hysterical, it usually means that the person is in a state of being very upset, is expressing his feelings dramatically, and without exercising much self-control. This may be quite unlike the behavior of a patient with hysterical pain.

Traditionally, patients with *hysterical pain* appear calm and relatively unconcerned about their pain. They also have less anxiety and depression but more *hypochondriasis* (Pilling et al., 1967) and a tendency to seek multiple surgical procedures (Spear, 1967). Merskey (1978, p. 115) says that these features combined with persistence of intractable complaints in spite of a variety of treatments "are parts of the stereotype nowadays of the chronic pain clinic patient with or without a physical basis for the illness." Thus, three entities—hysterical behavior described by the layman, hysterical neurosis, and hysterical personality—are very different but often are confused. Walters (1961) studied 430 patients with intractable pain, many of whom had hysterical conversion symptoms. His belief was that although the conversion mechanism definitely contributed to the pain it was neither the only nor usually the principal cause for the inception of the pain.

Hypochondriacal Pain

As a state, *hypochondriacal pain* is somewhat more difficult to discuss. The literature does not seem to differentiate it clearly from hysterical pain, depression, or the personality trait of hypochondriasis (Merskey, 1968; Mastrovito, 1974; Pilowsky, 1978; Pinsky, 1979). Again, the picture is complicated by the layman's loose usage of the term "hypochondriac."

Apparently, hypochondriacal pain may be a form of "pure" psychogenic pain, that is, pain caused solely by mental events. An acceptable definition of hypochondriacal pain of this sort seems to be lacking. However, there is general agreement that the person with hypochondriacal neurosis is characterized as having a preoccupation with his body and a constant fear of disease and body malfunction. This intense focus on the body, often accompained by depression, may result in the sensation of pain (Mastrovito, 1974). Pilowsky (1978, p. 211) says that the patient with pain as a hypochondriacal symptom focuses a great deal on the pain and its origin but exhibits no marked anxiety or depression.

Hallucinated Pain

Hallucinated pain may occur in association either with schizophrenia or endogenous depression. It is relatively rare and most psychiatrists have seen only one or two instances of it in their careers. Occasionally pain is the only symptom, but usually the pain occurs along with other delusional experiences, such as the feeling that the body is changing in size (Merskey, 1968).

Munchausen and Couvade Syndromes

There are two other syndromes in which pain may be a part of the symptomatology: the Munchausen syndrome and the Couvade syndrome. The patient presenting with *Munchausen syndrome* wanders from hospital to hospital feigning very convincing, often dramatic, signs and symptoms and at times presents falsified documentation of diagnostic studies associated with serious acute illness. The patient can very convincingly replicate almost any illness or injury from acute myocardial infarction to idiopathic pyrexia or hematemesis. At times the individual may self-mutilate, including amputation of an extremity. The syndrome is not simple dishonesty but represents a serious personality disorder and requires psychiatric treatment. Sale & Kalucy (1980, p. 61) suggest this syndrome may be due to the physician denying the patient the sick role. Because patients with Munchausen syndrome present themselves in acute care settings, often to the emergency room, pain may be one of the many symptoms requiring meticulous assessment (Berkow & Talbott 1977, p. 1491; Ireland et al, 1967).

The *Couvade syndrome* is a psychophysiologic syndrome occurring in the male partner of a pregnant female. The male may suffer from any of the symptoms accompanying pregnancy from conception to delivery. These include any of the pain syndromes from rib discomfort to labor pains (Trehowan & Conlan, 1965; Wilson, 1977).

In summary, we agree with Davis et al. (1980, p. 229) who "strongly recommend discarding formerly useful terms like 'psychogenic' because what is really meant is *cryptogenic*, or unknown." However, occasionally, a person's mental processes and emotions may be the only causes of a localized sensation of pain. In these instances, there are no physical findings to account for the origin or persistence of the pain and a diagnosis of psychogenic pain is made. In clinical practice, it is important to realize that if a patient receives such a diagnosis the pain is very real—the person is not lying about having pain. This pain is felt and it does hurt. This openess in approach is vital to deciding on and instituting appropriate therapy for the pain.

Guidelines have been recommended to assist in differentiating psychogenic pain from somatogenic pain or other types of pain from mental mechanisms (Brena, 1970; Hackett, 1976). However, it is more important when we see a patient with pain that we try to gain some understanding of what he is experiencing and why and to remember from a conceptual viewpoint that all pain has a physiological component. Even though physical stimuli for the pain may be absent in psychogenic pain, the emotional stimuli are present and recall that they are conveyed by physiological mechanisms to the level of consciousness or awareness along the nervous system. Therefore using both physical and psychological languages often will be the most profitable approach to pain assessment.

When it is suspected that a patient does have a pain problem resulting from mental processes, extreme respect and diplomacy must be consciously employed during the assessment process. Failure to approach the patient in such a manner may result in his or her feeling blamed for the pain problem, alienating him or her and having him or her abort an attempt to find a solution for the pain problem.

We must heed Mastrovito's (1974) caution that we do not become moralistic and disdainful in our conclusions about the patient with functional, idiopathic or psychogenic pain.

PERSONALITY CHARACTERISTICS

"Pure" organic pain, pain sensations that result only from physical stimuli, are as unlikely as *"pure" psychogenic pain*. As soon as pain occurs, and at times before, emotions such as anxiety, anger, or depression arise to influence the total pain experience. Pain changes a person in significant ways. Emotions and feelings that are more or less situational or "state," that is, closely related to the immediate circumstances surrounding the pain sensation, will be discussed with the effects of pain on the patient in Chapter 7.

Here attention is directed at those emotional and mental states that seem to be relatively stable and enduring within the person. They distinguish one person from another. These attributes are referred to as *personality*. Are there preexisting personality traits that influence the occurrence of pain? The expression of pain? Sensitivity to pain? Tolerance for pain? In general, the answer is yes.

Personality characteristics may be measured and labeled by a variety of psychological tests such as the Taylor Manifest Anxiety Scale, Eysenck Personality Inventory (EPI), and the Minnesota Multiphasic Personality Inventory (MMPI). In pain clinics, psychological testing of some form tends to be used. Sternbach (1978, p. 256) points out that although objective tests are used and are the best indicators of abnormality and quantify information so that it is more useful with various clinical populations "only the MMPI has a clinically useful profile with sizeable medical and psychiatric patient norms, and with each passing year it is becoming more outdated." His opinion is often verbalized by others in the field of dolorology. Unfortunately these objective tests provide information relative to character traits that is often used against the patient. Yet the information gleaned from a diagnostic interview is considered to be problematic also. Sternbach (p. 255) says that because patients are focused on their pain, they ascribe all associated difficulties to it often not acknowledging the anxiety or depression at all, insisting that when the pain is gone so will the other symptoms be. Even though the patient may be correct there is a distinct possibility that it may not be possible to eliminate the pain.

In general clinical practice, patients with pain rarely have psychological testing. The patient's preexisting personality usually is a guess made by the practitioner on the basis of the patient's present behavior, and random comments made by the patient and his family concerning his life before he had pain or became ill. Although this approach to personality assessment has limited validity, it may be somewhat useful by shedding light on why a patient responds to pain in a particular manner. At least it may be helpful in understanding and accepting the patient.

Some characteristics will be described here in a manner as easily recognizable. Emphasis will be placed on how a person with a certain personality trait may respond to pain. This is for the purpose of gaining a better appreciation of the basis for individual differences.

Algesic Types

One of the most interesting preexisting personality characteristics studied in relation to pain is perceptual style. It is possible that people exposed to the same stimuli differ greatly in their estimation of the intensity of that stimuli. *Algesic type* refers to a person's general tendency in perceiving the intensity of pain. Specifically, some people may perceive pain at lower levels of stimulation than others. Although this difference may be biologically determined rather than learned as was discussed in Chapter 2, it will be considered here as a personality characteristic because information in relation to it is most often found in the psychological literature.

One of the *perceptual responses* that has been correlated with pain responses is *magnitude estimation*. If an individual makes errors in the estimation of size, for example, he tends to be consistent in the direction of his errors. Thus, one person will almost always overestimate size while another repeatedly underestimates size. *Relationships* have been found between the direction of error and the person's *tolerance* for *pain* and *sensory isolation*.

On the basis of these findings three algesic types were identified: reducers, augmenters, and moderates. *Reducers* tend to decrease subjectively what they perceive. Therefore reducers tolerate pain well because they underestimate the intensity of pain. On the other hand, they are intolerant of sensory isolation because they apparently diminish even further the minimal sensory input. It follows that *augmenters*, because they tend to overestimate input, do not tolerate pain well but tolerate sensory isolation. *Moderates* alter only slightly what they perceive and tend to be moderately tolerant of both pain and isolation (Petrie et al., 1960).

While the inverse relationship between the ability to endure pain and the ability to tolerate sensory isolation has not been supported by others (Peters, et al., 1963), the importance of these findings is that a person may have a consistent *perceptual style*. That is, an individual's judgments of external stimuli, including pain, may consistently err in one direction or the other.

If a patient appears to be reporting higher intensities of pain or more incidences of minor pain than other patients with similar physical problems, it may be that the patient is an augmenter. Further exploration may reveal that this patient seeks quiet environments for work or leisure or that he is bothered more than usual by noise or crowds of people.

Other personality characteristics are sometimes related to an increased sensitivity to pain. Examples are *hypochondriacal neuroses* and *introversion*. However, once we understand that some people may indeed be more sensitive than others to potentially painful stimuli, it seems more relevant for clinical practice to begin examining how different personality traits may be related to the patient's *response* to the sensation of pain.

Neuroticism and Trait Anxiety

A person who is emotionally labile, overly responsive, usually anxious, and who frequently reports minor aches and pains is said to be high in *neuroticism* as measured by the EPI. This is similar to "trait" anxiety, that is, anxiety as a persistent personality trait rather than anxiety that results from a specific situation (Jacox & Stewart, 1973). Persons high in neuroticism may be more sensitive to pain and have more difficulty tolerating pain (Jacox, 1977).

Hypochondriasis

Some patients respond to pain with a high degree of *hypochondriasis*. As previously mentioned, a person is said to be hypochondriacal if he is preoccupied with his body, often afraid of disease and body malfunction, and/or convinced that disease is present in spite of reassurance that it is not (Pilowsky, 1967). "There are no actual losses or distortions of function" (Pinsky, 1979, p. 306). Conversation with such a patient seems to revolve around pain, other symptoms, and various body functions. Even in the presence of a known illness, "*fascinated absorption* by the experience of impairment" is considered hypochondriasis (Sternbach, 1974, p. 32). Both acute and chronic pain normally will precipitate some degree of hypochondriasis (Sternbach, 1978, p. 255). Thus, there is a spectrum of hypochondriasis, ranging from healthy concern to delusion.

People who respond to pain with an excessive amount of hypochondriasis are thought to have a preexisting tendency, probably learned in childhood. Hypochondriasis often is associated with depression and may mask anxiety or depression. For example, if an upsetting event occurs, instead of experiencing feelings of depression, the patient may focus on a headache. Focusing attention on the headache may increase the discomfort. Along with this, the patient may begin to worry about the seriousness of the headache. Handling emotional stress by focusing on body functioning is called *somaticizing* and few individuals have not had such an experience at some time during their life.

In clinical practice, it is important to understand that pain and illness naturally cause some degree of bodily concern in most people. To some extent the person pays closer attention to his body, is more concerned about disease, and may be unresponsive to casual reassurance that "everything is okay," and there is "no need to worry." Sometimes we are too quick to label a person a hypochondriac. Even when the term is justified, a derogatory meaning should be avoided.

Occasionally, it seems to us that too much emotional maturity is often expected in others, and we are too ready to criticize a lack of it. Perhaps we should consider the fears and sorrows that are hidden by the pain. Anyone who has grieved the loss of a loved one should readily appreciate how much easier it would have been to feel a stomachache than to feel the grief. Apparently, the hypochondriac defends himself against such intolerable feelings by focusing on bodily symptoms. He attends to, and perhaps perpetuates, symptoms that another person would ignore.

Introverts and Extroverts

Patients also have different *expressive styles*, that is, they differ in the way they report pain. As previously described, some cultures allow more expression of pain than others, but personality characteristics also influence the expression of pain. Some people tend to be introverts; others, extroverts. By definition, *introverts* are less expressive and outgoing than extroverts. It is not surprising that introverts are less expressive about their pain than are extroverts (Sternbach, 1976). *Extroverts* probably complain of pain more readily and freely, and they may tend to use more descriptive phrases. Sternbach (1978, p. 244) illustrates this point through serial documentation in relation to patients with advanced cancer. He says that introverts may suffer in silence, there being little relationship between their pain severity and pain complaint, whereas extroverts have little difficulty communicating their pain.

"Pain Patient," "Painful Person," "Painful Family," and "Painful Home Life"

Along with attempts to classify pain according to characteristics such as its cause and duration, mention is usually made of the "pain patient." Actually *pain patient* is difficult to define. The label is most often reserved for the patient with chronic benign pain. Gorrell (1975) has suggested what it *is not*: "If you can function with chronic pain and are not a complainer, you are not a "pain patient." Szasz (1975) says a *painful person* is one "whose humanity is intimately related to, or wholly dependent upon, his being in pain and suffering." Sternbach (1974) says that the label *pain patient* refers to those who present themselves to doctors with a complaint of pain, seeking relief from it" (p. 3). Thus, the patient with acute pain, such as myocardial infarction, is by definition a pain patient if he comes to the physician for the relief from his pain. However, he is rarely referred to as a pain patient.

Painful families are families in which one or both parents, more frequently the mother, and sometimes more distant relatives such as cousins or grandparents, suffer from recurrent pains and psychological problems, recurrent illnesses, and pseudo-illnesses. Parents in these families are excessively preoccupied with their children's health and it is unlikely that the children will grow up symptom-free (Craig, 1978, p. 85). Further, children often develop symptoms in the same body structures as their parents (Apley, 1975). Oster (1972) indicates that rather than proneness to a specific body structure, the family tendency is toward pain proneness.

Lastly, Harwood (1981) says that when role responsibilities and social activities are interferred with illness may be precipitated. He refers to this as a *painful home life.*

"Pain-prone" Patients

The patient's own special personality affects his experience of pain in complicated ways that are not yet well understood. For years reference has been made to the *pain prone* patient, a person who suffers repeated or prolonged pain. Often attempts are made to relate personality characteristics to this type of patient. So far, very little progress has been made. In reviewing the literature, Sternbach (1974) finds that the gist of the psychodynamic theories is that the pain-prone person is exposed to certain forms of abusiveness in childhood. As a result, the person adopts a lifestyle in which suffering is a major factor.

Discussing constitutional differences in relation to pain sensitivity, Terenius (1981, p. 166) reports that low endorphin levels result in a "vulnerable personality" because the individual is not well-protected by his endorphin system. Further, malfunction of the serotonin and endorphin systems, important in pain modulation, result in low levels which seem to be of etiologic significance for the "pain-prone patient." That is, there is biochemical support for the existence of this particularly vulnerable patient (p. 170).

In these patients the organic pathology underlying pain very often is identifiable as is childhood abuse. By what mechanism physical abuse in childhood results later in various physical problems is unknown, and perhaps there is no connection. Coincidences are sometimes misunderstood when we are searching for possible cause and effect relationships. As has been pointed out by Terenius (1981), however, low endorphin levels result in vulnerability to illness and childhood abuse is frequently correlated with decreased resistance and increased frequency of illness in adulthood.

PAST EXPERIENCE WITH PAIN

A person's *past experiences with pain* seem to have a profound effect upon his total response to a current painful event. Here we are not discussing the pain-prone patient nor the patient with a history of childhood abuse or extreme neglect. Rather, we are focusing on the normal range of experiences with pain.

Upon first consideration of the effects of past painful experiences upon the patient's behavior and attitude, it is tempting to believe that the more experience a patient has the more "used to it" he will be. It would seem that he would be less sensitive to pain and less threatened by it. While this may be true for some patients, for most patients it is *not* true.

Numerous experiences with pain during childhood appear to have a rather generalized effect on the patient's response as an adult. The fact that lower socioeconomic status is a frequent correlate of increased pain sensitivity has been interpreted as meaning that increased experience with pain during childhood results in increased pain sensitivity in adulthood. It is likely that children from the lower socioeconomic levels have more painful experiences than children from higher socioeconomic levels. Varni et al., (1980, pp. 375–376) say that chronic pain in adults more frequently is correlated with painful childhood experiences than it is for children. Further, adults who have had greater experience with pain in childhood are most likely to perceive pain as threatening and to be more sensitive to painful stimuli (Collins, 1965; Schluderman & Zubek, 1962). As discussed in Chapters 2 and 6, central pattern-generating, neural mechanisms can be activated to produce pain even when there is no nociceptive input. It is based on neural substrates of the memories of past pain experience (Melzack & Loeser, 1978, pp. 195–210). Therefore even remembering or imagining pain can result in physiological arousal.

In another study, it was found that patients who estimated they had experienced above average amounts of pain in their lifetimes tended to anticipate more pain than did patients with lower estimates of previous pain (Petrovich, 1958).

Some people never have experienced severe pain; others have had one or several instances of severe pain. Although little systematic study has been done, talking with patients with pain reveals a strong relationship between past and present pain.

A patient who has never had severe pain may have relatively little fear of pain. He may not realize how intense the sensation of pain can become. The patient simply does not know that severe pain can occur; therefore he cannot fear it. This lack of knowledge is testified to by patients who say, following a painful event, "I never knew anything could hurt so much." On the other hand even if the patient has had repeated episodes of severe pain, such as angina, he may be relatively unafraid of the current episode, especially if he received immediate and adequate pain relief for it in the past. He may feel in control of the painful experience saying that he knows what the pain is and what will relieve it whether or not the treatment is immediately available. Still another patient who has felt very severe pain may now be very frightened of impending pain or of the possibility that mild to moderate pain may escalate in intensity. If the patient also has had inadequate relief from pain in the past, he may be fearful that this will happen again.

A prolonged and uninterrupted bout of pain may also have adverse effects on the patient's response to the continuing pain. One woman with mild to moderate pain of only several months' duration associated with endometriosis commented, "You'd think I'd get used to it [the pain]. But it seems that the longer this goes on the more and more grouchy I get and the harder it is to stand it." Indeed, the longer pain lasts, the more demoralizing it is and the more the patient seems to suffer.

Misunderstanding of the effect of past experience with pain can produce some well-intentioned but counterproductive approaches to patients with pain. For example, one nurse who cared for patients with sickle cell crisis felt that only partial alleviation of pain would be most helpful to the patients. She reasoned that if the patients continued to feel some degree of pain it would help them build up a tolerance to pain. The result was that one man eventually said he was unwilling to experience even the slightest amount of pain. He wanted total pain relief immediately. Perhaps a more productive method of handling the painful crises would be to provide reasonably satisfactory relief as soon as possible. In that way, the patient might develop less anticipatory fear and anxiety about each impending crisis. Further, when the crisis occurred, the patient might be less anxious because he or she could feel confident that the pain would be satisfactorily relieved. With anxiety at a low level, less potent pain relief measures might be needed.

To understand the present pain, a patient may use information about a previous but different pain experience. For example, David, 11 years old, was about to receive a preanesthetic injection and acknowledged that he thought it would hurt. The nurse asked when and what was his last injection. He said it was penicillin about a year ago. She told him this injection would not hurt as much, and David then proceeded to get into position for the injection. After it was over he told the nurse she was correct. It is interesting to speculate whether or not he would have found the present injection as painful as the penicillin if the nurse had not introduced additional information as a positive suggestion.

It is possible, but probably infrequent, that past experience with pain can condition the sensation of pain. In classical conditioning two stimuli are paired. For example, Pavlov (1927) found that alarm or defense reactions could be initiated by any stimulus that had been previously associated with injuries, dangerous threat situations or frustrations. Dogs were conditioned to experience a pain response at the mere sight of the symbol for infliction of pain. As has been documented repeatedly in this book, clearly, once pain has been experienced, psychic stimuli are capable of triggering the mechanism for pain in the absence of peripheral stimulation. This is illustrated by Mr. Armstrong, 24 years old, who received the wrong anesthetic for an appendectomy. The surgery was cancelled and he was taken to the recovery room. Upon awakening he complained of abdominal pain. He may have been conditioned to experience pain on the basis of his past experiences or as a result of his knowledge or observations.

COGNITIVE PROCESSES

Cognitive processes are critical determinants of the pain experience because "The individual in pain tends to interpret its source and *personal meaning* in terms of the immediate environment, his or her past history, and the future implications of an injury or disease" (Craig, 1978, p. 78). Cognitive ability involves how a person thinks and is, reflected in the extent to which the individual organizes what he knows. In other words, it is the extent to which the patient possesses symbols (of reality) and manipulates them internally. Language is a symbolic means of communication. Thus a person's cognitive ability, irrespective of age, is one determinant of the existence of language and the effectiveness of language as a means of communication.

In working with children with pain it is important to know the child's level of growth and development especially in relation to cognitive ability. Kauffman (1980) and McCaffery (1968; 1969; 1979) point out that it is very important to know the child's level of cognitive development to effectively assist him or her with pain experience and hospitalization. Isler's (1976) reference is limited to utilizing knowledge of the child's cognitive development to assist him in coping with hospitalization. In addition to pain assessment and hospitalization, such knowledge facilitates the assessment of possible fears that a child may have during these experiences. Other possible positive results of the nurse's assessment of the child's cognitive level may provide the child with an opportunity to increase his trust, decrease his anxiety, maintain his emotional equilibrium, minimize possible long-term emotional trauma, and help the child improve his behavior.

Infants and young children below about the age of two years have a limited vocabulary and concept of pain. They are less likely to be able to let you know the cause of their pain or fears. They also are less likely to present behavior problems when they are in pain. Children in this age group communicate their pain primarily through nonverbal behaviors such as crying, irritability, changes in eating patterns, erratic sleep patterns, or changes in normal sleeping habits, and such physiological changes as diaphoresis and tachycardia. Kaufman (1980) warns that these symptoms are nonspecific to pain and may be due to other causes. However, both in the absence and in the presence of other symptoms the possibility that pain may be causing the behavioral changes must be assessed. For example, if an infant suddenly refuses to take fluids pain should be considered and his mouth should be inspected for the possibility of "thrush" and his throat for tonsilitis. Tactile stimulation such as cuddling and rocking may provide the most comfort to the infant and young child with pain.

Children ages two-to-four years still do not have a well-developed concept of pain. Although their verbal skills are significantly improved they are generally too limited to communicate thoughts and feelings.

On the other hand, it is easy to be misled by the language of a four- or five-year-old child who usually has a large vocabulary and may be able to construct organized sentences. This barrage of language encourages the listener to believe that the child understands what she or he is saying. A careful listener will find that the child often contradicts himself or herself, that he or she fails to see or understand important aspects of a given topic, and that the meanings ascribed to words are not necessarily those shared by adults.

Preschool children between the ages of about two to four or five years of age usually express their pain and displeasure through withdrawal, temper tantrums, and other regressed behavior such as feeding problems, thumbsucking, and bedwetting. When painful procedures are explained to them, they usually are quite capable of comprehending them even though they may not be able to verbalize well themselves. Role playing, and allowing children to handle things, especially related to procedures, may effectively assist with decreasing pain perception.

Discrepancies between the perceptions of a child of four years of age and adults related to pain and pleasure were reported to us by the mother of a child following his discharge from the hospital for second- and third-degree burns of his leg which required multiple painful procedures. The child vividly described how terrified he was by practitioners who he felt were receiving pleasure from inflicting pain on him. The first memory he described was the happiness of a nurse who was successful in doing a venipuncture on him after several others had failed. The second was when the plastic surgeon had successfully completed a very painful debridement. The third occurred when the plastic surgeon was viewing a new skin graft.

Between the ages of two and seven years the child's cognitive processes involve *centering* on a single striking feature to the exclusion of other important aspects of a situation. This is demonstrated by John, 4½ years old, who had painful dressing changes involving the use of saline on cotton balls to cleanse the outer area. When the nurse tried to acquaint him with the equipment by handing him a cotton ball, he began to cry and pushed the cotton away. Apparently he had centered on the cotton balls as the cause of pain. When the cotton touched his hand he reacted as he had during the dressing change. It was impossible to tell whether he had been conditioned to feel pain on contact with the cotton ball, or simply anticipated pain when he saw one. In any event he appeared to have focused on the cotton balls as an important factor in the cause of pain.

Also between two and seven years of age the child's tendency toward *artificialism* affects the meanings he ascribes to pain. Artificialism is defined as "regarding things [as the] products of human creation" (Piaget, 1959). One seven-year-old boy told the nurse who had just given him an injection that she was "mean" for doing that. He seemed to believe that the infliction of pain was deliberate and hostile and that the nurse had control over whether or not it was done. Sometimes it helps to orient the child to reality by emphasizing the injection is given along with acknowledging that it hurts and that you are sorry.

Children, ages four-to-eight, have an adequate vocabulary and concept of pain. They usually are able to provide information regarding their pain such as its severity, quality, location and duration. It is very important not to underestimate this child's communication ability and to provide him with adequate explanations that he can understand. Children of this age group often enjoy conversing. It is very helpful to offer them any options possible especially related to pain experiences. Children four to eight years old respond to pain and stress by verbally complaining, temper tantrums and outbursts and assaultive behavior. Anger at the child's behavior by the staff may be perceived as retaliation, further decreasing his trust and intensifying the child's unproductive behavior, which may be as disturbing to him as it is to the staff.

Children over the age of eight years have a well developed cognitive level and usually have more experiences related to illness and pain either with themselves or others. If the pain and/or illness was not threatening and was well-handled, the child usually will be able to face his present situation with less fear. Teenagers have an especially difficult time admitting that they do not know things or are afraid. Common fears with older children related to pain and illness often revolve around changes in body image, role changes, and their sexuality. Their fears are often evidenced in very frightening night dreams, anxiety, depression, manipulation, assaultive behavior, and sexual acting-out. Frustrations relative to changes in body image and role include being forced into a dependent position involved in the patient role, limitations which curtail their natural boisterousness, high activity level, loud volumes on radios, stereos, and televisions, and the use of obscenities. In spite of their seeming confidence, these children need thorough explanations, reassurance, the opportunity to participate in as many decisions especially relevant to pain and their illness, activity to minimize boredom, and, when possible, the opportunity to be assigned to their favorite staff member.

Artificialism, centering, and other characteristics of the various cognitive levels in children are also seen in adults. The adult may regress to a lower cognitive level for a variety of reasons including pain, anxiety, fear, depression, fluctuations in the level of consciousness, and from physical and mental illnesses. For example, the patient who has had a massive cerebral vascular accident may have a thalamic pain syndrome and expressive and receptive aphasia. All three may interact with the resulting stress significantly decreasing his cognitive ability.

There are two aspects of one's cognitive processes that have been cited as having special significance for the patient with chronic pain—vigilance and cognitive dissonance. *Vigilance* is what one selects to respond and pay attention to. Selective attention allows the individual to interact efficiently with his environment through emotional arousal and stimulation of the autonomic and central nervous system and the endocrine system (Chapman, 1978, p. 178). *Cognitive dissonance* may be defined as an awareness "that there is inconsistency, or lack of agreement, between actions, beliefs, opinions or values" (McCaffery, 1979, p. 30).

The patient with pain can be either *hypervigilant* or *hypovigilant* as well as *normovigilant*. The patient's state of vigilance may alter his tolerance for pain. For example, during a natural disaster such as a fire, a patient may suffer burns in the process of attempting to escape. At this time he is hypervigilant to survival and usually hypovigilant to the immediate pain. It is believed that part of the problem for patients with chronic benign pain is that they are hypervigilant to their pain experiences. Therefore, one goal of therapy for these patients may be to help them learn to become less anxious and hypovigilant about their pain experience.

Pinsky (1979) discusses the role of cognitive dissonance in maintaining the suffering for the patient with the chronic pain. He says that because the object loss is less acute it may be more difficult for the individual to cognitively identify physical and psychosocial concomitants of the pain experience as losses (p. 312). Further, he feels that the patient with chronic pain has been unable to develop a cognitive system allowing for coping mechanisms that would minimize the suffering of the pain experience (p. 314). Cognitive focusing on painful conflictual material is one of the beginning steps that enables a person to gain better control of his pain and suffering (Pinsky & Malyon, 1979, p. 319).

One of the major treatment approaches for patients with pain involves the use of *cognitive strategies* to manipulate one's cognitive processes. Webb (1978, pp. 80–81) says that a patient can employ guided imagery and hypnosis to reduce anxiety, restore a sense of mastery and raise the pain threshold. Cognitive strategies to alter the perception of pain may be directed at focusing on or away from the pain or imaginatively transforming it. These uses of one's cognitive processes for pain relief is consistent in the literature.

The next chapter commences Part B of this book. The focus of chapters in this section is on the components, communication, and assessment of the patient's pain experience. Specific information will be presented on the important behaviors, both signs and symptoms, which indicate that the patient is having pain; the major variables that may influence the patient's pain experience including some of the more common pain syndromes; and finally, methods and tools which we hope will facilitate and encourage the nurse to systematically and thoroughly assess and reassess the patient's pain experience. Chapter 5, the first chapter in this section, presents information on the sensation and experience of pain including the phases, characteristics, and classifications of pain.

REFERENCES

Apley, J. The Child with Abdominal Pains. Oxford: Blackwell, 1975.

Apley, J., & Naish, N. Recurrent abdominal pains: A field survey of 1,000 school children. Arch Dis Child 33(168): 165–170, 1958.

Barber, T.X. Toward a theory of pain relief: Relief of chronic pain by prefrontal leucotomy, opiates, placebos, and hypnosis. Psychol Bull 56: 430–460, 1959.

Beecher, H.K. Generalizations from pain of various types and diverse origins. Science 130: 267–268, 1959.

Berkow, K., & Talbott, J.H. Munchausen Syndrome. The Merck Manual. 13th Ed. Rahway, N.J.: Merck, Sharp & Dohme Research Laboratories, 1977, p. 1491.

Bonica, J.J. Introduction to the first World Congress on Pain. Goals of IASP and the World Congress. In J.J. Bonica, & D. Albe-Fessard (Eds.), Advances in Pain Research and Therapy, Vol. 1. New York: Raven Press, 1976, pp. xxvii–xxxix.

Brena, S. The pain prone patient. Northwest Med 69: 573–575, 1970.

Caghan, S., McGrath, M.M., Morrow, M.G., & Pittman, L.D. When adolescents complain of pain. Nurse Pract July–Aug.: 19–22, 1978.

Chapman, C.R. Pain: The perception of noxious events. In R.A. Sternbach (Ed.), The Psychology of Pain. New York: Raven Press, 1978, pp. 169–202.

Collins, L.G. Pain sensitivity and ratings of childhood experience. Perceptual Motor Skills 21: 349–350, 1965.

Craig, K.D. Social modelling influences on pain. In R.A. Sternbach (Ed.), The Psychology of Pain. New York: Raven Press, 1978, pp. 73–109.

Crue, B.L., Jr. Some philosophical considerations of pain—Suggestion, euthanasia and free will. In B.L. Crue, Jr. (Ed.), Pain: Research and Treatment. New York: Academic Press, 1975, pp. 401–413.

Crue, B.L., Pinsky, J.J., Agnew, D.C., et al. Observations on the taxonomy problem in pain. In B.L. Crue (Ed.), Chronic Pain: Further Observations From the City of Hope National Medical Center. New York: SP Medical and Scientific Books, 1979, pp. 13–27.

Davis, G.C., Buchsbaum, M.S., & Bunney, W.E. Pain and psychiatric illness. In L.K.Y. Ng, and J.J. Bonica (Eds.), Pain Discomfort and Humanitarian Care, Proceedings of the National Conference held at the National Institutes of Health, Bethesda, Md., Feb. 15–16, 1979. New York: Elseiver/North-Holland, 1980, pp. 221–231.

Freud, S., & Breuer, J. Studies on Hysteria. Studien Über Hysterie Leipzig: Vienna Deuticke, 1895. From Ref-Index of Psychoanalytic Writings by Grinstein. London: Pelican, 1974.

Gorrell, R.L. The chronic pain patient: Victim of villain? Arizona Med 32: 821–822, 1975.

Hackett, T.P. Psychogenic pain evaluated: A guide to diagnosis and management. Paper presented at American Association of Family Physicians, Boston, 1976. Reported in Pain, Current Concepts on Pain and Analgesia 4: 10–11, 1976.

Harwood, A. Introduction in A. Harwood (Ed.). Ethnicity and Medical Care. Cambridge, MA.: Harvard University Press, 1–36, 1981.

Ireland, P., Sapira, J.O., & Templeton, B. Munchausen's Syndrome. Review and report of an additional case. Amer J Med 43: 579–592, 1967.

Isler, C. The fine art of handling a hospitalized child. RN March: 41–45, 1978.

Jacox, A.K. Pain alleviation through nursing intervention. Unpublished findings, 1975. Reported by Shawyer, M.M., Pain associated with cancer. In A.K. Jacox (Ed.), Pain: A Source Book for Nurses and Other Health Professionals. Boston: Little, Brown, 1977, p. 387.

Jacox, A.K., & Stewart, M. Psychosocial Contingencies of the Pain Experience. Iowa City: Univ. of Iowa, College of Nursing, 1973.

Kaufman, R.E. Pain. In H.C. Shirkey (Ed.), Pediatric Therapy, (6th ed.) St. Louis: C.V. Mosby, 1980, Chap. 23. pp. 283–287.

Mastrovito, R.C. Psychogenic pain. Amer J Nurs 74: 514–519, 1974.

McCaffery, M. Cognition, Bodily Pain, and Man-Environment Interactions. Los Angeles: University of California Student Store, 1968. (Out of print.)

McCaffery, M. Brief episodes of pain in children. In B.S. Bergsen, E.H. Anderson, M. Duffey, et al. (Eds.) Current Concepts in Clinical Nursing, vol. 2. St. Louis: C.V. Mosby, 1969, pp. 181–182.

McCaffery, M. Nursing Management of the Patient with Pain. Philadelphia: J.B. Lippincott, 1979.

Melzack, R., & Dennis, S.G. Neurophysiological foundations of pain. In R.A. Sternbach (Ed.), The Psychology of Pain. New York: Raven Press, 1978, pp. 1–26.

Melzack, R., & Loesser, J.D. Phantom body pains in paraplegics: Evidence for a central "Pattern Generating Mechanism." Pain 4: 195–210, 1978.

Melzack, R., & Scott, T.H. The effects of early experience on the response to pain. J Compar Physiol Psychol 50: 155–161, 1957.

Merskey, H. An Investigation of Pain in Psychological Illness. D.M. thesis, Oxford University, 1964.

Merskey, H. Psychological aspects of pain. Postgrad Med J 44: 297–306, 1968.

Merskey, H. Pain and personality. In R.A. Sternbach (Ed.), The Psychology of Pain. New York: Raven Press, 1978, pp. 111–127.

Merskey, H., & Spear, F.G. Pain: Psychological and Psychiatric Aspects. London: Bailliere, Tindall & Cassell, 1967.

Oster, J. Recurrent abdominal pain, headache and limb pain in children and adolescents. Pediatrics 50: 429–436, 1972.

Pavlov, I.P. Conditioned Reflexes. G.V. Anrep (Ed. and Tr.). Oxford: Oxford University Press, 1927.

Peters, J., Benjamin, F.B., Helvey, W.M., et al.: Study of Sensory Deprivations, Pain and Personality Relationships for Space Travel, NASA TN D-2113. New York: Republic Aviation Corp. for NASA. Washington, D.C., Sept., 1963.

Petrie, A., Collins, W., & Solomon, P. The tolerance for pain and sensory deprivation. Amer J Psychol 73: 80–90, 1960.

Petrovich, D.V. The pain apperception test: Psychological correlates of pain perception. J Clin Psychol 14: 367–374, 1958.

Piaget, J. Judgement and Reasoning in the Child. Patterson, N.J.: Littlefield, Adams, 1959.

Pilling, L.F., Brannick, T.L., & Swenson, W.M. Psychologic characteristics of psychiatric patients having pain as a presenting symptom. Can Med Assoc J 97: 387–394, 1967.

Pilowsky, I. Dimensions of hypochondriasis. Brit J Psychiatr 113: 89–93, 1967.

Pilowsky, I. Psychodynamic aspects of the pain experience. In R.A. Sternbach (Ed.), The Psychology of Pain. New York: Raven Press, 1978, pp. 203–207.
Pinsky, J.J. Aspects of the psychology of pain. In B.L. Crue, Jr. (Ed.), Chronic Pain: Further Observations from the City of Hope National Medical Center. New York: SP Medical & Scientific Books, 1979, pp. 301–314.
Pinsky, J.J., & Malyon, A.K. The intractable pain and suffering process—Facilitating change. In B.L. Crue, Jr. (Ed.), Chronic Pain: Further Observations from the City of Hope National Medical Center. New York: SP Medical and Scientific Books, 1979, pp. 315–320
Sale, I., & Kalucy, R. An observation on the genesis of Munchausen Syndrome: A case report. Aust. New Zealand J Psychiatr 14: 61, 1980.
Schluderman, E., & Zubek, J.P. Effect of age on pain sensitivity. Perceptual and Motor Skills 14: 295–301, 1962.
Spear, F.G. Pain in psychiatric patients. J Psychosom Res 11: 187–193, 1967.
Sternbach, R.A. Pain: A Psychophysiological Analysis. New York: Academic Press, 1968.
Sternbach, R.A. Pain Patients: Traits and Treatments. New York: Academic Press, 1974.
Sternbach, R.A. Psychological factors in pain. In J.J. Bonica & D. Albe-Fessard (Eds.), Advances in Pain Research and Therapy, Vol. 1. New York: Raven Press, 1976, pp. 298–299.
Sternbach, R.A. Clinical aspects of pain. In R.A. Sternbach (Ed.), The Psychology of Pain. New York: Raven Press, 1978, pp. 241–264.
Szasz, T.S. Pain and Pleasure. New York: Basic Books, 1975.
Terenius, L. Endorphin and pain. In L.R. Rees, & T.B. van Wimer sma Greidanus (Eds.), Frontiers of Hormone Research, Vol. 8, 1981, pp. 162–177.
Tretowan, W.H., & Conlan, M.E. The Couvade Syndrome. Brit J Psychiatr 111: 57–66, 1965.
Varni, J.W., Bessman, C.A., Russo, D.C., et al. Behavioral management of chronic pain in children. Arch Phys Med Rehab, 61: 375–378, 1980.
Walters, A. Psychogenic pain alias hysterical pain. Brain 84(3): 1–8, 1961.
Webb, W.L. The therapy of psychosomatic pain. Curr Psychiatr Ther 18: 73–84, 1978.
Weiner, C. Pain assessment, pain legitimation, and the conflict of staff-patient perspectives. Nurs Outlook, 23: 508–516, 1975.
Wilson, L.G. The Couvade Syndrome. Amer Family Physic 15: 157, 1977.

SUGGESTED READINGS

Aronson, E. The rationalizing animal. Psychol Today 6 (May): 46–52, 1973.
Asberg, M., Thorén, P., Träskman, L., et al.: "Serotonin depression"—A biochemical subgroup within the affective disorders? Science 191: 478–480, 1976.
Barsky, A.J. Patients who amplify bodily sensations. Ann Intern Med 91: 63–70, 1979.
Bonica, J.J. Letter to the editor—re: The relation of injury to pain. Pain 7: 203–207, 1979.

Cohen, F., & Lazarus, R.S. Active coping processes, coping dispositions and recovery from surgery. In M. Weisenberger (Ed.). Pain: Clinical and Experimental Perspectives. St. Louis: Mosby, 1975, pp. 291–302.

Eland, J.M. & Anderson, J.E. The experience of pain in children. In A. Jacox, (Ed.) Pain: A Source Book for Nurses and Other Health Professionals. Boston: Little Brown, 453–473, 1977.

Elton, D., Stanley, G.V., & Burrows, G.D. Self-esteem and chronic pain. J Psychosom Res, 22: 25–30, 1978.

Engel, G.L. Psychogenic pain and the pain-prone patient. Amer J Med 26: 899-918, 1959.

Fink, B.K. (Moderator). Floor discussions: Chronic pain behavior. In J.J. Bonica, (Ed.), Advances in Neurology, Vol. 4. New York: Raven Press, 1974.

Freidman, R. Some characteristics of children with "psychogenic" pain. Clin Pediatrics 11(6): 331–333, 1972.

Jaffee, W.G., & Sandler, J. On the concept of pain with special reference to depression and psychogenic pain. J Psychosom Res 11: 69–75. 1967.

Johansson, F., Almay, B.G.L., von Knorring, L. et al.: Personality traits in chronic pain patients related to endorphin levels in cerebrospinal fluid. Psychiatr Res 1: 231–239, 1979.

Kanfer, F.H., & Goldfoot, D.A. Self-control and tolerance of noxious stimulation. Psychol Rep 18: 79–85, 1966.

Kanfer, F.H., & Seidner, M.C. Self-control: Factors enhancing tolerance of noxious stimulation. J Personal Social Psychol, 25: 381–389, 1973.

Kapp, F.T. Psychogenic pain. In M.A. Freedman, & H.I. Kaplan (Eds.), Comprehensive Textbook of Psychiatry, II. Baltimore, Md.: Williams & Wilkins, 1975, pp. 1704–1708.

Kubler-Ross E. On Death and Dying. New York: Macmillan, 1969.

Maltbie, A.A., Cavenar, J.O., Hammett, E.B., et al. A diagnostic approach to pain. Psychosomatics 19(6): 359–366, 1978.

McMahon, M.A., & Miller, P. The influence of psycho-social-cultural factors. Nurs Forum 17(1): 58–71, 1978.

Mechanic, D. Social psychologic factors affecting the presentation of bodily complaints. N Eng J Med 286: 1132–1139, 1972.

Mechanic, D. Correlates of psychological distress among young adults: A theoretical hypothesis and results from a 16-year follow-up study. Arch Gen Psychiatr 36: 1233–1239, 1979.

Merskey, H. Pain, learning and memory. J Psychosom Res 19: 319–324, 1975.

Ng, L.K.Y. Pain and well-being: A challenge for biomedicine. In L.K.Y. Ng & J.J. Bonica (Eds.) Pain, Discomfort and Humanitarian Care. Proceedings of the National Conference held at the National Institutes of Health, Bethesda, Md. Feb. 15–16, 1979. New York: Elseiver/North-Holland, 1980, 353–365.

Pennebaker, J.W., & Skelton, J.A. Psychological parameters of physical symptoms. Personal Social Psychol Bull 4: 524–530, 1978.

Pennebaker, J.W., & Skelton, J.A. Cognitive processes influence the interpretation of bodily state. Charlottesville, VA: University of Virginia, 1978. (Duplicated).

Pilowsky, I. Abnormal illness behavior. Brit J Med Psychol 42: 347, 1969.

Price, D.D., Barrell, J.J. & Bracely, R.H. A psychophysical analysis of experimental factors that selectively influence the affective dimension of pain. Pain, 8: 137–149, 1980.

Reich, T. Principles of pathophysiology, diagnosis and management of pain—Psychiatry and pain. In R.E. Wilson (Ed.), The Management of Pain in Surgical Practice. Plainfield, N.J.: Chirugecom, 1979, pp. 9–13. Copyright, Pfizer Laboratories, Inc., 1979.

Robinson, G., & Merar, A. Informed consent: Recall by patients tested postoperatively. Ann Thoracic Surg 22(3): 209–212, 1976.

Scott, J. & Huskisson, E.C. Graphic Representation of Pain. Pain, 2: 175–184, 1976.

Shealy, C.N. The Pain Game. Millbrae, CA: Celestial Arts, 1976.

Simonton, O.C., & Simonton, S.S. Belief systems and management of the emotional aspects of malignancy. J Transpers Psychol 7: 29–47, 1974.

Staub, E., Tursky, B., & Schwartz, G.E. Self-control and predictability. J Personal Social Psychol 18: 157–162, 1971.

Sutherland, A.M. Psychological impact of cancer and its therapy. Classics in oncology. CA—Cancer Journal Clin, 31(3): 159–171, 1981. Reprinted from Med Clin North Amer 40: 705–720, 1956.

Szasz, T.S. Pain and Pleasure. New York: Basic Books, 1975.

Szasz, T.S. The painful person. Lancet 88: 18–22, 1969.

Violon, A. Pain as a disease: Psychological investigations. Headache 13 (Apr.): 25–28, 1973.

Wolfer, J.A., & Davis, C.E. Assessment of surgical patients' preoperative emotional conditions and postoperative welfare. Nurs Res 19: 402–414, 1970.

Woodforde, J.M., & Merskey, H. Personality traits of patients with chronic pain. J Psychosom Res 16: 167–172, 1972.

PART B

Components of the Pain Experience

5

Sensation and Experience of Pain

CHARACTERISTICS AND CLASSIFICATIONS

Assessment of the patient with pain involves determining certain parts of the overall picture. The nurse needs to know the phase or phases of pain with which the patient must deal; the characteristics of the pain sensation, that is the onset, duration, location, intensity, quality variations, and chronology; the general types of pain or pains, according to acuteness and chronicity; and the stage of adjustment to pain and/or pain relief. This chapter considers these components of the pain experience.

PHASES OF THE PAIN EXPERIENCE

Briefly and simply, the experience of pain usually occurs in three phases: (1) anticipation of pain, (2) sensation (or presence) of pain, and (3) the aftermath of pain. All three phases may occur in a matter of seconds, or they may extend over a period of years. The phases may also occur in cycles over a period of hours or years. For example the spasmodic pain of renal colic which occurs during the passing of a kidney stone may last hours and recur over the years. In addition to nursing assessment and interventions for specific signs and symptoms of pain, there are interventions which may be more specific during a given phase of the pain experience.

Anticipation

The *anticipation phase* is that period prior to the actual onset of the sensation of pain. The person knows that the pain will occur. The anticipatory phase is a very important period of time for the pain patient. As we have seen in Chapter 2, what happens during that phase profoundly affects all of the dimensions of the pain experience and may affect the aftermath experience. The patient may utilize the anticipation phase to learn about his pain and its relief. Anticipation of pain does not always occur, however, since some injuries and painful procedures are unforeseen. Sometimes information about impending pain is withheld from the patient and sometimes patients deny information that they receive about forthcoming pain. For example, a very controlled man was scheduled for a bone marrow aspiration. As part of the explanation of the procedure the physician informed the patient of the type and length of pain associated with the procedure. During the procedure, the patient became very angry with the physician about the pain he was experiencing and asked the physician why he had not been honest and told him he would have pain. Later the patient was discussing the painful procedure with the nurse who also was present when the explanation was given by the physician. The patient told the nurse this was the first time he realized that cancer (leukemia) was being considered as his diagnosis. He said that he became so concerned about the possible outcome of the procedure that he did not hear anything after the reason the bone marrow aspiration was necessary. Patients who fear pain may suffer from lack of knowledge for an entirely different reason—a feeling that the less they know, the better.

A common misconception is that frequent painful experiences favorably condition or desensitize the individual to pain and that consequently the patient is "used to" pain or less bothered by it. Quite the opposite is true in the majority of patients. Katz's (1979, p. 4) research with children undergoing repeated painful procedures found that children did not habituate to these painful procedures nor were the nurses very sensitive to their nonverbal distress such as anxiety and fear. "Nurses appeared to be most sensitive to crying, screaming, and measures of cooperativeness (e.g., needs to be restrained), and less so to more subtle behaviors that were harder to observe (seeking emotional support)" (p. 3). Because the nurses' ratings correlated highest during the procedure phase of the child's pain experience, Katz concluded that "nurses were apparently less sensitive to anticipatory behaviors" (p. 3).

Two other experimental pain studies have been done that have relevance for nursing assessment and interventions during the anticipatory period. Johnson (1973) studied the responses to the qualitative component of the pain experience using ischemic pain. He found that individuals who had received a description of the sensations of ischemia were less distressed than individuals who had only received a description of the procedure resulting in the ischemia. More recently Price et al. (1980) studied both the sensory component and the affective component of the pain experience. Their findings were that, although the degree of noxious input administered was not changed, the subjects perceived the pain as less unpleasant when it was preceded by a warning signal. The subjects accomplished this by decreasing their expectations of being able to avoid pain or by changing how they evaluated the pain sensation. These studies are helpful in alerting nurses to the fact that they can structure nursing interventions during the anticipatory period which will assist patients with their pain experience. It seems likely that nursing interventions devised for the anticipatory phase can have an impact during all three phases of the pain experience and with all three dimensions of pain. With adequate assistance and based on success in utilizing techniques patients may mobilize their cognitive processes to desensitize them thus elevating their pain tolerance by decreasing the affective cyclical anxiety component through activation of neurophysiological processes.

Sensation

The *sensation phase* of pain obviously can be defined as that time when the pain is felt. Most discussions of the pain experience revolve around this phase, although there are increasing numbers of references to the anticipation phase of pain. Interviews with patients reveal that suffering in response to pain "seemed to begin even before the pain and included many anticipatory fears that sometimes were even more acute than the eventual pain" (Copp, 1974, p. 492). Most of us are personally familiar with the dreaded fear of the unknown or of the fear of uncertainty. Indeed, we all have probably heard patients after anticipating a painful experience say that the pain was not as bad as waiting for it and not knowing when it would occur. Possibly because the pain sensation is precise, known and certain it seems easier to bear than the anticipation of it. This is often seen in patients who have multiple venipunctures each day such as patients with electrolyte imbalances or blood dyscrasias. Venipuncture sites soon become painful and veins become sclerosed. This necessitates increased needle probing for veins. Each subsequent blood aspiration becomes a dreaded experience. When the technician succeeds in obtaining the specimen the patient often verbalizes relief and almost immediately the visible signs of anxiety decrease. When the patient starts to anticipate the next venipuncture he may again verbalize his fear of pain and exhibit behaviors associated with increased anxiety.

Aftermath

The *aftermath phase*, the third phase of the patient's pain experience, occurs when pain ceases or is substantially reduced. This period has received less attention in the literature. However, there is little doubt that it is an equally important phase and warrants as complete an assessment as the others. Because pain may present a crisis situation to the patient, it is not uncommon that after the painful experience the patient may experience many symptoms in response to both the pain and the stress including chills, tremors, nausea, vomiting, anger, depression, and nightmares, or even a complete grief response. The effects of pain on the patient will be discussed in Chapter 7.

During the aftermath phase, helping the patient assimilate the most recent pain experience may provide an opportunity to reestablish self-esteem and decrease fear about future possible painful experiences. If the patient believes he or she has acted "out of character" or his or her behavior during the pain experience was negatively commented on by the staff, assuring him or her that this behavior was not unusual and discussing pain relief strategies that may be used in the future are often beneficial. This is as important for children as for adults. One report indicated that children between the ages of two and four years of age may remain disturbed for up to six months postoperatively (Vaughn, 1957).

For the patient with almost constant pain, the three phases of pain usually exist in a modified form. For example, the patient may be experiencing a mild sensation of pain but for all practical purposes may be in the anticipatory phase, expecting the onset of severe pain. Likewise, when the severe pain subsides, he or she may be in the aftermath phase in spite of having some residual pain.

Many patients with chronic pain including cancer report that they only obtain partial relief from analgesics. Therefore, they may always be in one or more phases of the pain experience. For example, if the patient is receiving narcotic analgesia he or she may report it produces only 60 percent pain relief during the peak of its action. As the analgesic is being metabolized, the patient may say that the pain decreases from 60 percent relief to 0 percent relief within a matter of minutes. Thus, these patients are constantly anticipating severe pain—an important reason to use a preventive around-the-clock (ATC) approach to pain relief.

In summary, assessment of the phases of the pain experience involves determining which phase of the experience exists at that moment and which ones can be expected. Does the patient anticipate pain? Is pain present right now? Has the patient experienced a sensation of pain that continues to concern him in some way? We have already stressed the fact that many patients are reluctant to communicate their pain. Hence, determining the existence of the anticipation, presence, or aftermath phases of pain may require considerable effort by the nurse.

CHARACTERISTICS OF THE PAIN SENSATION

Once the nurse has carefully determined that pain is present or that the patient is in the anticipation or aftermath phase, the nature of the pain must be examined. Certain characteristics of pain are almost universally recognized as being important to assess: location, intensity, quality, onset, duration, and variations. Each is discussed here separately. Careful assessment of these characteristics of pain are important both to establish the medical and nursing diagnoses and to determine pain relief measures.

Because pain threshold and pain tolerance are often used interchangeably and frequently in a negative judgmental manner when assessing a patient's pain, defining these terms may be helpful. *Pain threshold* is the sensory component of the pain experience and refers to that point at which the sensation of the pain stimulus is first perceived. It has been repeatedly demonstrated that the pain threshold *does not* vary significantly from individual to individual and remains consistent at different times in the same individual. What varies greatly, however, is the individual's pain tolerance. *Pain tolerance* is just that—the patient's ability or willingness to tolerate a given intensity of pain or to endure it for a given duration. It is the affective and cognitive component of the pain experience. Because of our psychocultural uniqueness some individuals are willing to tolerate a great deal of pain and others are unwilling to tolerate almost any pain.

Sometimes the health team may not only expect and value a high tolerance for pain, they enforce it. It is not unusual for a nurse to convey to the patient that he should tolerate more pain. For example, if a patient requests an analgesic for pain, the nurse often asks "Do you really need it?" or "Can you wait or hold off for just a little while longer?" One nursing team leader responsible for a patient who had very extensive resection of a deeply invasive malignant melanoma and reconstructive skin grafting was overheard, on the patient's second postoperative day, to say:

> Is he asking for something again? What is he going to do tomorrow when he can't have any more injections? He had better get used to it. Just give him 30 mg of codeine and aspirin.

The nurse was not only unconcerned about the patient's pain experience, but felt no responsibility to assess the patient considering the possibility that his pain was atypical, that he may have had a wound infection, let alone that she had a responsibility to obtain an order for more potent analgesia if that was determined through an assessment of the patient. The fact that poorly controlled pain and suffering impede recovery and rehabilitation is often not considered. Pain tolerance is not a matter of good or bad nor is it a sign of bravery or cowardice (McCaffery, 1979, p. 19).

Onset, Duration and Time Sequence

Onset, duration, and *time sequence* of pain may provide one of the earliest clues to the diagnosis. For instance, a slow constant but increasing pain may be indicative of a progressive inflammatory process such as appendicitis. If the pain suddenly becomes very severe and persistent it may be an indication that the appendix has ruptured. When the pain is sudden and severe, the onset is relatively easy to identify. However, some types of pain are gradual in onset, beginning with very mild intensities of sensations that might not initially be considered uncomfortable or painful. Thus, it is not unusual for the patient to find it difficult to answer the simple question, "When did the discomfort or pain begin?"

When someone is unable to state how long the pain has lasted, it is often possible for the nurse to help the patient associate the onset of pain with a particular event. One patient who did not have a watch told the nurse that he had been experiencing pain for about three hours. When she asked him when it had begun he said that it was after lunch. Since it was 1:30 p.m. and the nurse knew he had finished his lunch at 12:30, she was able to determine more accurately the duration of the pain. Time tends to pass slowly for the person with pain, so its duration may be overestimated by the patient.

Helping the patient associate the onset of pain with an external event not only helps in establishing exactly when pain began, it is also valuable in determining possible causes of the pain. Assessment may reveal a *pain pattern* such as the onset of pain always being associated with the physical exertion of climbing two flights of stairs to return home from work at the end of each day.

The child has special difficulty giving information about the duration of pain because of his undeveloped concept of time. Also, the child may not be consciously aware of the onset of pain if the intensity of pain is mild initially and only gradually increases.

The assessment of the onset and duration of pain includes both the total period of pain beginning with the first twinge of pain to the present and, as far as possible, each individual episode of pain during that period. For example, the patient may have experienced a sharp abdominal pain for the first time at noon two days ago. For two days he has experienced this pain, but it has not been constant. He has had five episodes, each lasting between three and four hours.

Location

Pain is assigned some *location* in the body, although there may be difficulty in determining the precise site. The location of pain includes the body parts, the extent of the area and whether the pain is superficial or deep. Frequently the patient has pain in more than one location.

Having the patient point to the area of pain is one of the best ways to assess location. Especially for children, marking the location of the pain on a doll or a figure drawing is very useful. A sample figure drawing is presented in Figure 10.1, the initial pain assessment tool.

Superficial Pain *Superficial pain*, sometimes called *cutaneous pain*, usually refers to pain in the skin and mucous membranes. Pain in superficial tissues can be identified fairly easily and precisely by the patient because of its rich innervation. Also, their superficial location exposes them to all types of stimuli including chemical, thermal, mechanical, and electrical. The characteristic quality of superficial pain is sharp and pricking or burning. Pricking usually describes the sensation experienced when the skin or mucous membrane is punctured in contrast to burning.

Deep Pain—Visceral and Somatic *Deep pain* involves structures deep in the body and is anatomically divided into splanchnic and deep somatic. *Splanchnic pain* refers to pain in viscera. *Deep somatic pain* refers to pain which involves deep structures other than viscera. These include such structures as periosteum, muscles, tendons, fascia, and joints.

The location of deep pain is more difficult to determine than is the location of superficial pain. There are at least three neuroanatomical and physiological reasons that make localizing and diagnosing the cause of deep pain more difficult. Guyton (1981), Seiden (1981), Adams (1980), Jensen (1980), Mountcastle (1980) and Schwartz (1979) describe these reasons. First, there are few nociceptors in most viscera. This may result in a higher threshold for pain. Second, spinal segments receive nociceptive signals from more than one structure. This means that innervation is multisegmental and overlapping. Therefore, with deep pain the margins enveloping the painful part are not distinct and the pain usually cannot be localized closer than two to three spinal segments above or below. Third, neuronal pools may be partially depolarized by preexisting conditions. This in turn would result in new nociceptive signals further depolarizing the neuronal pools causing the pain to spread, which also may lower the pain threshold.

Other factors resulting in the vague or diffuse representation of internal sensation in deep pain may be due to the fact that, by virtue of their location, deep structures are less accessible to chemical, thermal, mechanical, and electrical stimuli. Therefore, sensitivity to these stimuli has not developed. Consequently there is a general lack of experience in localizing deep pain. Also, one is unable to use vision to assist with localization. Further, laymen, both adults and the children, have much less knowledge about the internal aspects of their bodies than about the external parts.

We will now consider some of the differences between visceral and deep somatic pain. Most of the viscera are supplied by C fibers. Thus, the quality of visceral pain is described as aching or burning. Viscera do not respond to stimuli that are applied to the skin. Nor do viscera react to stimuli which excite somatic structures such as cutting, burning, or pressure. What may be surprising is that viscera do not even always react to their own pathology. When pathology in the viscera is highly localized it rarely causes pain. Yet severe visceral pain does occur when there is diffuse stimulation of nerve endings. Normal contractions of viscera are not painful either. Yet in the presence of inflammation or ischemia the pain threshold of viscera is decreased and normal contractions may then be experienced as painful.

Nociceptive signals in the viscera and parietal walls are carried by both visceral and somatic afferents. The visceral afferents, sometimes referred to as the true visceral pathway, regulate visceral motility and secretions in reflex response to stimulation by mechano- and chemo- receptors. Visceral afferents transmit sensory signals in the autonomic nervous system. The signals travel along the visceral sympathetic pathways and the cardiac and splanchnic nerves to their respective spinal segments. There are a few exceptions to this route of visceral innervation. Some of the nociceptive signals from the pharynx, trachea, and upper esophagus are transmitted in the glossopharangeal and vagus nerves. Some stimuli from the center at the diaphragm and lower esophagus are transmitted in the phrenic nerve. Some of the nociceptive impulses from the colon, rectum, and bladder enter the spinal cord through the sacral parasympathetic nerves. The somatic pain of the parietal walls and the distal portion of the diaphragm are transmitted by branches of the thoracic and lumbar spinal nerves.

Due to this dual innervation intense visceral pain may also evoke concommitant autonomic responses. These may include restlessness, tachycardia or bradycardia, hypotension, diaphoresis, nausea and vomiting: a response similar to shock. Obviously, these autonomic responses from visceral pain may significantly complicate the underlying causative pathological state. A fairly common example of this autonomic response is seen in patients who have had a myocardial infarction. Failure to treat their pain may place additional demands on an already compromised myocardium that could result in further myocardial damage and possibly death.

Diagnosis of visceral pain may also be made more difficult because visceral pain often spreads to the parietal wall of the peritoneum, pleura, pericardium, posterior mesentary, and retroperitoneal viscera such as the kidney. Deep somatic pain, which spreads with *parietal pain* may be experienced not only at areas distant to the viscera, but also on two body surfaces at the same time. For example, in kidney pathology the patient often experiences both aching abdominal and costoverterbral angle (CVA) pain and tenderness. In spite of these types of dual innervation, visceral and parietal pain remain as one of the best diagnostic indicators of visceral pathology.

The parietal wall is extensively supplied by the fast A-delta fibers very much like the skin is. Therefore the quality of parietal pain may be very sharp and pricking. It can usually be localized regionally directly over the area where the pain is experienced. When there is diffuse stimulation of the nociceptive parietal afferents, burning or aching pain is experienced. The mechanism of visceral and parietal transmission of pain is illustrated in Figure 5.1.

Following is an example of a patient who presented a "textbook picture" of highly localized visceral pathology which produced no pain, yet when it spread to other viscera and the parietal peritoneal wall it produced

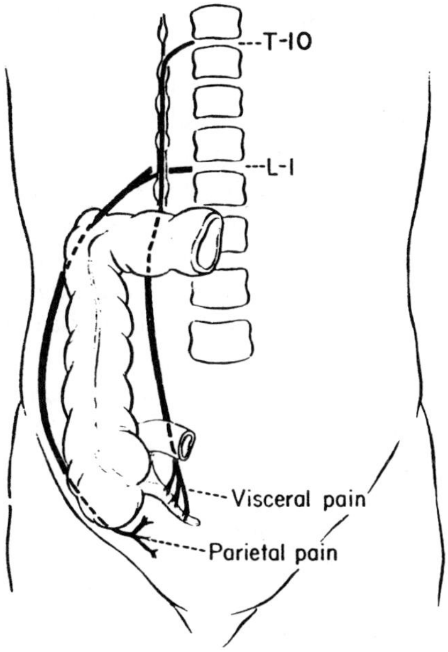

Figure 5.1. Mechanism of visceral and parietal transmission of pain from the appendix. *(Guyton, A. Textbook of Medical Physiology (6th ed.). Philadelphia: W.B. Saunders, 1981, Figure 50.7, p. 619, with permission.)*

severe pain and autonomic responses. A 27-year-old woman with rheumatoid arthritis had been receiving steroid therapy for one year. Suddenly one morning, she was awakened by severe, burning periumbilical pain and referred pain in her right shoulder. During emergency surgery, the presumptive diagnosis for this patient was confirmed, a small perforated gastric ulcer. This patient was totally asymptomatic, consistent with her very small localized gastric ulcer. Also consistent was the severe sudden burning pain due to spillage of the proteolytic gastric juices through the perforation resulting in diffuse stimulation of the surrounding viscera and peritoneum. One of the definitive diagnostic signs of a perforated ulcer is the muscular rigidity, referred to as a "board-like" abdomen which accompanied this patient's severe pain. The area of referred pain was also consistent and will be explained later in this chapter. Concommitant autonomic responses that this patient had were restlessness, tachycardia, hypotension, diaphoresis, and nausea.

Guyton (1981), Jensen (1980), and Mountcastle (1980) describe four primary mechanisms which result in deep visceral pain. Two of these initially are primarily chemical irritants and the other two primarily mechanical. The chemical irritants include ischemia and algoneic (pain-producing) chemical stimulation and the mechanical mechanisms include overdistention of viscera and spasm of a hollow viscera.

The events involved in *ischemic pain* basically are that algogenic substances such as metabolic wastes or end products of tissue degeneration accumulate in the tissues. When these substances come in contact with nerve endings, they cause pain. An example of this type of deep pain occurs in peripheral vascular disease. *Chemical stimulation* of viscera may result from visceral perforation and spillage of enzymes into the visceral cavity as was seen in the example of the patient with a perforated gastric ulcer. Chemical stimulation may also result from hypersecretion of digestive enzymes or aberrant pattern of secretion of digestive enzymes. This latter process is seen in acute pancreatitis. Normally some enzymes in the pancreas are secreted in an inactive form and become activated in the intestines. In acute pancreatitis, these enzymes are activated within the pancreas resulting in autodigestion of the pancreas. This condition causes a characteristically severe type of deep pain.

Visceral overdistention results in stretching the highly innervated visceral capsule. This tension on the nerve endings and highly innervated blood vessels causes deep pain. Some of us may have experienced this type of pain from excessively imbibing in food and spirits during festive occasions. *Spasm of hollow viscera* result partially in pain from a similar mechanism as from overdistention. However, if a viscera continues to spasmodically contract, especially if it does so against an obstruction, another mechanism is added. Stimulated viscera need additional nutrients to supply their accelerated metabolic activity. This compounds the insult caused by tension on nerves and blood vessels because it leads to a relative ischemia. This mechanism is commonly present in the deep pain of gastroenteritis and the pain of ureteral obstruction from renal calculi. When there has been severe spasmodic contraction of a hollow viscera the patient may continue to experience tenderness long after the cessation of the contractions. For example, the wretching that often accompanies vomiting may cause the individual to feel gastric tenderness long after the wretching and vomiting have ceased. The atypical use of associated abdominal muscles involved in vomiting may result in somatic pain.

The description of pain may vary depending on the intensity and the structures. Superficial pain can be described as to its height and width or circumference. Deep pain may have the third dimension, depth. For instance, superficial pain may be described as being as large as a silver dollar but deep pain may be described as being the size of a golf ball.

Referred Pain The problem of localizing deep pain, as was briefly mentioned, may be compounded by referred pain. *Referred pain* may be defined as pain which is present in an area that is removed or distant from its point of origin. The area of the body to which the pain is referred is *regional*. These regions are illustrated in Figures 5.2 and 5.3. This is in contrast to *radiating* or *radicular pain* which extends directly from the site of origin in known spinal nerve root segments. Such is the pain of nerve root compression. Radicular pain may greatly facilitate diagnosing the etiology of this pain.

There are several theories about the mechanism of referred pain. The

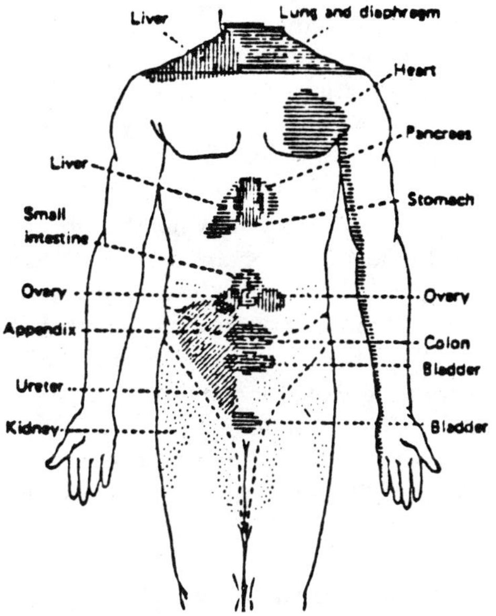

Figure 5.2. Referred pain, anterior view. This indicates the cutaneous areas to which pain in the various organs is referred. *(Chaffee, E.E. & Greisheimer, E.M. Basic Physiology and Anatomy. (3rd ed.) Philadelphia, J.B. Lippincott, Co., 1974, with permission.)*

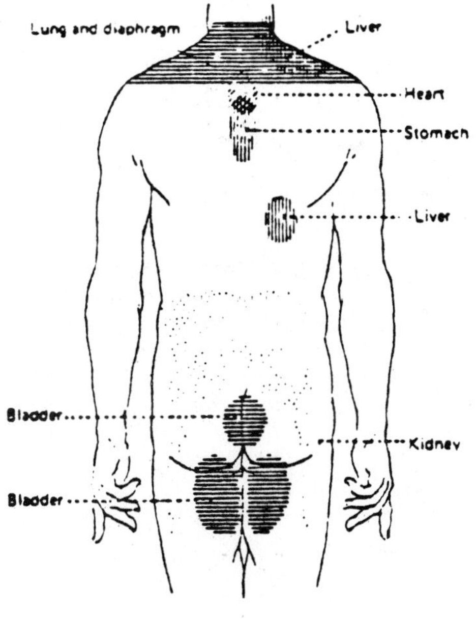

Figure 5.3. Referred pain, posterior view. *(Chaffee, E.E. & Greisheimer, E.M. Basic Physiology and Anatomy, (3rd ed.) Philadelphia, J.B. Lippincott, Co., 1974, with permission.)*

convergence theory (convergence-projection hypothesis) seems to be the most widely accepted. This mechanism of referred pain is illustrated in Figure 5.4. It proposes that pain in both viscera and somatic regions converge on the same spinothalamic neurons. These signals arrive in the sensory cortex as if they were identical. Somatic pain is much more common than visceral pain. Consequently the brain has had much more experience in interpreting afferent nociceptive signals as arising in somatic regions, thus misinterprets the incoming visceral signals. In practice, for example, when there is pathology in the deep structures, nociceptive signals in the afferents from the skin (dermatome) and viscera will converge on the same neuron at the same time. The brain interprets all of them as coming from the skin because the brain has had more extensive experience with input from cutaneous afferents. In pathological pain syndromes which will be discussed in Chapter 6, it has been suggested that, at least in part, it is the brain's misinterpretation of converging nociceptive signals that is responsible for the pain.

Referred pain most commonly is referred from viscera to parietal regions. As has been pointed out, however, pain can also be referred from one body surface to another or one viscus to another. Referred pain may occur in conjunction with pain in the anatomical part generating it or it may exist when there is no pain in that site. It is also well to remember that stimulation of the area of referred pain, as well as stimulation of the organ from which the pain is referred, may produce greater pain in the area of referral than at the pathological site.

Both deep visceral and somatic pain usually are referred superficially from the generating structures following known dermatomes. Therefore,

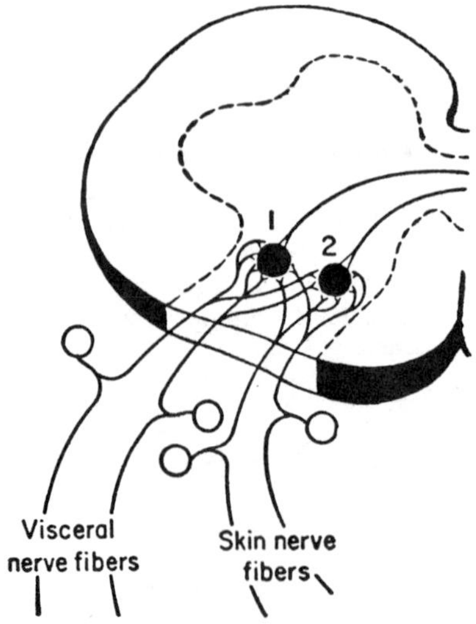

Figure 5.4. Mechanism of referred pain and referred hyperalgesia. *(Guyton, A. Textbook of Medical Physiology (6th ed.). Philadelphia: W.B. Saunders, 1981, Figure 50.5, p. 617, with permission.)*

the area of referred pain is supplied by the same spinal segment as the generating site. The genesis of dermatomal innervation was explained in Chapter 2. Figures 5.5 and 5.6 illustrate anterior and posterior dermotomes for the total body. In Chapter 6 dermatomes will be combined with motor and reflex illustrations for the neurologic levels most subject to pathology which produces many pain syndromes. This information can be seen in Figure 6.1.

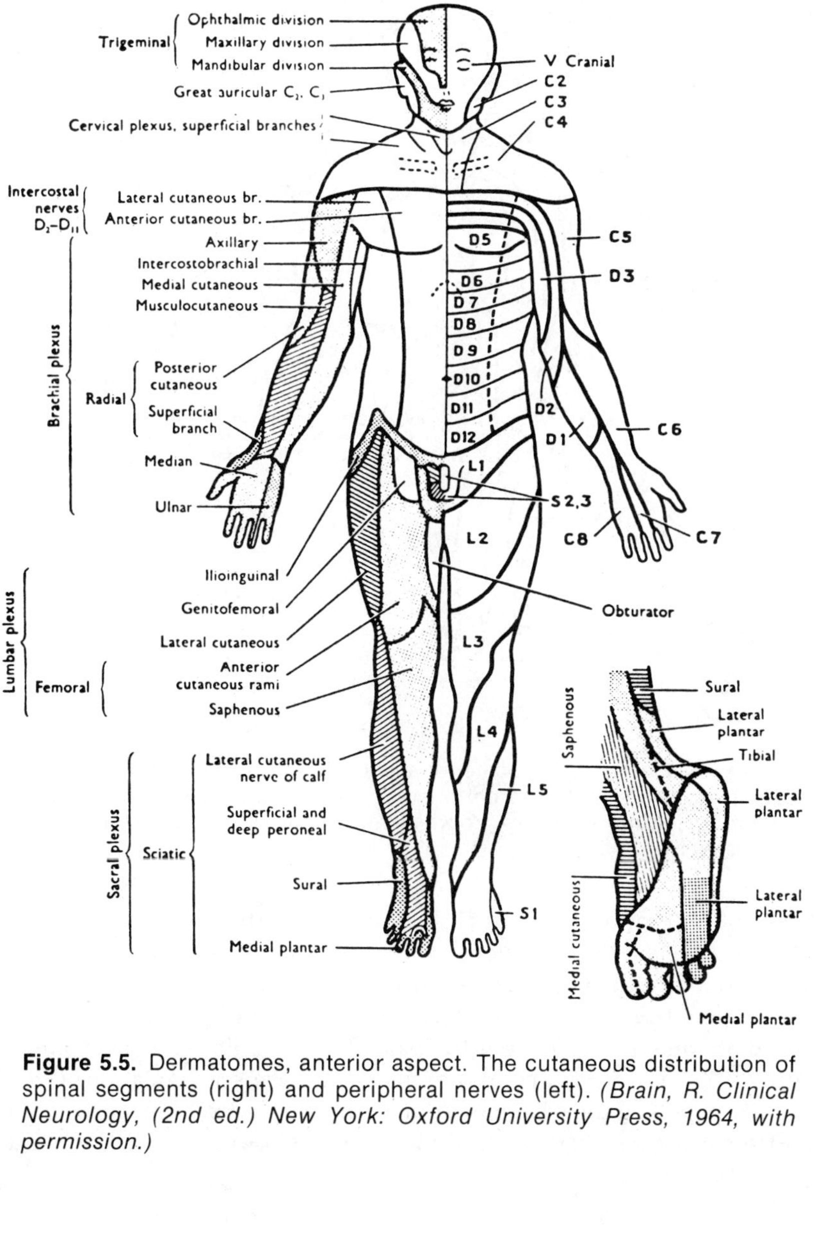

Figure 5.5. Dermatomes, anterior aspect. The cutaneous distribution of spinal segments (right) and peripheral nerves (left). *(Brain, R. Clinical Neurology, (2nd ed.) New York: Oxford University Press, 1964, with permission.)*

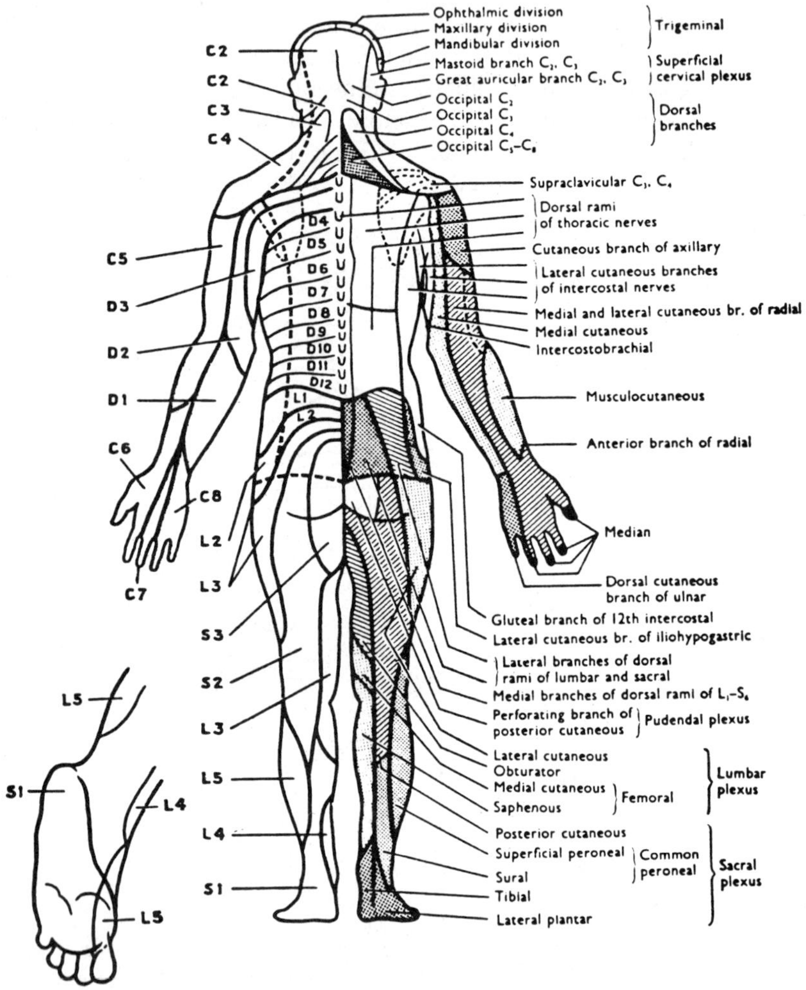

Figure 5.6. Dermatomes, posterior aspect. The cutaneous distribution of spinal segments (left) and peripheral nerves (right). *(Brain, R. Clinical Neurology, (2nd ed.) New York: Oxford University Press, 1964, with permission.)*

Another type of referred pain is associated with trigger points. Posner (1978, p. 728) and Bonica (1966, p. 119) discuss this type of referred pain. The *trigger point* is a small, hypersensitive region in the muscle or connective tissue. Some trigger points are located in the area of pain but others are located at some distance from the pain. Trigger points are illustrated in Figures 5.7–5.10. Trigger points are so named because stimulation of them is similar to pulling the trigger of a gun with the effect being experienced in another place, the *target area* (*reference zone* or *area of reference*). When the trigger

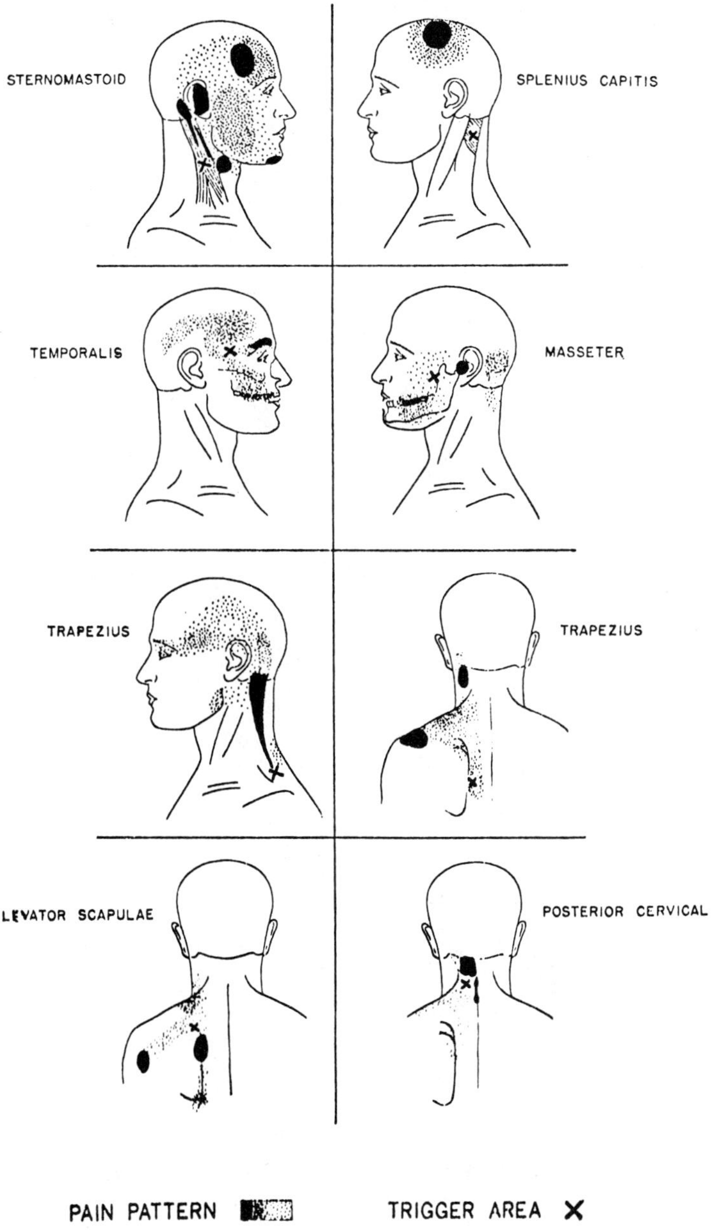

Figure 5.7. Trigger points associated with myofascial pain syndromes of head and neck. *(Travell, J. & Rinzler, S.H. The myofascial genesis of pain. Postgrad Med 11, 1952, p. 427, with permission.)*

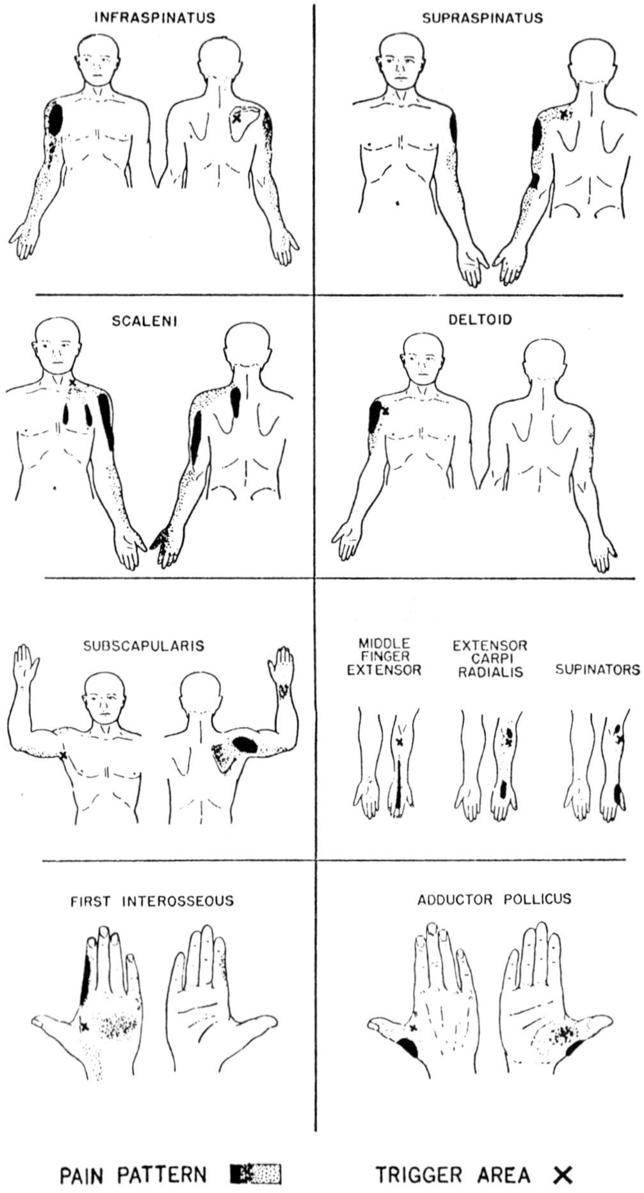

Figure 5.8. Trigger points associated with myofascial pain syndromes of the shoulder and arm. *(Travell, J. & Rinzler, S.H. The myofascial genesis of pain. Postgrad Med 11, 1952, p. 428, with permission.)*

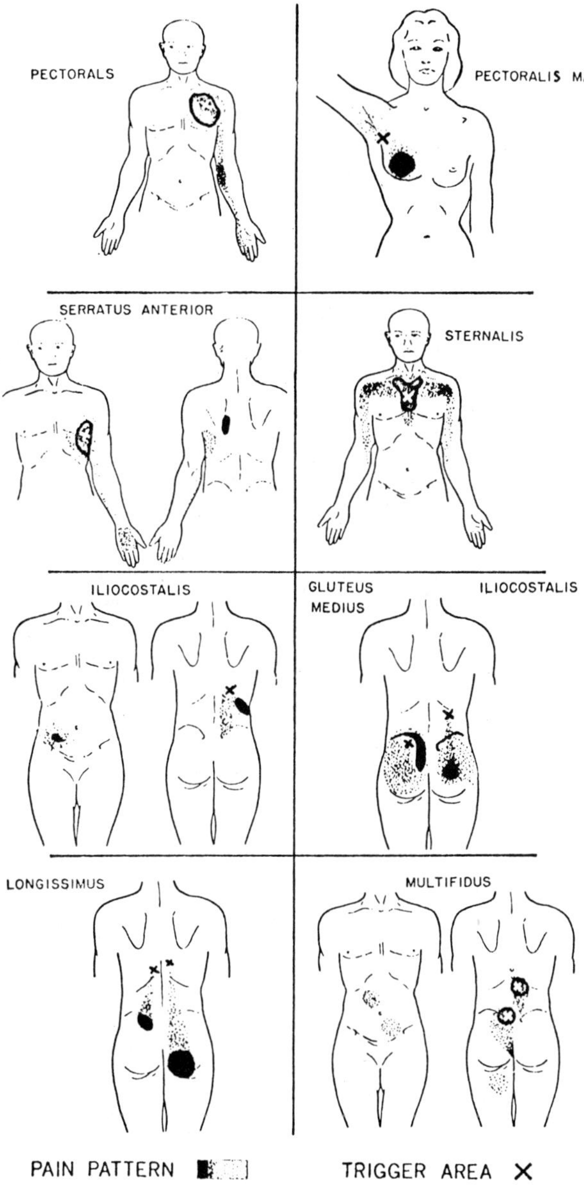

Figure 5.9. Trigger points associated with myofascial pain syndromes of the chest and back. *(Travell, J. & Rinzler, S.H. The myofascial genesis of pain. Postgrad Med 11, 1952, p. 429, with permission.)*

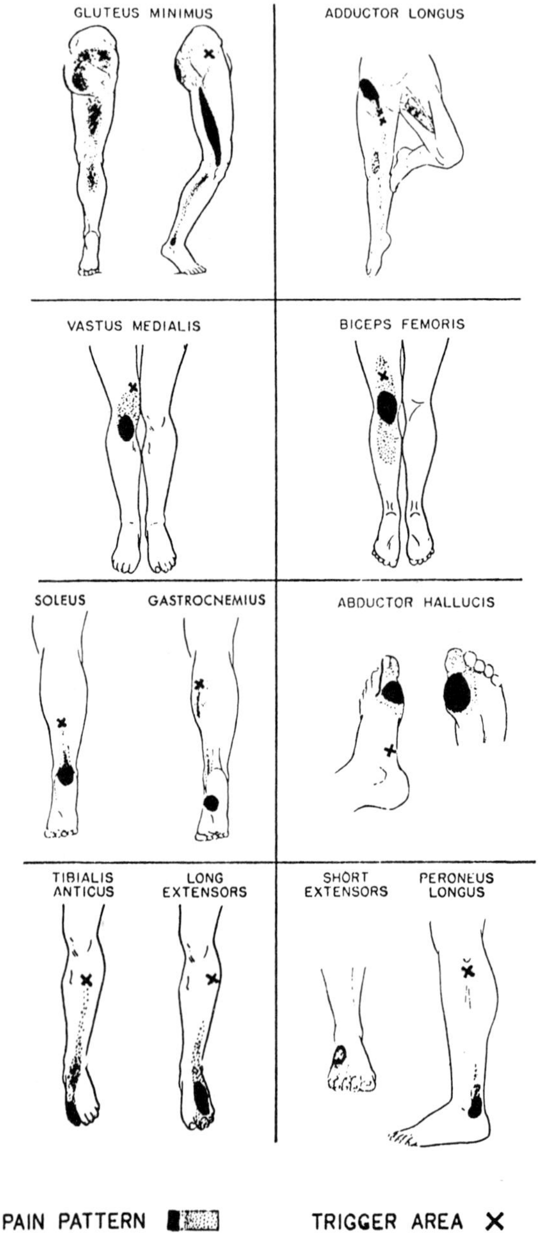

Figure 5.10. Trigger points associated with myofascial pain syndromes of the lower extremities. *(Travell, J. & Rinzler, S.H. The myofascial genesis of pain. Postgrad Med 11, 1952, p. 430, with permission.)*

point is stimulated impulses bombard the central nervous system and give rise to referred pain which may vary in intensity from a dull, aching, low-grade discomfort to pain which is severe and incapacitating. Sometimes rather intense pressure on the trigger point may be required to elicit the pain. In other instances the trigger point may be so sensitive that a breath of air will trigger pain. The more sensitive the trigger point the larger the area of referral.

Although the referred pain from trigger point stimulation does not follow known dermatomes, stimulation will produce pain in a relatively constant and predictable location. For this reason Bonica (1966, p. 109) believes that there are fixed anatomic pathways which are not known at this present time. In 1977 Melzack et al. demonstrated that *acupuncture points* correspond to a high degree with trigger points. A chart of acupuncture points is seen in Figure 5.11.

Trigger point injections, and electrical and mechanical stimulation of acupuncture points, both acupressure and needling, offer hope for pain relief for many patients with pain. Trigger points exist in a variety of diseases including myofascial (muscle and its fascia) pain syndromes and visceral diseases such as myocardial infarction.

Knowledge of referred pain is helpful to the nurse not only in assessing the patient's pain but in explaining to a patient with a common duct stone, for example, that the pain she feels between her shoulders is not necessarily indicative of an additional disease but most likely is referred pain.

Some patients do not report the location of pain because they assume the nurse knows or they think this information is relevant only to the physician in making his diagnosis. But location of pain is pertinent to nursing intervention, as the following example illustrates.

During the second day after his abdominal surgery, one patient requested medication for his abdominal pain. The nurse asked him to show her exactly where the pain was and in inspecting the area she discovered that adhesive tape had excoriated the skin. Further assessment through discussion with the patient identified this as the cause of his "abdominal pain."

Children may react differently from an adult with respect to localized pain. Following extensive surgery, a child often will refrain from moving even a finger, as if he thought the pain involved his whole body. A child who cuts his hand frequently refuses to move the entire arm. Because children do not have a complete concept of their anatomy, a child may tell you that his mouth hurts when the pain is obviously located in his inflamed and pustular throat.

Not uncommonly, an adult will report that he hurts all over. Naturally it helps to narrow it down a bit. No doubt some patients do in fact hurt all over; certain types of influenza seem to have this effect. However, such a

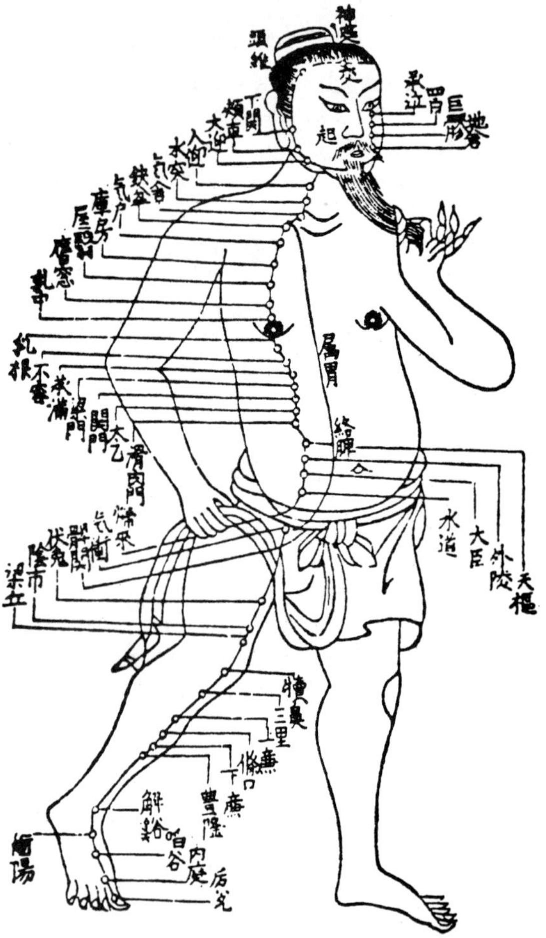

Figure 5.11. Acupuncture chart demonstrating that acupuncture points correspond to a high degree with trigger points. *(Melzack, R. & Jeans, M.E. Acupuncture analgesia. Minn Med Mar.: 161, 1974, with permission.)*

statement may be a reflection of the emotional component of the pain experience. When the patient says he hurts all over, in some instances he is really saying that the pain is a total and consuming experience. Possibly, though, the patient actually is having difficulty localizing the pain. The nurse can assist by beginning at the periphery of the body, touching each part, and asking if it hurts. The nurse might, for example, start with the fingers of the left hand, progress up the arm, and proceed to the next extremity. In this way, the patient and the nurse can discover what hurts as well as what does not hurt.

Intensity (Severity)

Hardy (1965) found that there is a maximal intensity of pain which can be perceived and that beyond that point an increase in stimulus will not cause greater pain as was discussed in Chapter 2 in relation to summation of signals.

A large number of methods have been developed to measure the *intensity* of the patient's pain. Most of the time we essentially rely upon the patient's verbal reports about his pain. This may be influenced by many variables including the patient's age, cognitive level at which he is functioning, his intelligence, vocabulary, what he believes about his pain, and the presence or absence of significant others.

Knowing the etiology of the pain may be a clue to the intensity of the pain, but usually it is not a very reliable predictor. Furthermore, the etiology of the pain is not always known. However, severe pain usually causes major disruptions to the patient's normal activities of daily living and life style, in contrast to mild pain which may not. Areas of the patient's life which need to be assessed include changes in the individual's ability to eat, sleep, work, participate in interpersonal relationships, and recreational activities. All of these variables will be considered more fully in subsequent chapters. Regardless of the etiology of the pain, the intensity can range from mild to extremely severe. In spite of these facts, it is not uncommon to hear members of the health team say "he shouldn't be having that much pain," implying that he does not and that there is a fixed pain intensity for a given diagnosis. Hence, we must somehow assess the intensity of the patient's pain directly from him.

Intensity of pain is usually assessed verbally, although sometimes paper and pencil evaluations are used particularly in research settings. Some tools are designed to measure only one component of the pain experience such as intensity. When one attempts to explain the tests and their purpose to the patient it is often somewhat difficult not to contaminate a "pure tool." For example, when asking a patient about his pain intensity for a variety of reasons it may be necessary to explain to him what you mean. Your descriptions then may represent some of the qualitive aspects. Obviously in clinical practice absolute precision is not as important as it is in research.

The following tools and methods are used primarily to measure the intensity of the pain sensation.

Currently, the most widely used rating scale for pain intensity probably is 0 to 10, 0 being no pain or least pain possible, 10 being the worst pain imaginable. An alternative is 0 to 100. The patient may be asked to rate his pain as: none, slight, moderate, severe, very severe. When pain is known to be present, some clinicians simply ask the patient to select from three categories: slight, moderate, severe (Houde et al., 1960). Another variation is: slight or little, moderate or medium, severe, or a lot (Beaver & Feise, 1977).

An example of combining numbers (*numerical scale*) and descriptive terms (*adjectival scale*) is: 0–normal, 2–uncomfortable, 4–very uncomfortable, 6–painful, 8–very painful, 10–very severe pain (Barber & Cooper, 1972). On the *McGill Pain Questionnaire* (Melzack, 1975), the intensity of pain is assessed with the following: 1–mild, 2–discomforting, 3–distressing, 4–horrible, and 5–excruciating. These terms are used to report present pain as well as variations in it in the past and comparisons with other types of pain experienced by the patient. This introduces quality with intensity.

A visual analogue scale (*VAS*) may be used. In this method a straight line may be drawn horizontally or vertically on paper. The ends of the line are defined as the extreme limits of the pain. The two ends of the line may be labeled as "no pain" and "pain as bad as it can be." The patient is asked to mark the level of his pain on this line:

No pain ____ Pain as bad as it could be.

Researchers prefer this type of scale because of its ease in use and repeated assessments of the pain can be accurately measured and mathematically computed.

A variation of this scale is to add to it a series of numbers, e.g., one through ten, at intervals along the line, or a series of descriptive terms such as those mentioned above. The patient may be asked to mark or state the number or term (Scott & Huskisson, 1976). For example, the line may be ten inches long with consecutive numbers marked at one-inch intervals. Zero may be labeled as no pain and ten as severe as it can be. The patient may then select a number to indicate the severity of his pain. Ordinarily, if he picks five, his pain is considered to be of moderate intensity.

Comparing the present pain with some pain that occurred in the past may be a useful way for the patient to describe the intensity of the pain. It may also be somewhat more understandable to the nurse, especially if the nurse has experienced the pain with which the patient is comparing his present pain. Of course, there is always the risk that the nurse and the patient will differ greatly in their perceptions of the pain they have in common. Nevertheless, especially with children, it is helpful to compare present pain to past pain regarding intensity. Language limitations and the level of cognitive development make the use of rating scales difficult with children. Making comparisons is often difficult for adults, especially those for whom English is not the primary language, who have limited language skills, or those who are especially anxious and depressed. In such instances, when the nurse can explain rating scales so that the patient can grasp them, these may be of more value.

As previously mentioned Katz (1979) studied iatrogenic anticipatory anxiety and pain in children undergoing painful procedures. The children rated both pain intensity and anxiety. Anxiety influences the qualitative aspect of the pain experience. The children's assessment of the pain intensity associated with the BMA, bone marrow aspiration, and LP, lumbar puncture, was done using a "Pain Thermometer," illustrated in Figure 5.12. The children's self-report of anxiety was done on a "Fear Face" scale, illustrated in Figure 5.13. At times these instruments may be preferable for some adult patients.

Rogers (1981) also reports the use of "Fear Faces" in measuring pain and pain relief in children eight years and younger. She has found that children over eight years of age are able to assess their pain and pain relief using some of the previously described rating scales.

There are numerous other methods of assessing the intensity of pain

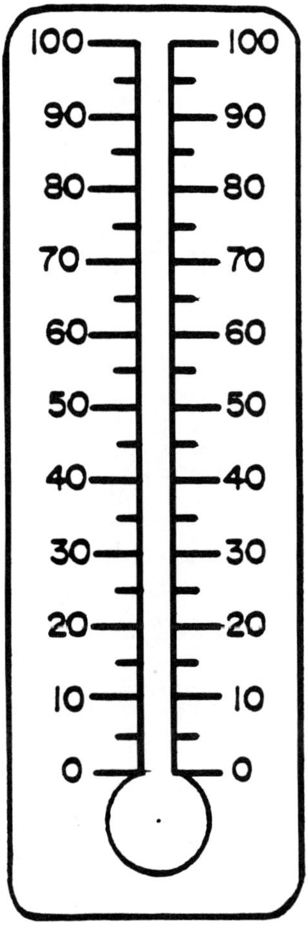

Figure 5.12. Children's pain self-report measure, pain thermometer. (BMA: Bone Marrow Aspiration/LP:Lumbar Puncture.) This thermometer tells how much you hurt during the BMA/LP.Zero (point) means you felt <u>no hurt</u>, and 100 (point) means you felt the <u>most hurt possible.</u> Point to the place that shows how much you hurt. *(Katz, E.R. Distress behavior in children with leukemia undergoing medical procedures. Paper presented at the meeting of the American Psychological Assoc., Symposium: Psychological strategies in the management of children with life-threatening illness, New York City, Sept., 1979, with permission.)*

SCARED

Now look at these faces. Think of the face marked one as not being scared at all. Think of the face marked seven as being the most scared possible.

Choose the face that shows how scared you were during the bone marrow procedure.

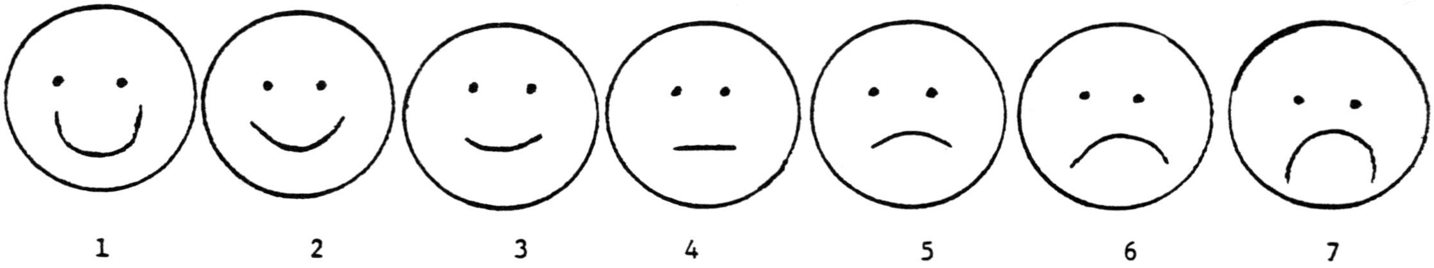

Figure 5.13. Fear faces. *(Katz, E.R. Distress behavior in children with leukemia undergoing medical procedures. Paper presented at the meeting of the American Psychological Assoc. Convention, Symposium: Psychological strategies in the management of children with life-threatening illness, New York City, Sept., 1979, with permission.)*

through the cooperation of the patient, both verbally and in writing. The patient may develop his own list of words to describe the intensity of his pain. In working with pain patients and studying their response to analgesics over a period of several days, we have seen the relevance of certain words for certain patients in describing their pain intensity and pain relief. At the beginning of the study patients are given ten words to categorize their pain from most severe to least severe. Consistently, in the 50 assessment sessions over four days, most patients select only three or four words. One elderly American man with a third-grade education found it very difficult to use most of the words normally supplied for the testing. Using a dictionary and much discussion, the words were translated into words which were more meaningful to the patient. For example, when asking him about how much relief the analgesic was still providing, the words that the patient had selected were formulated into the question "How much of the medication has not 'gone off in vapors?' " instead of the more frequent question, "Is your pain medication 'wearing off'? "

Some patients are simply unable or unwilling to use any type of multilevel rating scale for the intensity of their pain. As an example, one patient who appeared to have severe pain was only able to convey his pain intensity with the statements "I'm uncomfortable" or "I'm comfortable."

The best method to measure pain intensity for all types of patients is debatable. In one study measuring pain intensity with chronic pain patients, all patients used visual analogue, numerical, and adjectival scales. The findings were that although the patients preferred the adjectival scale their preference did not influence their reporting of their pain intensity. The intensity of pain ratings for these patients correlated significantly on all three scales (Kremer et al., 1981). These researchers believe, however, that in some clinical situations the numerical scale is likely to yield a better measurement of pain intensity. Wallenstein et al. (1980), working with cancer pain patients, have demonstrated superiority (increased efficiency and sensitivity) utilizing the visual analogue scales. They base their findings on the need for fewer patient observations to arrive at similar conclusions during analgesic assays.

Because no one method of assessing pain intensity for all patients has been found to be superior there seems to be only one logical solution: Find the method most suitable for the individual patient with whom you are working. Spare the patient by using it consistently with that patient. Communicate that method to others involved in assessing the patient's pain.

A more complete discussion of scales to measure the intensity and other qualities of clinical pain is provided by Stewart (1977).

Quality

Unfortunately, the quality of the pain sensation, per se, may be the most difficult to describe. Although the patient may easily relate the onset, location, and intensity of his pain, he may say frankly that the pain is indescribable. The varied and numerous lists of words used to communicate the quality of pain are a testimony to its illusive nature.

When the patient cannot find words to describe the quality of his pain sensation, the nurse can assist him by giving him some examples from which to choose. Since there are so many words that may be applicable, it may be difficult to know where to begin. It has been suggested that there are three main pain qualities: pricking, burning, and aching (Hardy, et al., 1952). We have found these terms very useful initially when the patient is not able to describe his pain. Usually the patient can reject one or two and elaborate on the other.

Words used to describe the quality of pain have been categorized into the three dimensions of the pain experience, by Melzack & Torgerson (1971), and are presented in Figure 2.15. One class describes the sensory aspects of pain, such as pounding (a temporal quality), radiating (a spatial quality), and hot (a thermal quality). A second class of words describes the affective aspects of pain, such as choking and cruel. A third class describes the evaluative aspects of pain, such as miserable and unbearable. Obviously, many words may overlap with other components of the patient's pain experience such as the meaning of the pain, the degree of suffering, and the intensity of pain.

As the pain becomes more severe, the patient may use a larger number of words or more complex ones. There is also a tendency for the word pain to be reserved for sensations that approach being intolerable and for words such as ache or hurt to be used for less intense pain.

The *McGill Pain Assessment Questionnaire*, Part 2, (Melzack, 1975, p. 281) is an example of a frequently used tool to assess the intensity and quality of pain. A completed copy of this tool is seen in Figure 9-2. Melzack (1975b) reports that patients respond positively to these pain descriptors. He has observed that patients are usually highly selective, rejecting many words until they find the right ones. Sometimes the patient smiles and says, "that's it." Patients also seem grateful and relieved to be provided with words to describe their pain.

Another method of assessing the quality of the pain sensation is used at the University of Washington Pain Clinic and was reprinted in a report by Isler (1975). This tool lists pairs of opposite descriptions such as hot and cold or steady and throbbing. The patient checks a space to show how closely (or whether or not) his pain resembles one of the words.

Another question that may assist the patient to describe the quality of his pain is, "What would you do to me to make me feel the pain you have?" This question was helpful in assessing phantom limb pain in an elderly woman. The patient was unable to describe the quality of her severe pain, but when that question was asked she responded without hesitation—"I'd take all the ice I could get and pile it on your leg."

Information about these areas of pain may be obtained from a variety of sources. Most often we attempt to obtain the information verbally from the adult, but in some cases written records by the patient are also very helpful. In both adults and children direct observation of nonverbal behaviors also provides valuable clues about these characteristics of pain. The patient's family and friends are additional sources of information, as well as the patient's medical record and other health team members.

Associated Factors, Variations, and Chronology

Other variables to be assessed in helping to diagnose the cause of pain include associated factors, variations, and chronology. Many types of pain, such as backache, arthritis, postoperative wound pain, and headaches will wax and wane for unknown reasons or in relation to identifiable factors. Associated factors include the history of a precipitating event such as trauma or infection; exposure to foods, drugs, or toxins; and a family history of a similar problem. Adams (1980) discusses factors such as body functions and other movements which may result in a variation in the pain. Of importance is that these variations may be diagnostically definitive in themselves. Visceral functions such as swallowing, breathing, and peristalsis are not normally painful. When pathology is present they may become painful such as the painful swallowing with tonsillitis, painful breathing with pleurisy, and the abdominal cramping with constipation. Alteration in posture, for example, which results in pain or pain relief often will be indicative or bone, muscle, or ligament conditions. Ischemic and neural pain usually increase with general body movements and subside with cessation of the movement. Further, asking the patient to cough or do a strenuous movement may more clearly delineate the pain. Such functions may reproduce radicular pain because they change the position of or stretch nerve roots, muscles, tendons, and blood vessels. Pain may be relieved by minimal treatment. For example, ingestion of food or an antacid may relieve the pain of gastritis by diluting or neutralizing gastric juices.

Variations in the patient's pain may include any or all of the characteristics previously discussed, that is, onset, duration, intensity, and quality. When variations occur in these characteristics of the patient's pain it is useful to organize the data in relation to time. Thus, we may develop a chronology of events over a 24-hour period or over a longer span of time. This may enable us to begin to identify what causes the pain or makes it worse and when pain relief would be most important.

Questions that we find especially revealing include "When (or under what circumstances) was your pain the most severe since its onset?" "When was it the least severe since its onset?" "Is there anything that you find increases your pain?" "What have you tried to do to decrease your pain?" "What have you found does decrease your pain?" "Does the time of day influence your pain?" The answers often provide a myriad of clues as to the causes of the pain and the pain relief measures most likely to be effective with that individual patient.

In general, we find that whether the pain is acute or chronic, planning nursing intervention for pain relief is greatly facilitated by having a 24-hour picture of the patient's pain. This does not always have to be based upon the patient's report. If the patient has acute pain of recent onset, he has no past experience on which to base a 24-hour report of variations in pain. However, the nurse can be alert to such possibilities as fatigue making the pain more intense at the end of the day. Whatever the variations may be, such information often suggests that pain relief is needed at certain times and not at others. Also, some pain relief measures may be more appropriate at night than in the morning.

We find the use of a pain diary in which the patient or nurse records this information very helpful. Figure 9.3 is a sample form for a pain diary. Figure 9.4 is a pain diary a patient devised and completed. Also helpful is the nurse's recording of information on a flow sheet regarding pain and its effect on the patient. A sample flow sheet with directions can be seen in Figure 10.2. Figures 10.3 and 10.4 are samples of completed flow sheets.

TYPES OF PAIN ACCORDING TO DURATION AND CAUSE

Classification of pain according to its duration and cause seems helpful since it is suggestive of the treatment for the pain and its effect upon the patient. Most attempts at such classifications of pain are rather brief with overlapping categories. Classification of a syndrome is arrived at by identifying a complex of symptoms that either result from a single cause or occur together so frequently that a definitive clinical picture is seen. It is usually based on the knowledge of the etiology and mechanism of the presenting problem. Crue et al. (1979, p. 14) state that "the *etiology* of the pain complaint is often multivariate and idiosyncratic. Furthermore, *pain mechanism* remains too complicated [in their opinion] to be presently considered a basis for classification in a useful taxonomy." For the most part, then, pain continues to be relegated to the state of being a symptom, not a definitive primary diagnosis.

This is all very unfortunate for patients with pain and those who attempt to assist them with their pain. For instance, many practitioners whose scientific orientation is not to treat symptoms until the etiology has been identified are confronted with an ethical dilemma when such information is not available for many patients presenting with a pain problem. Consequently, the patient's treatment for the pain problem may be severely deficient. Another group affected by the lack of a taxonomy for pain is the third-party carriers. Crue et al. (1979) describe attempting to get third-party carriers to pay for pain treatment often as "gamesmanship" or "one-upmanship." Illustrating this, they say that "not only are most diagnoses starting with the word 'pain' unacceptable, but 'headache' in recent years has likewise been rejected by most insurance companies. However, 'migraine' will still get through some of the time; and 'cephalgia' is still a 'winner' the majority of the time" (p. 15). Nurses are also experiencing a need for a taxonomy of pain problems (Gebbie, 1976). One nursing author, Campbell (1978, pp. 1813–1818), has formulated 57 nursing diagnoses related to pain.

"Normal" Pain

Adams (1980) points out that not all pain is indicative of injury or disease. He describes and differentiates normal and abnormal pain. *Normal pain* occurs "by the thousands as a part of daily sensory experience" in otherwise healthy individuals of all ages. The duration of these pains is brief. Common examples of normal pains include the sudden hard momentary pain felt with pressure over the temporal area over the eye, aching pains in muscles such as the "growing" pains common in children, and the fleeting precordial pain which may induce fear of heart disease. They only assume significance if the individual seeks medical care for them or if they are identified during the physical assessment for another unrelated health problem. The types of pain that we will concern ourselves with at this time are those pains which are considered as *abnormal pains*—indicative of disease or injury and those which are considered the primary diagnosis themselves. Normal and abnormal pains must be differentiated during the assessment of the pain problem.

Most authors describe pain problems in relation to a *temporal component* such as acute (brief) or chronic (prolonged). Although there are semantic differences in the use of such words, nevertheless, the temporal component serves as a springboard for communicating about pain problems. Agnew et al. (1979, p. 84) believe that the temporal component of pain is crucial and have recently proposed a classification of pain complaints based on the temporal component. Their classification is seen in Figure 5.14.

Acute Pain

Typically, *acute pain* refers to pain which has a rapid onset, which may vary in intensity from mild to severe, and which lasts from a very brief period to pain which lasts for any period of time less than six months. (Six months or more is the time frame used most often for pain research purposes.) Depending on the circumstances, acute pain has peripheral nociceptive input which serves the biologic function of warning the individual of impending or actual tissue damage or organic disease even though the cause may remain idiopathic. As healing of the causative factor occurs, pain resolves. In other words, there is an end in sight to the suffering. The time sequence in acute pain, and the fact that the pain is resolving usually results

1 *Acute*—(up to a few days); mild or severe—cause known or unknown
2 Sub-acute—(few days to a few months); though no longer an emergency, in most ways treat like acute
3 *Recurrent Acute*—Examples: Arthritis (either rheumatoid or osteoarthritis); Migraine; Primary Trigeminal Neuralgia
4 *"Chronic"*—Due to uncontrolled *malignant* neoplastic disease
5 *Chronic-Benign*—(non-neoplastic) but with seemingly *adequate coping* by the patient (usually over 6 months)
6 *Chronic Intractable Benign Pain Syndrome* (CIBPS)—Chronic pain with *poor* patient *coping.*

Figure 5.13. Temporal classification of pain complaints. *(Agnew, D.C., Crue, B.L. & Pinsky, J.J. A taxonomy for diagnosis and information storage for patients with chronic pain. Bull LA Neurol Soc 44: 84-86, 1979, with permission.)*

in more willingness by the health team to treat patients' pain with whatever seems indicated such as narcotic analgesics, sedatives, hypnotics, and general medical or surgical procedures. The patient may also be better able to cope and more willing to endure acute pain. The patient knows that there is an end in sight and is receiving treatment for the pain which is reducing it. Common examples of acute pain occur daily. Some require no treatment and are time limited such as the pain which results when one accidentally sticks his finger with a pin. Other types resolve as healing takes place, after medical or surgical treatments such as antibiotics for an ear infection or suturing of a laceration. The time sequence of the patient's reactions to acute pain is seen in Figure 5.15.

Subacute Pain

Subacute pain, sometimes referred to as *limited pain,* exists when there is known pathology but for some reason healing may be prolonged. It is that period between acute and chronic pain. Subacute pain is treated very similar to acute pain. However, there may be concern by the health team about tolerance and addiction when narcotic analgesics are being used for the control of the pain. During the subacute pain period the current practice is usually to attempt to decrease or eliminate the use of narcotics. There is usually more flexibility with other pain relief modalities especially when their liability potential is believed to be low. One example of subacute pain is a musculoskeletal injury such as crushing injury with extensive soft tissue damage and fractures. With solid fracture healing and muscle reeducation, pain usually resolves.

Recurrent Acute Pain

Recurrent acute pain, sometimes referred to as *intermittent pain,* may or may not have well-defined pathology. The frequency and duration of recurrent acute pain may vary. During the time interval between the pain episodes

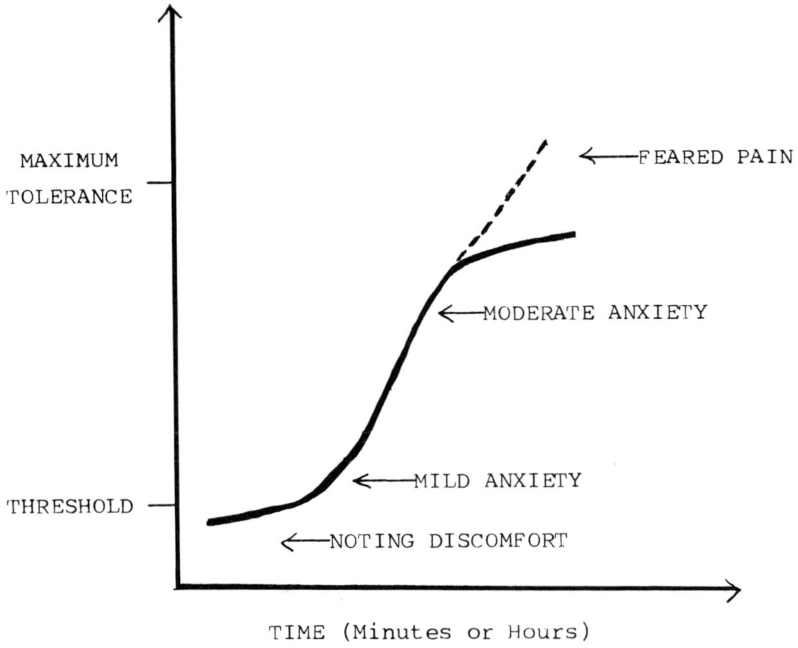

Figure 5.14. Sequence of the patient's reactions to acute pain. *(Sternbach, R.A. Pain Patients—Traits and Treatment. New York: Academic Press, 1974, p. 6, with permission.)*

the patient is pain-free, or at least has significantly diminished pain. Examples of this type of pain include Saturday morning migraines and sickle cell crisis.

Chronic Cancer Pain

Chronic pain due to *uncontrolled cancer* sometimes referred to as *intractable pain* or *limited pain,* is most often treated very much like acute pain. The health team usually is more willing to use potent narcotic analgesics and to titrate them upward or downward. Surprisingly cancer patients and their families may be the ones who are reluctant to use narcotics. Their usual reasons include not only the annoying undesirable side effects of lethargy and constipation, but very common are their fears of addiction and suppression of the immune system. Another often heard reason from patients and their families is that they are afraid that analgesics will interfere with the efficacy of their chemotherapy or radiation treatments. More information on cancer pain is presented in Chapter 6, when cancer pain is considered as a pain syndrome.

Chronic Benign or Resistent Pain

Another major classification of pain is *persistent* or *chronic benign pain*. *Chronic benign* pain refers to pain which usually lasts for more than six months and in which there may or may not be known active pathology to account for the suffering that the individual is experiencing. It often connotes pain which exists long after healing of the involved part and cessation of pain for that condition are expected to have occurred. However, the patient continues to report the presence of pain, and, in fact, he may report that the painful area has extended.

The life of the patient with chronic pain usually becomes quite constricted as he experiences a variety of changes. Indeed chronic benign pain is anything but benign. Common reports from patients with chronic pain include significant disruptions and changes in all of their normal functions such as their personal relationships, ability to think, concentrate, sleep, work, and eat. Kapp (1975, pp. 1704–1708) in defining pain as a "fusion of mind and body" says that the experience of pain requires conscious attention and self-concern. Maltbie, et al. (1978, p. 360), in discussing *ongoing pain*, add that it can destroy the individual's will to live and that suicidal preoccupation is frequent in patients with protracted pain. The sequence of the patient's reactions to chronic pain is illustrated in Figure 5.16.

Agnew, et al. (1979, p. 84), Pinsky (1978), Pinsky (1979, pp. 301–314) and Pinsky & Malyon (1979, pp. 315–327) further categorize chronic benign pain into *chronic benign pain (CBP)* and *chronic intractable benign pain syndrome (CIBPS)*. In their classification, the differentiating feature is the patient's ability to cope with his pain. Accordingly, patients with CBP usually exhibit adequate coping mechanisms, whereas patients with CIBPS usually exhibit poor coping mechanisms. At any rate, the belief by the health team is that the patient could conceivably function better in spite of his pain. Although their differentiation seems to be a helpful one, it is not frequently in use at this time. Because chronic benign pain is the more common term in the literature we will use it more globally to include both categories except when further discussing the work of Agnew, Crue, Pinsky, & Malyon.

The onset of chronic pain may be acute such as injuries or gradual such as degenerative joint disease. *Pain* itself becomes the patient's *pathology* and is considered a *syndrome*, the *primary diagnosis* and not just a symptom. Patients presenting with chronic benign pain problems include patients with low back pain, phantom limb pain, and the neuralgias, such as postherpetic neuralgia. Because there is no predictable point at which CBP will terminate, and it is often doubtful that it ever will, or that it may even become worse, there is much controversy over the treatment and rehabilitative goals for CBP patients. The value of narcotic analgesics and surgery are perhaps the two most controversial areas of treatment for these patients since, if used improperly, they may do more harm than good.

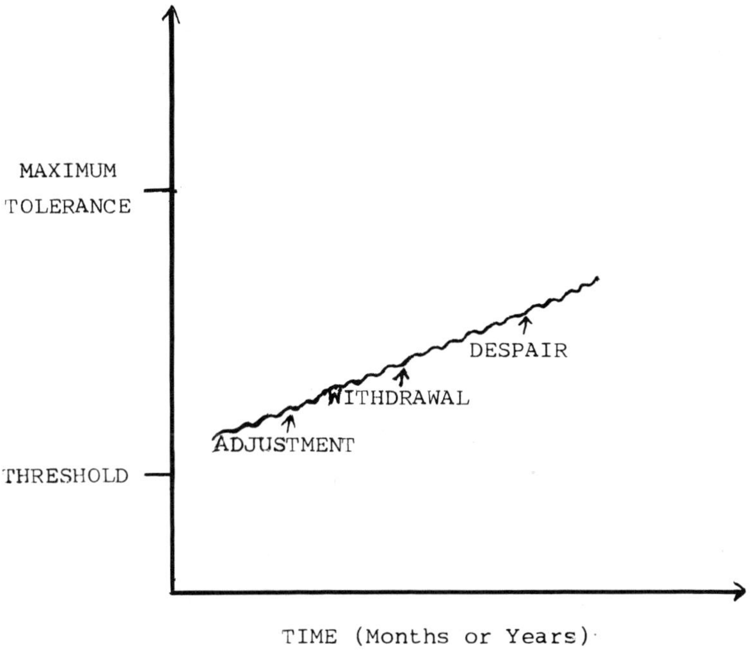

Figure 5.16. Sequence of the patient's reactions to chronic pain. *(Sternbach, R.A. Pain Patients—Traits and Treatment. New York: Academic Press, 1974, p. 8, with permission.)*

Peripheralists Versus Centralists Although the exact etiology or mechanism of chronic benign pain is not known, there are primarily two philosophical views of the problem, the peripheralists and the centralists. This does not mean to imply that either school does not acknowledge both organic and psychological mechanisms as being involved nor employ a more eclectic or holistic approach to assessment and treatment of the patient with chronic benign pain. Rather it indicates their primary approach.

The *peripheralists* use the traditional acute medical model for assessing and treating chronic pain. In doing so, they view the major portion of the patient's chronic pain as "real" or organic. The lesser mental component of the pain problem is considered psychogenic or the psychological overlay. Chronic pain is viewed the same as acute pain is in relation to etiology, that is, it is due to neurophysiologic and endocrine processes. Peripheralists believe that the pain is caused by ongoing peripheral nociceptive input from either an area of inadequate or abnormal healing (Bonica, 1979, pp. 203–207). Treatment of the chronic pain problem then is directed at stopping the peripheral cause of the pain. The patient can expect to be treated with the traditional medical and surgical approaches for his chronic pain. First line efforts are directed at resolving the underlying problem and if this is not possible, treatment is then directed at blocking or in some way interrupting the nociceptive input.

The *centralists,* on the other hand, believe that chronic pain is primarily due to psychogenic or *central mechanisms,* more of a psychosomatic process. These central nervous system (central) mechanisms include such things as one's affect and mood, the attention one pays to pain and the meaning attributed to pain and suffering. Pinsky (1979, p. 305) says that chronic pain cannot be attributed to a biologic function of tissue damage or continued peripheral stimulation because they rarely exist. Crue (1979, pp. 7–8), another centralist, says that even acute pain is a subjective experience and, therefore, better considered as a perception than a sensation. According to Crue nociceptive input from A delta and C fibers constitute only a small part of the overall patterning in pain perception. *Spatial* and *temporal summation* and *amplitude* or *intensity factors* also contribute to the "readout" of *pain perception*. Crue believes that the "peripheralists do not give due heed to the power of suggestion in light of the knowledge that even the placebo effect works through the neurophysiological endorphin mechanism" (p. 7). He hypothesizes at least three factors which may predispose an individual to chronic pain from a centralist's standpoint: (1) there may be a primary or secondary neuroanatomical or physiological lesion in the central nervous system; (2) an individual may be neuroanatomically and physiologically genetically predetermined; (3) environmental programming either prior to the onset of the chronic pain problem or acquired, as a reactive process to pain may be the predisposing culprit (pp. 8–9).

Pinsky & Malyon (1979) also approach the problem of chronic benign pain more psychologically. They say that with ongoing pain the major predisposing or perpetuating factors are unresolved and often unrecognized intrapsychic and interpersonal conflicts. They feel that the chronic benign pain patient is an individual who is generally threatened by intense affective experiences and copes maladaptively, utilizing denial, repression, and somatization. They view the individual's chronic pain problem as another example of a partial failure of an already maladaptive coping strategy resulting in inadequate or displaced attempts at gratification. According to Pinsky & Malyon, CIBPS patients are inclined to seek total relief from their suffering from sources and techniques totally outside themselves. They negate any possibility of the role of psychological events in their pain experience. Believing that an organic dysfunction is the cause of their pain problem they go to get "it fixed" (pp. 316–317). When techniques or procedures such as hypnosis and acupuncture are done to them by others in standard medical settings, they produce unsuccessful results. Although the patients appear to voluntarily cooperate in their treatments for some reason they are seen as *treatment failures* in reducing their own pain.

One speculation on why they are treatment failures is that they are unable or unwilling to accept that they in any way can modulate their own pain. Therefore, they do not really collaborate with the health team. Physical hypoactivity, dysphoric feeling states, and regressive psychosocial interactions characterize the CIBPS patients according to Pinsky & Malyon.

The idea of a patient being a *treatment failure* is, of course, an opinion that must be expressed with qualification and great caution. In some instances it is undoubtedly the treatment which has failed because it was improperly chosen or carried out. Care must be taken not to blame the patient simply and only because he did not improve as a result of a certain treatment. Many patients with prolonged pain eventually feel guilty, saying that they must somehow have caused the problem or that something must be wrong with them because they did not benefit from therapy and recover. It is not helpful to increase this guilt by blaming the patient for a treatment failure.

Livingston (1943) and Melzack (1973) propose the view that chronic benign pain is due to physiologic process even though there is no evidence of active tissue damage. They hold that a central nervous system mechanism is the culprit in the pain problem and suggest that a reverberatory or other self-sustaining neural circuit is at work. Melzack & Loeser (1978) refer to this concept as a *pattern generating mechanism*. This mechanism may be activated by even low-level input. Melzack & Dennis (1978) believe that the neural memory-like mechanism can be convincingly supported by human and animal research. One study cited was that of Reynolds & Hutchins (1948) with dental patients. Patients had teeth filled without anesthesia. Up to 70 days following this procedure, when the patient's nasal mucosa was stimulated by pinprick, pain was produced in the treated teeth. In another project a patient had four teeth extracted with nitrous oxide anesthesia. Thirty-three days following the procedure, referred pain was experienced in the jaw when the mucous membrane was stimulated with pinprick. Melzack & Dennis (1978) conclude that the input and *not* conscious awareness resulted in the abnormal neural activity. Cohen's (1944) work with angina patients, Frankstein's (1947) work with decerebrated cats, and Chamberlain, et al.'s. (1963) work with cats following transection of the spinal cord are other studies cited as producing similar evidence to that of Reynolds and Hutchins. The work of Chamberlain et al. lead Melzack & Dennis to another significant conclusion applicable to the chronic pain patient. *Permanent* changes capable of producing pain in spinal neuronal networks occurs after only 45 min. (p. 17).

There are two other views at more extreme ends of the continuum of the dilemma of the CBP problem that the nurse may encounter. Black (1980) characterizes the CBP patient as one whose condition is stable—rarely becoming worse and rarely improving. He describes the patient as one who is excessively preoccupied with multiple inappropriate complaints of pain for which he receives multiple nonproductive diagnostic procedures and treatments including the iatrogenic complications of multiple surgical procedures and drug abuse. Black (1980), quoting himself (1975) and Swerdlow (1972) say "All sufferers of the 'Chronic Pain Syndrome' have an audience for their suffering and in a most skillful manner play to that audience to obtain their immediate gains. Features of depression, anxiety, and neuroticism are present" (p. 210). Black (1980) goes on to say that the victim of this syndrome lacks realistic future plans and is impatient with any therapy requiring his active participation and time.

A seemingly contrasting view of the CBP patient is held by LaFia (1974). He characterizes these individuals as people who have been materially, spiritually, and socially fortunate in life who have been victimized and robbed of the "good life" by "chronic pains that throb and beat against their nerves, night and day" (p. 69). Their life becomes one in which their mind must constantly focus on devastating realities of their lives caused both because of the constant "agony" and the concomitant losses. These include loss of employment, income, being on a medical merry-go-round of appointments and possible litigation. Tremendous resentment is evoked in the patient and he may develop "an attitude of 'I'm a loser. What's the use? Life is passing me by.' " (p. 69).

Melzack & Dennis (1978) say "that pain therapy at present is often predicated on a one cause–one effect relationship." Because sympathetic activity, sensory input from distant areas and psychoneural activities (e.g., mood, meaning of post and present pain experiences, personality, etc.) also influence pain perception, once the pain pattern is produced any input is capable of triggering the pain mechanism. Treatments for pain then should be multimodal aimed at modulating the specific input causing the pain. CBP has been successfully treated with such techniques as trigger point injections TENS and acupuncture. It is believed that these treatments interrupt the neural memory-like mechanism for pain perception. Although the results of such pain relief measures vary in time from no pain relief to pain relief just during the treatment to permanent relief in the same patient they certainly widen the pain relief horizons for most CBP patients.

In addition to the obvious increased comfort there are other reasons that such pain relief measures are warranted and of value to the CBP patient. Melzack & Dennis (1978) say that when the pain is blocked patients resume normal physical activities and these activities may prevent pain by preventing resumption of the abnormal nociceptive input. This is based on the fact that if the other neural input, such as propriception, is more intense and travels the same neural circuitry it overrides nociceptive impulses. In addition, distinction of the mechanism of CBP may prevent patients from inadvertently receiving psychiatric diagnosis such as conversion hysteria or hypochrondriacal neurosis or even more derogatory labels such as malingerer or "crock." Although the theory is still speculative, they believe, nevertheless, it is still useful.

Compounding the patient's pain problem and belief system may be the ensuing medical and surgical efforts and the subsequent communications, all of which may further decrease the patient's ability to function with CBP. As treatment failures occur, physicians often recommend that the patient decrease activity and impose other physical restrictions. The consequences of this may be to inadvertently increase the patient's pain and reinforce feelings of futility about his or her situation. Pain and suffering become a hallmark of this patient's adaptive style causing marked psychosocial disruptions. Szasz (1975) says that these repeated treatment failures with resultant ineffective coping may cause the *painful person* not to want to relinquish his suffering and chronic pain becomes a career. The patient becomes totally consumed with pain and attempting to cope with it. All of this process is based on unconscious mechanisms according to Pinsky & Malyon (1979, p. 317). The tragedy is that the quality of the patient's life may be totally and permanently destroyed.

The information available on children with chronic pain is more limited than that for adults. However, the same conflict regarding treatment seems to exist. According to Varni et al. (1980), most treatment approaches for children with chronic pain stress the importance of allowing children to express the emotions associated with their pain. The benefit of this empathetic approach may have important psychiatric benefits for the child, however, the therapeutic effectiveness in relation to accomplishing rehabilitation goals is still unproven. They believe that pain behaviors during the chronic pain experience *may* be used by the children for secondary gains of staff attention and avoidance of therapy thus extending the time for optimal rehabilitation. They make two major recommendations regarding the treatment plan for children with chronic pain. First, assessment must be made of what the pain behaviors are, when they occur and the effect they have on the therapeutic goals. Second, using an operant conditioning approach to treatment, the goals should not be the total suppression of pain but the encouragement of well behaviors when *pain behaviors* previously interferred with the long-term rehabilitation process.

Bonica (1979) believes that the across-the-board generalizations about chronic pain patients is unwarranted. He documents his conclusion with two studies in which he participated. In the first study (Pilowsky, et al., 1977, pp. 183–192), the relevant finding was that the majority of chronic pain patients fell into a "nondepressive syndrome category." Only a minority were found to have endogenous depression, a symptom frequently used as a hallmark of the chronic benign pain patient. In the second study, Chapman, et al. (1979, pp. 1–7) studied patients both in private practice and multidisciplinary pain clinics. One relevant finding of this study was that the characteristics of the patients in these two settings differed. An important point that Bonica makes is that much of the work reported with chronic pain patients has been reflective of patients treated in multidisciplinary pain clinics. He notes that patients who are treated in these clinics represent a highly select group of patients who present with a high percentage of psychologic or operant mechanisms for their pain problem, thus a very skewed population has been studied. Bonica says that the recent trend to believe that most, if not all, patients with persistent pain develop chronic pain behaviors due to reinforcement from those in their environment is not valid. He goes on to say that this belief results in injustice to many patients with chronic pain syndromes whose persistent pain complaints are due to dysfunction of the nociceptive system (p. 206).

During the experience in working with patients with all kinds of pain problems, the nurse will undoubtedly come across other individuals on the health team who represent divergent philosophies on the assessment and treatment of pain. We maintain that the greatest service that the nurse can provide to any patient is to listen and believe what the patient says about pain. After all he or she remains the only authority about it. In assessment, the bottom line is acknowledging the subjectivity of the pain experience. It is the patient's pain. Psychogenic versus organic may be irrelevant. This was so succinctly stated by one patient reported by Crue et al. (1979). A physician was attempting to convince a patient of the possibility that there may be some psychogenic component to her pain experience and that this component was considered to be "suffering." The patient's retort was "Doctor, that is just plain foolishness. It is all suffering."

In the next chapter we will consider some of the most common pain syndromes.

REFERENCES

Adams, R.D. Pain general considerations. In K.J. Isselbacher, R.D. Adams, E. Braunwald, et al. (Eds.), Harrison's Principles of Internal Medicine (9th ed.). New York: McGraw-Hill, 1980, pp. 12–26.

Agnew, D.C., Crue, B.L., & Pinsky, J.J. A taxonomy for diagnosis and information storage for patients with chronic pain. Bull LA Neurol Soc 44: 84–86, 1979.

Barber, T.X., & Cooper, B.J. The effects on pain of experimentally induced and spontaneous distraction. Psychol Rep 31: 647–651, 1972.

Beaver, W.T., & Feise, G.A. Comparison of the analgesic effect of oxymorphone by rectal suppository and intramuscular injection in patients with postoperative pain. J Clin Pharmacol 17: 276–291, 1977.

Black, R.G. The chronic pain syndrome. Surg Clin North Amer 55(4): 999–1011, 1975.

Black, R.G. The clinical syndrome of chronic pain. In L.K.Y. Ng & J.J. Bonica (Eds.), Pain, Discomfort and Humanitarian Care. Proceedings of the National Conference, National Institute of Health: Bethesda, MD, Feb. 15-16, 1979. New York: Elsevier/North-Holland, 1980, pp. 207–219.

Bonica, J.J. Management of pain in general practice—Practical therapeutics. GP Jan.: 107–123, 1966.

Bonica, J.J. The relation of injury to pain (Letter to the Editor) Pain 6: 203–207, 1979.
Brain, R. Clinical Neurology, 2nd. ed. New York: Oxford University Press 1964.
Campbell, C. Nursing Diagnosis and Intervention in Nursing Practice. New York: Wiley, 1978.
Chaffee, E.E. & Greisheimer, E.M. Basic Physiology and Anatomy, (3rd Ed.) Philadelphia: J.B Lippincott, 1974.
Chamberlain, T.J., Halick, P., & Gerard, R.W. Fixation of experience in the rat spinal cord. J Neurophysiol 26: 662–676, 1963.
Chapman, C.R., Sola, A., & Bonica, J.J. Illness behavior and depression compared in pain center and private practice patients. Pain 6: 1–7, 1979.
Cohen, H. The mechanism of visceral pain. Trans Med Soc London 64: 65–69, 1944.
Copp, L.A. The spectrum of suffering. Amer J Nurs 3: 491–495, 1974.
Crue, B.L., Jr. A physiological view of the psychology of pain. Bull LA Neurol Soc 44(1–4): 1–13, 1979.
Crue, B.L., Jr., Pinsky, J.J., Agnew, D.C., et al.: Observations on the taxonomy problem in pain. In B.L. Crue, Jr. (Ed.), Chronic Pain. New York: SP Medical and Scientific Books, 1979.
Frankstein, S.A. One unconsidered form of the part played by the nervous system in the development of the disease. Science 106: 242–244, 1947.
Gebbie, K.M. (Ed.). Summary of the second national conference: Classification of nursing diagnosis. St. Louis, MO.: Clearinghouse—National group for classification of nursing diagnosis, 1976.
Guyton, A. Textbook of Medical Physiology (6th ed.). Philadelphia: W.B. Saunders, 1981.
Hannington-Kiff, J.G. Pain Relief. Philadelphia: Lippincott, 1974.
Hardy, J.D. The nature of pain. J Chronic Dis 4: 22–51, 1956.
Hardy, J.D., Wolff, H.G., & Goodell, H. Pain Sensations and Reactions. Baltimore: Williams & Wilkins, 1952.
Houde, R.W., Wallenstein, S.L., & Rogers, A. Clinical pharmacology of analgesics. 1. A method of assaying analgesic effect. Clin Pharmacol Therapeut 1: 163–174, 1960.
Isler, C. For severe pain, self-medication on demand. RN 38: 51–60, 1975.
Jacob, S.W., Francone, C.A., & Lossow, W.J. Structure and Function in Man (4th ed.). Philadelphia: W.B. Saunders, 1978.
Jensen, D. The Principles of Physiology. New York: Appleton-Century-Crofts, 1980.
Johnson, J.E. Effects of accurate expectations about sensations in the sensory and distress components of pain. J Personal Social Psychol 27: 261–275, 1973.
Kapp, F.T. Psychogenic pain. In A.M. Freedman & H.I. Kaplan (Eds.), Comprehensive Textbook of Psychiatry, II. Baltimore: Williams & Wilkins, 1975, pp. 1704-1708.
Katz, E.R. Distress Behavior in Children with Leukemia Undergoing Medical Procedures. Paper presented at the American Psychological Association Convention. Symposium: Psychological strategies in the management of children with life-threatening illness, New York City, Sept. 1979.
Keegan, J.J., & Garrett, F.D. The segmental distribution of the cutaneous nerves in the limbs of man. Anatom Record 102: 411, 1948.

Kremer, E., Atkinson, J.H., & Ignelzi, R.J. Measurement of pain: patient preference does not confound measurement. Pain 10: 241-248, 1981.

LaFia, D.J. New Hope for Relief of Pain. New York: Hawthorn Books, 1974.

Livingston, W.K. Pain Mechanisms. New York: Macmillan, 1943.

Maltbie, A., Cavenar, J., Hammett, E., et al. A diagnostic approach to pain. Psychosomatics 19(6): 359-366, 1978.

McCaffery, M. Nursing Management of the Patient with Pain (2nd ed.). New York: Lippincott, 1979.

Melzack, R. The Puzzle of Pain. New York: Basic/Harper Torchbooks, 1973.

Melzack, R. The McGill pain questionnaire: Major properties and scoring methods. Pain 1: 277–299, 1975.

Melzack, R., & Dennis, S.G. Neurophysiological foundations of pain. In R.A. Sternbach, (Ed.) The Psychology of Pain. New York: Raven Press, 1978, pp. 1–26.

Melzack, R., & Jeans, M.E. Acupuncture analgesia. Minn Med, 57:161-166, Mar., 1974.

Melzack, R., & Loesser, J.D. Phantom body pain in paraplegics: Evidence for a central "pattern generating mechanism" for pain. Pain 4: 195–210, 1978.

Melzack, R., Stilwell, D.B., & Fox, E.J. Trigger points and acupuncture points for pain: Correlations and implications. Pain 3: 3–23, 1977.

Melzack, R., & Torgerson, W.S. On the language of pain. Anesthesiology 34: 50–59, 1971.

Mountcastle, V.B. Med Physiol, Vol. 1 (14th ed.). St. Louis: C.V. Mosby, 1980.

Pilowsky, I., Chapman, C.R., & Bonica, J.J. Pain, depression and illness behavior in a pain clinic population. Pain 4: 183–192, 1977.

Pinsky, J.J. Chronic intractable benign pain: A syndrome and its treatment with intensive short-term group psychotherapy. J Human Stress 4: 17–21, 1978.

Pinsky, J.J. Aspects of the psychology of pain. In B.L. Crue, Jr. (Ed.), Chronic Pain. New York: SP Medical and Scientific Books, 1979, Chap. 22, pp. 301–314.

Pinsky, J.J., & Malyon, A.K. The intractable pain and suffering process—Facilitating change and the eclectic nature of psychotherapy in the treatment of chronic pain syndromes. In B.L. Crue, Jr. (Ed.), Chronic Pain. New York: SP Medical and Scientific Books, 1979, Chap. 23, pp. 315–327.

Posner, J.B. Pain. In P.B. Beeson, W. McDermott, & J.B. Wyngaarden (Eds.), Cecil Textbook of Medicine (15th ed.). Philadelphia: W.B. Saunders, 1979, pp. 720–728.

Reynolds, O.E., & Hutchins, H.C. Reduction of central hyper-irritability following block anesthesia of peripheral nerve. Amer J Physiol 152: 658–662, 1948.

Rogers, A. Personal communication, March 12, 1981.

Schwartz, S.I., & Storer, E.H. Manifestations of gastrointestinal disease—Pain. In S.E. Schwartz, G.T. Shires, F.C. Spencer, et al. (Eds.), Principles of Surgery (3rd ed.). New York: McGraw-Hill, 1979, pp. 1039–1042.

Seiden, M.R. Practical Management of Chronic Neurologic Problems. New York: Appleton-Century-Crofts, 1981.

Sternbach, R.A. Pain Patients: Traits and Treatments. New York: Academic Press, 1974.

Stewart, M.L. Measurement of clinical pain. In A.K. Jacox, (Ed.), Pain: A Source Book for Nurses and Other Health Professionals. Boston: Little, Brown, 1977, pp. 107–137.

Swerdlow, B. The pain clinic. Brit J Clin Pract 26(9): 403–407, 1972.
Travell, J. & Rinzler, S.H. The myofascial genesis of pain Postgraduate Medicine, 11: 427, 1952.
Varni, J.W., Bessman, C.A., Russo, D.C., et al.: Behavioral management of chronic pain in children. Arch Phys Med Rehab 61: 375–379, 1980.
Vaughn, G.F. Children in hospital. Lancet 1: 1117–1120, 1957.
Wallenstein, S.L., Heidrich, III, G., Kaiko, R., et al. Clinical evaluation of mild analgesics: The measurement of clinical pain. Brit J Pharmacol 10: 319S–3275S, 1980.
Wolff, B.B. Behavioural measurement of human pain. In R.A. Sternbach (Ed.), The Psychology of Pain. New York: Raven Press, 1978, pp. 129–168.

SUGGESTED READINGS

Bradley, L.A., Prokop, C.K., Gentry, W.D., et al. Assessment of chronic pain. In C.K. Prokop & L.A. Bradley (Eds.), Medical Psychology—Contributions to Behavioral Medicine. New York: Academic Press, 1981.
Brannon, M.E. The problem back. Amer J Nurs 75(18): 1295–1297, 1975.
Brena, S.F., Chapman, S.L., Stegall, P.G., et al. Chronic pain states: Their relationship to impairment and disability. Arch Phys Med Rehab 60: 387–389, 1979.
Copley, I.J. No matter what you call it, it's still pain to the patient. RN 41: 64, 1978.
Crue, B.L., Jr. Chronic Pain. Further Observations from City of Hope National Medical Center. New York: SP Medical and Scientific Books, 1979.
Eland, J.M. Living with pain. Nurs Outlook 26: 430–431, 1978.
Epstein, M.H., & Harris, J.J. Children with chronic pain—Can they be helped? Pediatr Nurse 4 (Jan–Feb.): 42–44, 1978.
Fordyce, W.E. A behavioral perspective on chronic pain. In L.K.Y. Ng & J.J. Bonica (Eds.), Pain, Discomfort and Humanitarian Care. Proceedings of the National Conference held at the National Institute of Health, Bethesda, MD, Feb. 15-16, 1979. New York: Elsevier/North Holland, 1980, pp. 233–252.
Gildea, J.H., & Quirk, T.R. Assessing the pain experience in children. Nurs Clin North Amer 12 (4): 631–637, 1977.
Graceley, R.H. Pain measurement in man. In L.K.Y. Ng & J.J. Bonica (Eds.), Pain, Discomfort and Humanitarian Care. Proceedings of the National Conference held at the National Institute of Health, Bethesda, MD, Feb. 15-16, 1979. New York: Elsevier/North-Holland, 1980, pp. 111–137.
Hackett, T.P. Pain and prejudice. Why do we doubt that the patient is in pain? Med Times 99: 130–134, 1971.
Jacox, A.K. (Ed.). Pain, A Sourcebook for Nurses and Other Health Professionals. Boston: Little, Brown, 1977.
deJong, R.H. Occasional notes. Prof. R. Hall's three phases of pain. N Eng J Med 20: 1129–1130, 1979.
Le Shan, L. The world of the patient in severe pain of long duration. J Chron Dis 17: 118–126, 1964.
Lewis, T. Pain. New York: Macmillan, 1942.

Luckmann, J., & Sorensen, K.C. Medical-Surgical Nursing—A Psychophysiologic Approach (2nd ed.). Philadelphia: W.B. Saunders, 1980.

Mankin, H.J., & Adams, R.D. Pain in the back and neck. In K.J. Isselbacher, R.D. Adams, E. Braunwald, et al. (Eds.), Harrison's Principles of Internal Medicine (9th ed.). New York: McGraw-Hill, 1980, pp. 38–48.

McCaffery, M. Intelligent approach to intractable pain. Nurs 73 3: 26–32, 1973.

McCaffery, M. Pain relief for the child. Pediatr Nurs 3: 11–16, 1977.

McCaffery, M. Understanding your patients' pain. Nurs 80 10: 34–39, 1980.

Merskey, H. et al. (15 authors) IASP subcommittee on taxonomy Pain terms: A list with definitions and notes on usage. Pain 6: 249–252, 1979.

Pace, J.B. Helping patients overcome the disabling effects of chronic pain. Nurs 77: 38–43, 1977.

Pollin, W., Griffith, J.D., Gracely, R., et al.: (Panel). Understanding pain—Measurement and pharmacology. In L.K.Y. Ng & J.J. Bonica (Eds.), Pain, Discomfort and Humanitarian Care. New York: Elsevier/North-Holland, 1980, pp. 107–137.

Sternbach, R.A. Clinical aspects of pain. In R.A. Sternbach (Ed.), The Psychology of Pain. New York: Raven Press, 1978, pp. 241–265.

Twycross, R.G. The assessment of pain in advanced cancer. J Med Ethics 3 (4): 112–116, 1978.

Walker, H.K., Hall, W.D., & Hurst, J.W. (Eds.). Clinical Methods—The History, Physical and Laboratory Examinations (2nd ed.). Boston: Butterworth Publishers, 1980.

Wall, P.D. On the relation of injury to pain. The John J. Bonica Lecture. Pain 6: 253–264, 1979.

Wolff, B.B. Behavioural measurement of human pain. In R.A. Sternbach (Ed.), The Psychology of Pain. New York: Raven Press, 1978, pp. 129–168.

6

Pain Syndromes

Although pain from malignant and life-threatening conditions are usually agreed upon as capable of producing severe and/or prolonged pain, many other pain syndromes which are not life threatening often produce severe pain. In fact, suicidal ideation may not be an uncommon fantasied or acted upon solution for severe pain. This is especially true for individuals whose life becomes dominated by pain to the degree that the person's entire existence becomes riveted on minimizing and preventing pain and obtaining pain relief. Furthermore, when one develops a pain syndrome in response to treatment of a serious pathological state such as a neuropathy from vincristine therapy for cancer, it may be very difficult to convince the patient that his pain is not due to a recurrent malignancy. In addition, patients with severe pain may be more vulnerable to exploitation by and temptation to invest in quackery and gimmicks and charlatans because they desperately seek a miracle cure or treatment. As will be discussed later in this chapter, patients with chronic pain may also be victims of inappropriate polysurgery and polypharmacy by even well-meaning physicians attempting to respond to these patients' pleas to "do something."

It is impossible to cover all of the causes of pain therefore we will just consider some of the major pathological pain syndromes and some of the conditions which are most frequently associated with producing severe and/or prolonged pain. Some of the syndromes we will consider include pathological pain syndromes such as causalgia, trigeminal neuralgia, postherpetic neuralgia, myofascial pain, headaches, pain syndromes associated with cancer, and labor pain.

PATHOLOGICAL PAIN SYNDROMES

The first major category of pain syndromes we will address are those which Ruch (1979) refers to as pathological pain states. Ruch says that "all sensory pain-inducing processes are pathological but that some are more pathological than others" (p. 273). He categorizes pain processes into pain of pathology and pathological pain. He defines *pain of pathology* as pain that serves as a warning to the individual of impending or actual tissue damage which arise in nonneural structures such as the skin, viscera, and muscles. *Pathological pain*, on the other hand, is pain which arises in neural structures and occurs spontaneously without an apparent stimulus. Pathological pain has three hallmarks. First, the pain is accentuated by affective processes. Second, the pain *is not responsive* to medications including potent analgesics, which ordinarily are effective against severe pains of pathology. And third, neurosurgical procedures done to relieve pathological pain often result in an even more agonizing pain syndrome (p. 275). The acuity of the pain determines whether or not Ruch considers it pain of pathology or pathological pain. For example, an acute nerve injury is pain of pathology, whereas, to have pathological pain, chronic injury to the nerve is necessary. Pathological pain is sometimes divided into peripheral pain and central pain. The dichotomy is not "pure" because the mechanism of the pain syndromes are not completely understood and there may be more than one mechanism involved in different pain syndromes. Rather, peripheral and central pain refer more to the site in the nervous system where the pathology originated.

When one attempts to discuss spontaneous pain syndromes, one is again acutely reminded of the confusion caused by the lack of a taxonomy of pain problems. Almost every author uses their own system. In our discussion, we will use the classifications of peripheral and central pain syndromes. About these pain syndromes, Mountcastle (1980, p. 417) says "these pains are among the most severe known to man and they completely dominate the behavior of the sufferer and they present extraordinarily difficult therapeutic problems."

Peripheral Pain Syndromes

Reflex Sympathetic Dystrophies A picture of the reflex sympathetic dystrophies is provided by Bonica (1966, pp. 121–122,) and Posner (1979, pp. 727–728). Reflex sympathetic dystrophies is a collective term descriptive of a variety of conditions which result from injury to a peripheral nerve or to an extremity. These disorders which we will consider include causalgia, postherpetic neuralgia, and phantom limb pain. In the reflex sympathetic dystrophies, whatever the diagnosis, the pathophysiology, clinical picture, and response to therapy are similar. Signs and symptoms may be present in varying degrees or one sign or symptom may so dominate as to obscure the others. Rarely is the entire syndrome seen in one patient. The *reflex sympathetic dystrophies* are characterized by continuous severe pain, usually burning in quality, *hyperalgesia*, excessive sensitivity to pain (primary and secondary hyperalgesia were discussed in Chapter 2), *hyperesthesia* (excessive sensitivity to stimuli); or *hypoesthesia*, decreased sensitivity to stimuli. Other terms used may be *dyesthesias*, abnormal responses to stimuli, and *hyperpathia*, the affective response to stimuli is abnormally disagreeable. Hyperalgesia and hyperesthesia may be so severe that movement or touching the involved extremity may be considered unbearable by the patient. Pain is initially located at the site of the injury or in the injured nerve. Later it may spread and involve the entire extremity. In addition to the pain there is other sympathetic hyperactivity. This includes vasospasm and vasomotor changes. Initially there is vasodilatation, the skin being warm and dry. Later there is vasoconstriction with the skin being cool, cyanotic, and edematous. Other autonomic changes include *sudomotor disturbances*, (exerting an influence on the sweat glands), either *hyperhidrosis* (excessive sweating) or *hypohidrosis* (absence of sweating), *trophic, cutaneous*, and *skeletal muscle changes*. If the problem goes untreated one can expect that there will be a minimum of delayed functional recovery of the extremity or a maximum loss of function of the extremity. It may be so severe as to necessitate the amputation of the extremity. Considering that a sympathetic response is already involved in these reflex dystrophies, it is not surprising that with physical and emotional stress the syndrome is usually exacerbated. The etiology of the reflex sympathetic dystrophies varies and may result from a seemingly trivial injury or to a major injury of an extremity that may or may not involve a peripheral nerve. The suggested pathophysiology is the generation of afferent nociceptive impulses from the injured site resulting in disturbances in the internuncial pools of the spinal cord triggering widespread excitation in the central nervous system.

Causalgia The *causalgia syndrome* usually referred to just as *causalgia*, follows the above general picture of reflex sympathetic dystrophies. More specifically, however, there is pain in the area of a partially injured peripheral nerve. Although it is possible, rarely is the nerve completely transected. Causalgia may be due to injury of the ulnar or radial nerves, but most commonly lesions are of the brachial plexus, median, or sciatic nerve. The onset of the causalgia is usually within one to two weeks after the injury. The pain is described as burning, severe, diffuse, and persistent. The most common areas of pain are in the palms of the hand, soles of the feet, and in the digits. Occasionally, there are spontaneous episodes of more acute pain. Hyperalgesia and hyperesthesia are often so severe that almost any stimulus is capable of triggering the much dreaded pain. For example, the patient may be unable to tolerate contact of clothing and he may constantly protect and immobilize the involved limb. The pain may be increased by almost any peripheral sympathetic activity. Heat, noise, and emotional stress are very commonly reported as the triggering sources. Skin changes vary and the skin may be shiny and smooth or scaly and discolored. There may be excessive growth of the nails. Also, swelling, and stiffness of joints may occur. When there are sudomotor changes, the most common change is hyperhidrosis in the palms of the hands or soles of the feet. When the extremity is at rest, vasomotor changes may cause the limb to be either warmer or cooler than usual. There may be spontaneous recovery from the causalgia syndrome.

Several pathophysiological mechanisms are proposed: Activity in large myelinated afferent nerves may impinge on and increase the controlling action of the central regulating system. Another possibility is that anoxia within the injured nerve alters the transmission of impulses. That is, the normal or subthreshold afferent impulses in the C fibers at the site of the injured nerve are damaged so that transmission of impulses is prolonged or becomes repetitive.

Brechner (1982), describes three progressive stages of the causalgia syndrome. The acute stage is a stage of severe pain and paresthesias; the second stage, the chronic stage, occurs three to six months following the onset of the injury. In this stage, the painful state is accompanied by vasomotor changes especially marked edema and color changes (reddish-purple coloring) of the involved extremity. The third stage, called Sudeck's atrophy (Sudeck's-Leriche syndrome), is a disuse syndrome consisting not only of muscle atrophy but also of osteoporosis. The end result is a severely painful hyperesthetic dysfunctional extremity. The pain may be so severe that the patient requests amputation of the extremity which in some cases is indeed done. Of course, this offers the patient the possibility of another pain problem, phantom limb pain, which will be discussed later.

Brechner is emphatic when discussing the necessity of early treatment of causalgia in the prevention of both physical progression and the development of a chronic benign syndrome. Unfortunately, causalgia may become a vicious cycle pain problem for the patient. That is, the patient is unwilling to use the involved extremity due to the severe pain and paresthesias and the disuse phenomena results in increased pain and paresthesias. Rehabilitation involves early treatment aimed at having the patient use the extremity. To accomplish this nerve blocks followed by intensive physical therapy are usually necessary. Brechner believes that causalgia is at least partially caused by central mechanisms involving psychological variables. She illustrates her view by describing one 12-year-old girl who developed causalgia following a rather minor fracture of the ulnar. Following the divorce of her parents, the child's father failed to visit her unless a specific need heralded him. According to Brechner this child had learned that sick-role behavior yielded results from her father. Indeed, he became very involved in this patient's care. The patient was successfully treated by a nerve block, intensive physical therapy, and individual and family psychotherapy.

Unfortunately, all patients do not recover as well. Causalgia is often misdiagnosed and treatment comes all too late. Nurses may make a very valuable contribution in the assessment of this difficult pain problem.

Postherpetic Neuralgia *Postherpetic neuralgia* is a pain syndrome which follows an acute central nervous system infection primarily of the dorsal root ganglia, by the varicella-zoster virus, the same virus that causes chickenpox. The *herpes syndrome* is characterized by a vesicular eruption and neuralgic pain in the radicular distribution of the peripheral nerves arising from one or more of the involved dorsal root ganglia. Because of the distribution of the nerves, the vesicular eruption and pain is usually unilateral and encircles the body in band-like clusters. The areas most frequently involved are the thoracic, cervical, lumbar, and sacral areas and the opthalmic division of the trigeminal nerve. Pain often precedes the herpes zoster eruption by several days. The severity of the pain may vary from mild to severe. The quality may be burning, sharp, or dull. Occasionally, motor paralysis also occurs in the affected areas. Although hyper- and hypoesthesia may linger after the lesions have cleared, by far the most difficult residual problem is the severe intractable pain sometimes with episodes of lightning-like pain in the area of the original skin eruption. Young patients may experience the pain syndrome for a short period following the disappearance of the lesions. However, the elderly and the immunosuppressed patients may experience the postherpetic syndrome for months and years. When the syndrome becomes disseminated or does not resolve in two weeks a search must be made for an underlying malignancy which may be predisposing the patient to the syndrome. The cause of the postherpetic pain syndrome is not fully understood. Possible considerations include degenerative changes in the spinal cord, dorsal root ganglia, or nerve trunks.

Phantom Limb Pain *Phantom limb pain* must be differentiated from phantom limb sensation and stump pain. *Phantom limb sensations* include tingling, itching, and sweating in the illusionary limb. Phantom limb sensations occur in almost all patients who have had a body part amputated either surgically or traumatically and in those who have had any interruption or denervation of sensory pathways in the spinal cord or brain. *Phantom limb pain* occurs with significantly less frequency than phantom limb sensations. Estimates vary from 2 percent (Sternbach, 1968) to 35 percent (Melzack, 1973), depending on the criteria used. For example, Seiden (1981, p. 54) says that temporary phantom limb pain occurs in 30 percent of the patients but only 5 to 10 percent of the patients experience permanent phantom limb pain. Phantom limb pain most frequently occurs immediately following the amputation, but occasionally the "limb" may gradually become more painful with time.

Although a patient may have *stump pain*, postoperative discomfort in the surgical site, in addition to the phantom limb pain, they are not necessarily related to each other. The quality and characteristics of phantom limb pain may vary. The pain may be described as a severe burning fiery sensation, crushing, cramping, a sense that the limb is edematous, or a sensation that the limb is being twisted or is in a distorted position that the patient is unable to change. Craig (1978, p. 86) reports four rather unusual features associated with phantom limb pain. First, phantom limb pain is more likely to occur if the patient has had pain in the limb prior to amputation. Second, if pain was present prior to the amputation, the phantom limb pain will be qualitatively similar to the preamputation pain. Third, individuals experiencing traumatic injuries, especially those who do not regain consciousness, prior to their amputation, rarely experience phantom limb pain. Fourth, the individual may experience the limb as being in the same position that it was in immediately prior to the amputation.

Phantom limb pain may be triggered by many things including touching the amputated stump, the occurrence of another illness, fatigue, atmospheric changes, and emotional stress. Phantom limb pain that does not resolve with time may be evoked by touching other healthy areas of the body. The pathophysiology of phantom limb pain is not fully known. Because transecting the spinal cord, sympathectomy, and other surgical procedures to interrupt the sensory pathways may not completely eliminate phantom limb pain other possible mechanisms for the pain have been proposed. Melzack & Loeser (1978, pp. 195–210) postulated *pattern generating mechanisms*. These mechanisms include the entire gating system in the dorsal horn, the homologous in the brain and the regions in the brain which subserve pain. Once the phantom limb pain pattern generating mechanism has been established almost any stimulus is capable of triggering it.

Central Pain Syndromes

According to Ruch (1979, p. 287) the *central pathological pain syndrome*, or *central pain*, is thought to be due to pathological central neurons which may spontaneously produce high-frequency bursts of impulses. "Denervation hypersensitivity has been suggested as the cause of this abnormal neuronal discharging." We will consider two pain syndromes that are commonly considered in the central pathological pain syndrome category—the thalamic pain syndrome and the trigeminal neuralgia pain syndrome.

Thalamic Syndrome The *thalamic syndrome* is described by Guyton (1981, p. 672) and Mountcastle (1980, p. 419). Typically the thalamic syndrome is characterized by severe, spontaneous, and often continuous pain and hyperesthesia on the contralateral side of the lesion in the thalamus. The location of the pain is described as varied with the pain sometimes spreading to areas of the body that are quite distant to that stimulated. Although the pain threshold is considered normal or even elevated the pain intensity may be so severe that it cannot be adequately controlled by narcotics. In addition, stimuli that are considered normal are capable of producing this severe pain.

The mechanism responsible for the thalamic syndrome is not fully understood. The most common cause of this syndrome is an acute irritative lesion or process that destroys the central or lateral nuclear complexes of the dorsal thalamus resulting in the discharge of high-frequency central neurons concerned with pain transmission. It is believed that, because the medial nuclei of the thalamus are not involved, they then become hypersensitive which facilitates transmission of nociceptive input. One rather common example of a patient who may experience the thalamic syndrome is the patient who has suffered a cerebral thrombosis. The vascular lesion causes the degeneration of the thalamic nuclei and thus the thalamic syndrome also.

As mentioned in Chapter 2, the thalamus is the relay station in the brain and one of its major roles is to maintain tonic activation of the central nervous system. Therefore, another possible cause of the thalamic syndrome could be anything that interrupts the transmission of afferent impulses to the thalamus. Such causes may include degeneration of myelinated fibers or peripheral nerves. Because of the major relay function of the thalamus, any disturbance in the thalamus can be expected to produce a myriad of symptoms in addition to the possible pain syndrome. For instance, all contralateral sensory transmission may be lost. *Proprioception* and *kinesthetic senses* may be lost so that the patient is ataxic. He may experience *asterognosis* (the inability to recognize familiar objects by feeling their shape). Another very disturbing problem for the patient is that he may have marked *affective changes* which most often are extremely unpleasant, often terminating in emotional tirades.

After a period of several weeks or months, the patient may regain some sensory abilities. Unfortunately, their return may be even more problematic for the patient because they may increase the hyperesthesia and result in a lancinating type of pain. In the presence of a known thalamic insult, the thalamic syndrome is usually easily recognizable.

***Trigeminal Neuralgia** (Tic Doloreaux)* Bonica (1966, pp. 120–121) defines *neuralgia* as any type of pain which has a segmental or peripheral nerve distribution. *Trigeminal neuralgia* can be described as paroxysms of lancinating or lightning-like stabs of intense pain in the distribution of one or more divisions of the trigeminal nerve, the fifth cranial nerve. Pain most frequently is in the second and third divisions and only rarely is the opthalmic division involved. Therefore pain is experienced usually in the mouth, gums, lips, side of the nose, cheek, chin, and on the surface of the head.

Commonly, it is precipated by mechanical stimulation of areas, but in the absence of this, pain may still spontaneously occur. Everyday events "trigger" the painful episodes including talking, eating, washing the face, shaving, putting on lipstick, and brushing one's teeth. The pain may occur for only a few seconds or it may be almost continuous. Most typically scientists describe the pain of trigeminal neuralgia as bursts of pain lasting for a few seconds occurring in clusters, spontaneously remitting. However, the patients often describe their pain as lasting for hours. The severity may cause the patient to wince, thus the name, *Tic doloreaux*. The pain of trigeminal neuralgia is so severe that patients will refrain from anything which may trigger it including talking, washing their face or brushing their teeth. The more serious consequences of this pain syndrome include dehydration, wasting, and exhaustion, especially if the pain has been ongoing for a period of time.

Two interesting facts about trigeminal neuralgia are that the pain rarely occurs at night and the syndrome is most common in the spring and in the fall.

Trigeminal neuralgia, like other neuralgias, often is indicative of underlying pathology such as inflammatory, circulatory, degenerative, or neoplastic processes which are causing the neuritis. More specifically, trigeminal neuralgia may be indicative of multiple sclerosis, lesions in the posterior fossa, or dental problems. According to Mountcastle (1980, pp. 418–419) one theory for this pain syndrome is that there is damage to the fibers of the root or ganglion allowing for "cross-talk" between mechanoreceptive and nociceptive fibers.

PAIN WITH UNDERLYING PATHOLOGY SYNDROMES

Musculoskeletal Pain Syndromes

Musculoskeletal pain syndromes are among the most common causes of chronic pain although they also present severe acute problems. Many conditions are capable of causing severe pain in the musculoskeletal structures—the bones, joints, cartilate, synovial membranes, fibrous sheath, muscles, and tendons. Some of these painful conditions are due to fractures, intervertebral disc protrusions, tendonitis, bursitis, severe muscle spasm, acute and chronic arthritis. Of the most common are those that are classified as myofascial pain syndromes. One of the most common of the musculoskeletal pain problems is the low back pain syndrome.

Patients with musculoskeletal pain syndromes may present with an acute or chronic onset, which is local or referred (radicular or trigger point) and which varies significantly in intensity. All of these were discussed in Chapter 5. The patient with an acute process is most likely to present with localized pain and marked limitation of mobility and function. The patient with a chronic pain problem may present with less pronounced symptoms.

Of the musculoskeletal pain syndromes bone pain is usually one of the easiest to assess. It is usually described as being deep aching, poorly localized pain. Pain in other musculoskeletal structures is usually described as steady, sometimes intermittent, sharp or dull, sometimes diffuse with variations influenced by position and activity by the patient. Qualitative descriptors contribute to the diagnosis although they are not definitive in themselves. For example, pain which is described as aching and cold may be caused by nerve root compression, a vascular lesion or even severe muscle spasm. Characteristics of pain in musculoskeletal tissue are presented in Table 6.1.

Assessment of tenderness and referred pain often are very helpful when assessing musculoskeletal pain problems. Of course it is important to determine where the pain is being referred from, such as from another neuromuscular structure or a viscera. Referred pain in neuromuscular and skeletal structures may be that of a trigger point or radicular nature. Trigger points which are palpable with their unique pattern of referral are common in musculo-skeletal pain syndromes especially the myofascial ones. When radicular pain is present it is important to assess for other corroborating neurological findings. Important to assessment of musculoskeletal pain problems is knowledge of the sensory and motor levels of the spinal cord. Figure 6–1 illustrates common patterns for pain, areas to which

TABLE 6.1. Characteristics of Pain in Musculoskeletal Tissues

Issue	Characteristics
Bone	Slow pain; ache; poorly localized; often throbbing. Aggravated by forces of all attached muscles, aggravated by torque (applied manually) and percussion. Causes pseudoparalysis of all attached muscles. Tenderness, but localization of tenderness mediocre.
Muscle belly	Mostly slow pain at rest; aching, some fast pain on contraction. Aggravated directly by contraction of affected muscle and by passive stretch. Poor subjective localization. Affected muscle protected by pseudoparalysis. Tenderness with good localization. Wasting in pain of long duration, plus osteoporosis in activated bones, plus joint contracture.
Tendon, ligament, fascia	Mostly slow pain at rest: some fast pain on contractile force; localization poor; tender, and localization of tenderness is good.
Bony attachments of tendon, ligament, fascia	Mixed slow and fast pain; localization good; protected by pseudoparesis or pseudoparalysis; tenderness accurately localized.
Hyaline Cartilage	Totally insensitive.
Synovia	Slow pain; ache; poorly localized. May produce the gelation phenomenon.

(Frost, H.M. Musculoskeletal Pain. In Alling C.C., III (ed.), Facial Pain. Philadelphia: Lea and Febiger, 1968, p. 159, with permission.)

COMMON SINGLE NERVE ROOT SYNDROMES

LOWER CERVICAL

FIFTH CERVICAL

PAIN UPPER BORDER SCAPULA.

TENDERNESS OVER TRANSVERSE PROCESS C4–5 VERTEBRAE.

RADIATION OF PAIN TO ANTERO-LATERAL ARM.

NUMB SENSATION ANTEROLATERAL FOREARM.

HYPOALGESIA AS OUTLINED. MORE EVIDENT DISTALLY.

REFLEX OF BICEPS TENDON REDUCED.

MOTOR WEAKNESS & ATROPHY OF SERRATUS MAGNUS (WINGED SCAPULA) AND ANTERIOR DELTOID MUSCLES.

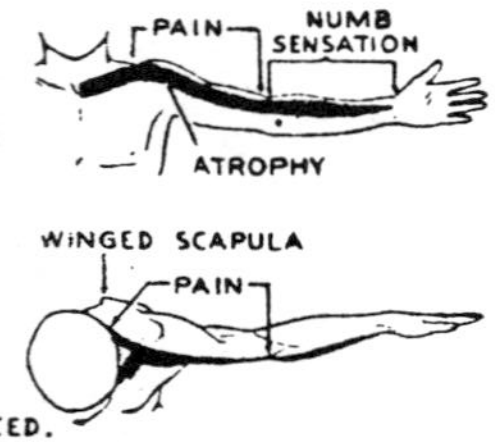

SIXTH CERVICAL

PAIN UPPER MEDIAL SCAPULA.

TENDERNESS OVER TRANSVERSE PROCESS OF VERTEBRA.

RADIATION OF PAIN TO LATERAL ARM.

NUMB SENSATION OF THUMB.

HYPOALGESIA AS OUTLINED.

REFLEX OF BICEPS TENDON REDUCED OR ABSENT.

MOTOR WEAKNESS & ATROPHY OF THUMB, BICEPS AND SCAPULAR MUSCLES.

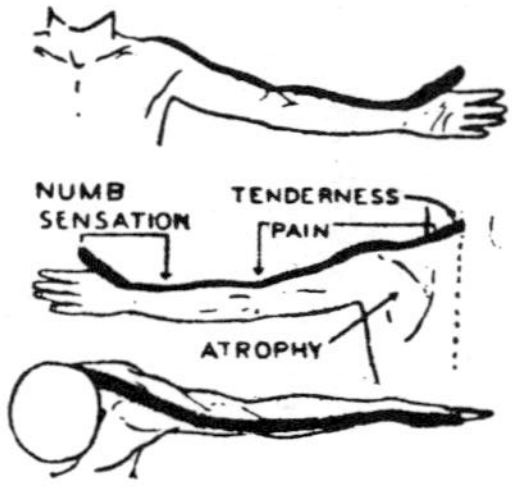

SEVENTH CERVICAL

PAIN UPPER MEDIAL SCAPULA.

TENDERNESS OVER TRANSVERSE PROCESS OF VERTEBRA.

RADIATION OF PAIN TO POSTERO-LATERAL ARM.

NUMB SENSATION 2ND & 3RD DIGITS.

HYPOALGESIA AS OUTLINED.

REFLEX OF TRICEPS TENDON REDUCED OR ABSENT.

MOTOR WEAKNESS & ATROPHY OF TRICEPS MUSCLE.

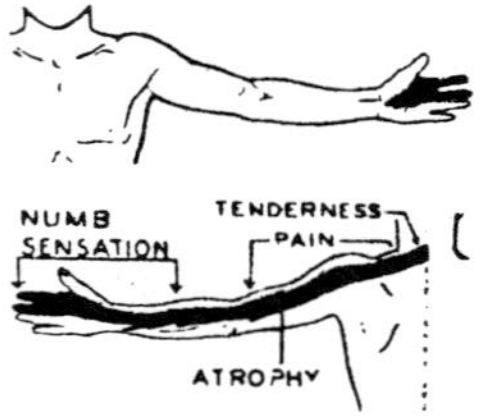

EIGHTH CERVICAL

PAIN OVER MEDIAL SCAPULAR SPINE.

TENDERNESS OVER TRANSVERSE PROCESS OF VERTEBRA.

RADIATION OF PAIN TO POSTERO-MEDIAL ARM.

NUMB SENSATION 4TH & 5TH DIGITS.

HYPOALGESIA AS OUTLINED.

REFLEX NO CHANGES RECOGNIZED.

MOTOR WEAKNESS & ATROPHY OF INTRINSIC MUSCLES OF HAND.

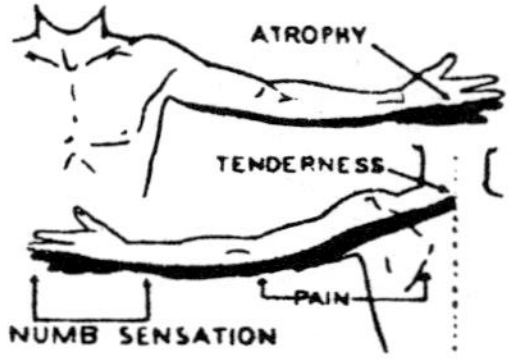

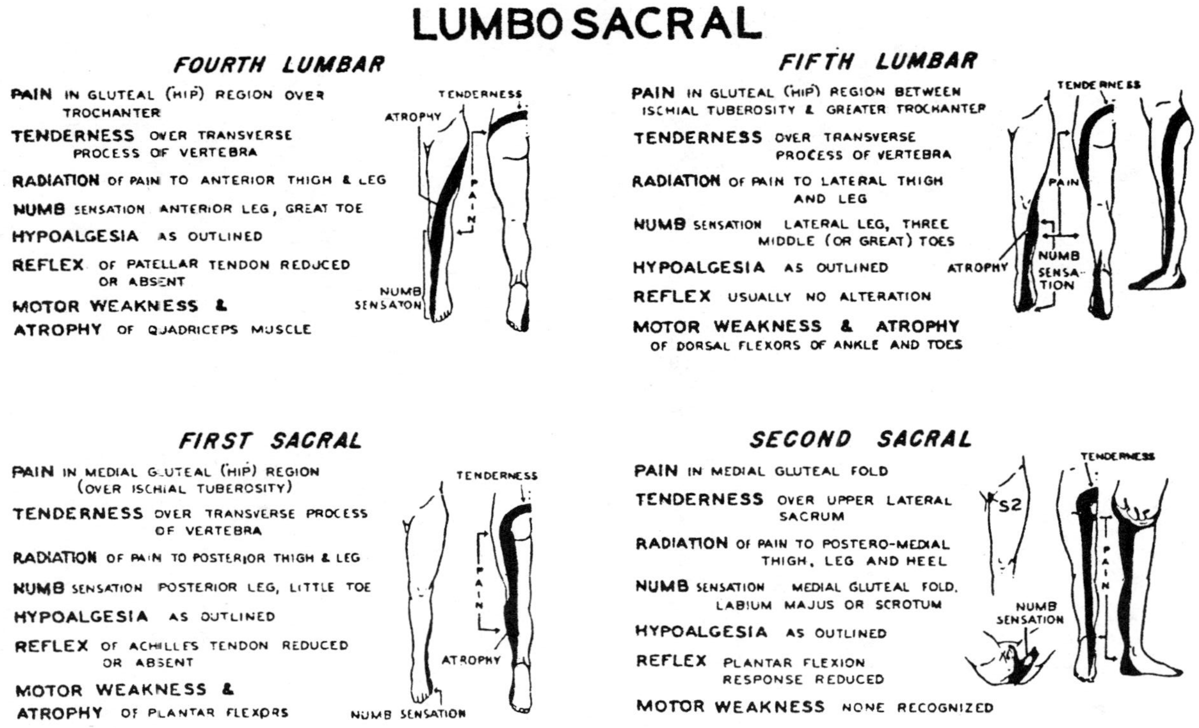

Figure 6.1. Common Single nerve root syndromes. *(Keegan, J.J. Variations of symptoms with herniation of intervertebral discs Nebraska Medical Journal, 1958, 43, Figure 2, p. 191, with permission.)*

the pain radiates, numbness, hypoalgesia, motor weakness, atrophy and reflex changes.

Unfortunately, pain assessment in musculoskeletal problems may be quite difficult for the patient and those assessing his problem. Considered to be of diagnostic significance is if the pain is increased by walking, standing, lifting, and the valsalva maneuver (sneezing, coughing, or straining at stool). These symptoms may be positive with both muscle spasm and nerve root compression. Sometimes of diagnostic significance is the fact that nerve root pain may come on a week or so after injury whereas muscle spasm most often comes on dramatically at the time of the injury or a day or two later. Also muscle spasm and nerve root compression pain frequently coexist and may be involved in bone disease.

Observation of the patient doing specific motions and functions which the patient reports aggravate his pain often are helpful. One patient, a 33-year-old man, had a history of a painful shoulder for many years. He had had innumerable consultations and followed all of the prescribed medication, treatment, and exercise regimes. However, he was never significantly improved nor was the improvement ever sustained. One day during an examination the patient moved his arm to remove his shirt for his shoulder to be inspected. With this movement his shoulder dislocated in the presence of the examiner. A diagnosis of congenital absence of tendons was made and confirmed at surgery.

Pain which markedly alters one's activities of daily living or one's life style usually is considered more indicative of a more serious pathological process than is pain which is less disruptive. The lifestyle and personality of the patient must be correlated with the assessment of any change presumed to be due to the patient's pain. One patient who had musculoskeletal surgery never reported multiple significant changes in her activities and life style. To compensate for her deficits the patient paid to have many things done for her such as cooking and cleaning. Although the patient had almost constant moderate pain, the criteria she had used about her ability to continue with her normal life was her ability to find other ways to continue working and doing other things which she enjoyed being involved in. When her limitations came to the attention of her physician her pain problem was reassessed and, indeed, the patient had a secondary treatable problem causing the pain.

In addition to listening to the patient, this situation illustrates another important point in the assessment of musculoskeletal problems. Many conditions are almost impossible to diagnose until a major structural or functional loss occurs. The patient and physician must be aware and willing to repeat, persistently, the assessment process as long as the problem occurs. Even if the pain problem is diagnosed as a chronic benign pain syndrome, a change may be indicative of an underlying pathological process.

When a patient presents with what seems to be a musculoskeletal pain problem one must keep in mind that the *single most important source of information is most likely going to be the patient*. Diagnostic procedures for musculoskeletal problems are limited and often inconclusive. Further, the validity of these reports is often dependent on the skill of the individual interpreting the results and, at best, often is equivocal. Misdiagnosing the patient's pain problem and possibly delaying treatment is likely if we fail to give credence to or lightly dismiss what the patient is telling us. This is even more problematic if the patient is presenting an atypical pain syndrome or one for which there is limited knowledge and experience.

Myofascial Pain Syndrome *Myofascial pain syndrome* is a broad term, descriptive of pain in the muscles and fascia. Conditions included in this syndrome are many which are similar or closely related such as myositis, fibrositis, myofibrositis, myalgia, and muscle strain.

Myofascial pain syndromes which are contrasted with intervertebral disc syndromes in Table 6-2 are among the most frequent causes of severe disabling pain. The most frequently involved structures are the shoulder girdle, neck, and low back. According to Bonica (1966, p. 119), myofascial

TABLE 6.2. Differential Diagnosis between Herniated Disk and Myofascial Syndrome.

Herniated Disk with Root Compression	Radicular Pain Secondary to Myofascial Syndrome or Postural Disorder
Increased pain with Valsalva (cough, strain) present	None or minimal
Focal neurologic signs present	None
Positive Lasègue, crossed straight-leg raising sign	Lasègue is sometimes present but crossed straight-leg raising sign negative
Tenderness in sciatic notch and along sciatic nerve present	Usually absent
Pain on lateral movement of spine present	Usually absent
Painful trigger points sometimes present	Painful trigger points and skin hypersensitivity present
Bladder and bowel function may be impaired	Sphincters not involved unless iatrogenically by drugs
Spasm of back muscles present	Spasm of back muscles present

(Seiden, M.R. Practical Management of Chronic Neurologic Problems. New York: Appleton-Century-Crofts, 1981, p. 60, Table 8, with permission.)

pain syndromes are often misdiagnosed and wrongly treated. These syndromes are characterized by the presence of trigger points in muscles or connective tissue together with a specific syndrome of pain–muscle spasm–tenderness–stiffness, limitation of motion, weakness, and occasionally autonomic dysfunction. Pain is described as dull and aching. The intensity varies from mild to severe and disabling. Initially it is localized to the affected muscle or muscle group. If the pain persists other muscle groups may become involved. This is more likely to occur if the patient assumes an abnormal posture, attempts to splint the involved muscles and an ongoing muscle imbalance results or there is repeated trauma. Tenderness is usually experienced in the affected muscles. Palpitation of trigger points which reproduce the pain in their distribution often confirms the diagnosis.

Myofascial pain syndromes are caused by acute trauma or prolonged sustained muscle contractions such as that resulting from poor posture, or too vigorously exercising muscles which are infrequently used, as with the weekend athlete or gardener.

Intervertebral Disc Syndrome Ruptured, herniated, or prolapsed intervertebral discs are another major cause of severe pain syndromes. The discs which are most likely to rupture are those between the fifth lumbar and first sacral intervertebral spaces. Although these discs constitute approximately 98 percent of the discs which rupture, according to Kraus (1970), they are not the major cause of *low back pain.* Only about 20 percent of patients with low back pain have an organic or structural basis for their pain. Fifty percent of patients with intervertebral disc disease in the low back have a history of major trauma. That the low back is most frequently involved does not seem surprising when one considers the demands placed on this area of our body. The low back assumes most of the burden of keeping us vertical and accommodates most of the activities in which we participate, such as walking, standing, and lifting.

The next most frequent discs to rupture are those of the cervical area. The most common intervertebral discs at the cervical level are those between the fifth and sixth interspace. Although trauma may cause a ruptured cervical disc the most common cause is degenerative arthritis.

With ruptured intervertebral discs there may be little or no relationship between the presenting signs and symptoms and the underlying pathology. Sometimes neurological deficits occur due to cord compression as the presenting symptom. Although the symptoms may be bilateral, unilateral symptomatology is by far more common and is due to unilateral displacement of a spinal nerve. Bilateral symptoms are more likely to occur if the extrusion of the nucleus pulposus (disc material) is large and it is centrally located and compresses the spinal cord or displaces bilateral spinal nerves.

The most frequent symptoms of ruptured intervertebral discs are pain and limitation. These symptoms often begin simultaneously and occur following trauma or stress on the involved disc. The onset of pain associated with disc syndrome may not occur for a week or so after the injury. Irritation or compression of nerve roots produces a well-defined mild to severe radicular pain in the area of the dermatome of the involved nerve root. This radicular pain is considered to be a reliable diagnostic symptom of intervertebral disc rupture. Pain is usually intensified with motion due to the stretching of the nerve root. To test for this, patients with low back pain are asked to do straight leg raising and patients with cervical root symptoms are asked to hyperextend or flex their neck. Corroborative neurological signs and symptoms of ruptured intervertebral disc include sensory and motor deficits in the distribution of the involved nerve root distribution. Sensory changes which are common include numbness, paresthesias, hypo- and hypersensitivity. Motor changes include fasciculations (spontaneous contractions of a number of muscle fibers, fascicles, supplied by a single motor nerve), weakness, flaccidity, and atrophy. Patients with lumbar and cervical ruptured discs may have involvement of the sphincters. Therefore it is important to assess any change in the patient's ability to defecate or urinate, including difficulty in initiating the process, retention, and incontinence. Figure 6–1 illustrates the most common single nerve root syndromes. Compression of the spinal cord may become an emergent situation. Patients with suspected ruptured intervertebral discs must be frequently and scrupulously assessed for this possibility.

Arthritis Arthritis is a chronic, systematic, often very painful disease of connective tissue. It is one of the major disabling chronic diseases in the United States. Approximately 10–15 percent of patients with arthritis are classified as totally disabled, unable to do most activities of daily living, some confined to a bed or wheelchair. The most common types of arthritis are rheumatoid arthritis (RA) and osteoarthritis. When rheumatoid arthritis occurs in children it is referred to as juvenile rheumatoid arthritis (JRA). Although the most common form of arthritis is osteoarthritis, by far the most potentially disabling form is RA. Osteoarthritis, sometimes referred to as degenerative arthritis, primarily occurs in weight bearing joints and is slowly progressive. It has been referred to as benign with a good prognosis.

Arthritis specifically refers to diseases of the joints, whereas *rheumatism* implies both joint and muscle involvement. *Nonarticular rheumatism* involves structures which are contiguous to joints such as tendons, muscles and fibrous sheaths. The cause of arthritis is unknown. Possible causes include viral, metabolic, and autoimmune processes. Arthritis sometimes is part of another disease complex or accompanies it such as psoriatic arthritis, and some veneral and viral diseases.

Rheumatoid arthritis is characterized by pain, inflammation, swelling, tenderness, and stiffness in the involved joints. Most frequently the onset is gradual with progressive joint involvement. However, it may also occur abruptly with simultaneous inflammation in multiple joints. Physical and emotional stress are often associated with the onset. There may be periods of unexplained exacerbations and remissions. Although arthritis may occur in any joint it most frequently occurs in the small joints of the hands, wrists, elbows, feet, and ankles. Joint involvement is usually bilateral. Stiffness in the joints is common on arising in the morning and may occur with any period of inactivity. As the patient becomes active, the stiffness gradually subsides. Joints and surrounding structures are progressively destroyed by the chronic inflammatory process. Normal tissue is replaced by granulation tissue. Deformities may develop rapidly due to both the proliferative inflammatory process in the joint and the painful spasms of flexor muscles and relaxation of the extensor muscles.

RA may be a difficult disease to initially or definitively diagnose. Patients may be required to undergo many repeated laboratory and other diagnostic procedures. Pain accompanies not only the disease but the treatment phase of arthritis. Often therapy is necessary when the acute process subsides to reverse some of the painful contractures which have occurred.

Headache

Headache is the most common type of deep somatic pain. It affects 90 percent of the population in one form or another (Plum, 1979, p. 728). Seiden (1981, p. 69) agrees and adds that "almost every individual experiences a headache at some time during their life." She adds that approximately 50 percent of the population regardless of sex report severe or disabling headaches. Some researchers classify headaches by their location, such as intracranial and extracranial (Guyton, 1980, p. 621; Plum, 1979, p. 729). Others classify headaches based on the causative mechanism such as dilation of vascular structures and changes in intracranial pressure (Adams, 1980, p. 19; Harvey, 1980, pp. 1255–1262; Mountcastle, 1980, pp. 415–417). The location, duration, onset, and associated factors of the most common types of headache are presented in Table 6.3.

Some headaches are symptomatic of underlying pathology while others represent the primary diagnosis. Headaches commonly caused by underlying intracranial pathology include intracranial infection, tumors, head injuries, hypoxia, and hypertension. Extracranial causes of headaches include systemic infections and conditions which affect proximal structures including eyes, ears, nose, sinuses, throat, and teeth. Other causes of headaches may include posttraumatic syndromes, psychogenic headaches, and conditions such as constipation and "hangover."

The quality of the pain and localized tenderness are important to the diagnosis of headache. The quality of the pain of headache is usually described as diffuse, dull, deep, and aching pain, although it may also be

TABLE 6.3. Common Forms of Headache

	Location	Duration	Onset	Associations
Muscle contraction	Occipital Posterior cervical	Hours to days	Gradual	Emotional stress Head and neck position
Migraine	Any area May be unilateral and repetitive	Hours	Gradual	Positive family history Aura secondary to vasoconstrictive events
Cluster	Temporal-ocular areas	Hours Groups of attacks	Abrupt	Homolateral vasocongestion and lacrimation Often nocturnal
Lumbar puncture	Occipital to frontal	Hours	Abrupt on standing	Relieved by lying down
Trigeminal neuralgia	One of more disease of 5th nerve (Unilateral)	Minutes to hours	Abrupt	"Trigger" areas often present Occur in attacks
Subarachnoid hemorrhage	Postcervical Occipital Frontal	Hours to days	Abrupt	Very severe Nausea, vomiting, Lethargy Localizing signs (Partial III nerve paresis)
Meningitis and encephalitis	Postcervical Frontal	Days	Gradual	Fever, lethargy, seizures
Cranial arteritis	Temporal areas	Weeks	Gradual	Painful vessels Systemic symptoms Increased E.S.R. Retinal arteritis Anterior optic neuritis
Hypertension	Occipital Frontal	Weeks	Gradual	Worse in A.M.

(McKhann, G. M. & Speed, III, W. G. Disorders of Sensation: Pain and Headache. In Harvey, A. M., Johns, R. J., McKusick, V.A. et al. The Principles and Practice of Medicine, 12th ed. New York: Appleton-Century-Crofts, Table 125-2, p. 1257, 1980, with permission.)

reported as sharp or throbbing. Still other patients may report their headaches as a feeling of pressure, tightness, or bursting. The severity or intensity of headaches varies. Intense pain is commonly reported by patients with significant organic pathology such as meningitis and subarachnoid hematoma. However, benign conditions such as the common migraine and cluster headaches are also often reported as severe. Yet, increased intracranial pressure may not cause any pain until it causes tension on proximal, pain-sensitive structures. The pain of headache often has a "self-intensifying" component. That is, the pain from the headache may result in reflex contractions of extracranial muscles not only of the head but also the neck and shoulders thus the mechanism discussed under "Extracranial Headaches" all come into play.

The location of the headache may be helpful in the diagnosis, but, it may also add to the confusion. For headaches which have a regional referral such as to the sinuses and teeth may be very helpful, whereas, headaches referred to the eyes and ears may not. Symptoms caused by headaches involving deep intra- and extracranial structures are usually diagnostically significant.

The onset, duration, frequency, time course (changing, unchanging, worsening, alternating in quality) of headaches often presents helpful information about the cause. For example cluster headaches usually have an abrupt onset, often occur following the ingestion of substances containing vasodilators such as alcohol, histamine, and nitrites. Their duration usually is a few minutes to a few hours. The patient may have several attacks over a period of a few days or weeks and then be asymptomatic for months.

Other important factors to be considered when assessing the patient with a headache include prodromal signs and symptoms which may be fairly specific for one type of headache, such as confusion or hemiplegia occurring with the vascular headaches. Sometimes the headache will be associated with other symptoms or phenomena such as nausea, vomiting, visual changes, mood, and personality changes. There may be a familial incidence as seen in both vascular and common migraine headaches. Biologic and environmental conditions may influence pain such as premenstrual tension and atmospheric conditions like cold weather.

Other factors to be considered are the history of previous trauma; exposure to drugs or industrial toxins; precipitating factors, coughing, sneezing, straining at stool, fatigue, excessive sleep; special foods; day of the week; posture; drugs, such as birth control pills; and emotional imbalance. Alleviating factors such as pressure on temporal arteries, ice packs, position, past and present drug regime, and a quiet dark room may also be informative.

Nociception of Headaches The general anatomy and physiology related to transmission of nociceptive impulses to the brain was presented in Chapter

2. Briefly, but more specifically, nociception related to headaches is as follows:

Both intracranial and extracranial structures may be responsible for headaches. Most of the intracranial structures are not pain-sensitive. Intracranial structures which are *insensitive* to pain include the brain parenchyma, most of the dura and pia–arachnoid, the ependymal lining of the ventricles, and the choroid plexuses. Obviously, then, most headaches are not specifically caused by brain pathology. The surrounding intracranial structures which are innervated by nociceptive afferents include the venous sinuses and their tributaries from the surface of the brain, arteries within the dura mater, the anterior and middle meningeal arteries, the cerebral arteries of the Circle of Willis, and portions of the dura mater at the base of the brain. Nerves which transmit nociceptive impulses causing headaches include cranial nerves V, the trigeminal nerve; VII, the facial nerve; IX, the glossopharyngeal nerve; and X, the vagus nerve. The upper first three cervical spinal nerves also transmit nociceptive impulses which can cause headaches. Nociceptors in the intracranial vault above the tentorium and including the upper surface of the tentorium and the anterior and middle fossa are transmitted in the fifth cranial nerve. Stimulation of these nociceptors evokes pain in the frontal, temporal, parietal, and supraorbital regions. Nociceptive impulses from subtentorial regions are transmitted in the second cervical nerve and the pain is experienced in the occipital area. The infradural and posterior fossa are innervated by the first three cervical nerves. Parts of the posterior fossa are also innervated by the ninth and tenth cranial nerves and pain may be referred to the ear and throat. The tentorium provides the boundary between the trigeminal and cervical nerves. As previously mentioned, proximal structures may cause referred pain to the head, however, pain in more distant areas of the body is not referred to the brain. Even though systemic processes such as infection may result in headache it is by a different mechanism.

Extracranial structures which are sensitive to nociceptive stimuli and which can cause headaches include skin, subcutaneous tissue, muscles, arteries, and periosteum of the skull. The cranium itself is not sensitive to pain. Pathology of the eyes, ears, nose, sinuses, teeth, and jaw often cause headache, as do musculoskeletal problems especially those involving the cervical spine.

Mechanisms of Headache *Changes* in *intracranial pressure* such as those due to brain tumor, abscesses, subdural hematoma do not in and of themselves cause pain. Pain results only when such conditions cause mechanical stimulation of nociceptive afferents by displacing or causing traction on pain-sensitive structures within the head. A common example of this mechanism is seen when a lumbar puncture is done to remove cerebral spinal fluid (CSF). The removal of fluid does not result in headache. Rather, the puncture site in the dura and arachnoid permit large amounts of CSF to leak out into the lumbar epidural space. This lowers the intraspinal pressure resulting in negative intracranial pressure. The brain, then, is no longer buffered by its normal floatation in the CSF. Consequently there is caudal displacement of the brain resulting in a downward traction on the unsupported pain-sensitive structures, particularly the veins, dural attachments and dural sinuses. Bringing the patient into an upright position causes a further increase in the negative pressure and increased headaches. The same mechanism occurs with significant fluid loss when there are tears and trauma to the coverings of the brain and spinal cord.

Increased intracranial pressure, per se, does not produce headache either. Rather, again, the mechanism is one of traction on pain-sensitive structures. Brain tumors cause increased intracranial pressure when they block the free flow of CSF through the ventricular system to the brain leading to mechanical traction or distortion of the pain-sensitive structures in the head. Escaping blood from cerebral vascular accidents, contusions, and lacerations may also cause increased intracranial pressure and headaches through the same mechanism. With horizontal shifts in body fluids, for example, during sleep an increase in intracranial pressure through the mechanism of cerebral edema may lead to symptomatology which is not present or decreased when the patient is in an upright position. An increase in intracranial pressure may also be caused by coughing, sneezing, etc. This increase is caused by decreasing venous outflow from the cranium.

Dilation and *distention* of *intracranial arteries* and *excessive pulsation* causes stretching of the surrounding pain-sensitive structures and headache. This type of headache may be precipitated by generalized vasodilation and a decrease in the systemic blood pressure. As recovery occurs, the passive intracerebral arteries distend with each heart contraction resulting in a severe throbbing headache. Headaches believed to be caused by this mechanism include vascular, septic, hypoxic and hypertensive crisis and those due to ingestion of nitrites and rapid infusion of epinephrine. As the blood vessels return to their normal tone and the pulsation subsides, the headache also subsides.

Infection or *hemorrhagic irritation* of meningeal vessels are two more causes of intracerebral headaches. A single mechanism is not at fault. Possible mechanisms include irritation of all the meninges including the sensitive area of the dura and around the venous sinuses; dilatation and congestion of inflamed meningeal vessels causing chemical irritation of nerve endings in the meninges leading to cerebral vasculitis; and increased intracranial pressure.

Extracranial headaches are caused by some of the same mechanisms that cause intracranial headaches: that is, traction, distention, dilatation and spasms of blood vessels; compression or irritation of sensory nerves; and irritation and inflammation of nerves and blood vessels.

Chronic muscle contraction headaches (tension headaches) are considered to be the most common type of headache in our society. Muscle contraction headaches are caused by prolonged reaction of skeletal muscles in the face, scalp, neck, shoulders, and upper back. Vasodilatation occurs in the associated cranial arteries. In addition, the sustained contraction causes local tenderness in the specific structures and trigger points may develop. The patient may further sustain the headache and painful muscle spasm by immobilizing the involved structures in an attempt to prevent pain. An example of this is seen when the sustained contraction is due to disease of proximal structures such as arthritis of the temporomandibular joint.

Temporomandibular joint (TMJ) syndrome is now being recognized as a major cause of headaches. One in every five people suffers this syndrome in their lives yet it is considered one of the body's best kept secrets. The diagnosis is frequently missed. The pain is caused by imbalance in the TMJ. The etiology may be due to a poor bite, bruxism, or any of the other joint problems such as inflammation, trauma, degenerative changes, and stress. The pain almost always is referred and experienced at a point distant to the TMJ. Headache in both adults and children is one of the most common sites of referral (Grummons, 1982).

Occular headaches are caused by disequilibrium of both intra- and extraoccular muscles. The disequilibrium results in sustained contractions and headache. Muscles involved in eyestrain include the frontal, temporal, and occipital muscles. Errors in refraction may also cause headaches. Intraoccular involvement resulting in headache occurs with glaucoma, infections, and problems of muscle accommodation. Inflammation of the iris may also be a source of occular headaches.

Nasal and *paranasal sinuses* cause headaches primarily by an inflammator response or changes in pressure. Pressure changes may occur from sneezing, stooping, movements of the head (particularly when the head is put in a dependent position), and blowing the nose too vigorously.

Posttraumatic headaches most often result from nonintracranial sources. Posner (1979, p. 732) cites four of the most common types of posttraumatic headaches as those resulting from "pain or tenderness from local tissue damage in a scar or at a site of impact; muscular contraction, vascular or delusional for which no cause can be found and no tissue abnormality exists."

Dental pathology may cause headache and the offending teeth may be difficult to determine. One possible technique involves blocking the area of the suspected teeth with novocaine. If the headache goes away the source may be confirmed.

Headache due to *ear pathology* is most frequently associated with an inflammatory or destructive process such as otitis media, osteomyelitis, or acoustic nerve tumors.

Cancer Pain Syndromes

Cancer patients may develop pain syndromes due to the progression of the disease, as a result of the therapy directed at the control or cure of the disease, or unrelated to their disease. All of these pain syndromes are considered to be capable of producing severe pain. "In almost all instances the complaint of pain in the cancer patient has an organic basis. The pain is rarely assigned to psychological influences alone" (Foley, 1981, p. 4). Further, the pain may occur for weeks or months before it can be detected on physical and neurological examination. One patient in the terminal stage of his disease who had severe inadequately controlled pain told us "coming to terms with cancer and then my imminent death have been easy in comparison to dealing with my pain. I doubt that I will ever be able to come to terms with my pain." The seeming lack of interest and concern about cancer pain were discussed in Chapter 1 and illustrated in Table 1-1. The incidence of cancer pain can be seen in Table 6-4.

Bonica (1980, pp. 15–16) in a well-documented article makes several comparisons between patients with chronic cancer pain and those with noncancer chronic pain. First, usually the physiologic and psychologic impact of cancer pain on the patient is greater than that of noncancer chronic pain. Second, cancer patients have greater physical deterioration due to loss of appetite, nausea, vomiting, and sleep disturbances. Third,

TABLE 6.4. Incidence of Cancer Pain.

Average Data			
Cartwright et al. (England) Terminal Cancer			87%
Foley (NYC) 38% of 397 Pts-In Terminal Pts			60%
Pannuti (Italy) Advanced Cancer			65%
Parkes (London) Advanced Cancer			65-70%
Twycross (St. Christopher's) 500 Admissions			80%
Wilkes (Sheffield) 300 Admissions			60%
Specific Lesions*			
Bone	85%	Male Gu	60-75%
Cervix	85%	Breast	55-68%
Stomach	70-75%	Intestine	58%
Lung	50-70%	Kidney	55%
Female Gu	70%	Colon-Rectum	50-60%
Pancreas	70%	Leukemia	5%

(Bonica, J.J. Pain research and therapy: Past and current status and future needs. In Ng L.K.Y. and Bonica J.J. (Eds.). Pain, Discomfort and Humanitarian Care. Proceedings of the National Conference, National Institutes of Health, Bethesda, MD, Feb. 15-16, 1979, New York: Elsevier/North-Holland, 1980, p. 14, with permission.)

cancer patients develop greater emotional reactions of anxiety, depression, hypochondriasis, somatic focusing, and neuroticism than noncancer chronic pain patients. Fourth, for several reasons, the effects of uncontrolled cancer pain are more serious than those of noncancer chronic pain. Many patients with uncontrolled cancer pain develop interpersonal problems with their family, friends, and co-workers. Further, the cancer patient's physical appearance due to disease progression, pain, and suffering are emotionally stressful for the significant others. Patients usually sense this and it aggravates their pain and suffering. Cancer patients usually have to terminate employment due to disease progression or pain which not only causes economic burdens but also increase the patient's feelings of dependency and uselessness.

Comparing cancer patients with and without pain Woodforde & Fielding (1975) found that cancer patients with pain were significantly more emotionally disturbed, responded more poorly to treatment of their cancer and died sooner. Bond (1979) and Bond & Pearson (1969) also studied cancer patients with and without pain. Patients with pain had elevated levels of hypochondriasis and neuroticism scales. Cancer patients who did not have pain had low scores on these test components. Following successful pain treatment their elevated personality factor scores returned to normal.

In a six-week outpatient cancer pain program utilizing multimodalities including pharmacologic tailoring, peripheral stimulation, afferent interruption and hypnosis, Ferrer-Brechner & Brechner (1981) reported acceptable pain relief was achieved in 89.5 percent of the referred cancer patients. Ferrer-Brechner and Gitelson (1981) found that successful pain treatment outcome correlated significantly with the pain physician's predictive and posttreatment ratings.

Reasons cited by Bonica (1980) for the ineffective treatment of cancer pain are ones which a thorough well-documented nursing assessment could significantly reverse. These include the "lack of appreciation of the deleterious effects of unrelieved pain on the patient" (p. 16) and the "improper application of available knowledge and therapies for pain relief which if properly applied would provide effective relief for most patients" (p. 23).

Foley (1981) and Foley et al. (1978) report that cancer pain due to the progression of the disease accounts for 78 percent of acute cancer pain syndromes. Of these pain syndromes 50 percent are due to either primary or secondary bone disease, 25 percent are due to nerve compression or infiltration and 3 percent are due to hollow viscus involvement.

Bone pain syndromes usually are described as constant and progressive in severity most commonly occurring in the spine, pelvis, and long bones. A not uncommon complication of bone metastases to the spine is *epidural invasion* and *vertebral dislocation* or *collapse.* The signs and symptoms from such a complication are similar to those discussed in the previous section on herniated intervertebral disks including the severe pain of nerve root and spinal cord compression. Dislocation and collapse may also cause an emergent paraplegia or quadraplegia. In addition, neoplasms may cause nerve root and spinal cord compression by *direct invasion*. Other *neurological pain syndromes* due to the progression of the disease may result from encroachment on *peripheral nerves*, the brachial, lumbar or sacral plexus, and meningeal carcinomatosis.

One patient with a slow-growing malignant intramedullary spinal cord tumor had pain and paresthesias for two years and was treated for chronic benign pain. Because the tumor is not completely resectable she now has had three surgical procedures to debulk the tumor. These procedures have minimized additional spinal cord damage, however this patient has been paraplegic since her first surgery and now suffers from a chronic benign pain syndrome in addition to pain caused by the recurrent tumor.

Disease progression often results in *visceral obstruction* causing varied pain syndromes. Some of the more common ones include those associated with pancreatic, colon, and bladder involvement. Often bypass procedures provide the best pain relief for these patients. Many patients with visceral involvement and bone metastasis could receive significant pain control by neuroablative procedures. However, when the patient's bladder and bowel are intact they may be unwilling to pay the price of incontinence resulting from neuroablative procedures which could provide pain relief. Obstructive lesions of the blood vessels and lymph system also cause severe pain syndromes.

Nineteen percent of cancer pain syndromes result from *iatrogenic causes* such as surgery, radiation, and chemotherapy (Foley, 1981). Cancer patients may experience pain in the postoperative period and also develop incisional neuritis from cutting sensory fibers during surgery and the development of traumatic neuromas. Examples of these pain syndromes are postmastectomy, postthoracotomy, and postradical neck dissection pain syndromes. Patients with these neuritic syndromes are also prone to develop a painful Sudeck's atrophy. Radiation may result in fibrosis of connective tissue, necrosis, and suppression of the immune system. Patients who receive some chemotherapeutic agents develop secondary pain syndromes. For example, some of the cytotoxic agents have an affinity for nervous tissue. During the course of the treatment and posttreatment, the patient may develop a painful neuropathy. Although it usually is reversible, sometimes it is not. Other types of chemotherapy and drugs used during procedures such as bone marrow transplants, for example steroids, suppress the immune system. Patients are left at high risk for infectious processes, pseudorheumatism, and aseptic necrosis of bones. A dormant herpes varicella may become activated and the patient may suffer from a postherapeutic neuralgia. Disuse contractures and decubiti may also cause pain problems for the cancer patient. Diagnostic tests are also often painful.

Pain syndromes that the general population experience and which are unrelated to cancer account for approximately 3 percent of the pain problems that cancer patients experience (Foley, 1981). These include arthritis, diabetic neuropathy, and myofascial pain syndromes.

Crue et al. (1979) say that many patients with advanced cancer have similar psychiatric mechanisms to those of patients with chronic intractable benign pain syndromes (CIBPS). They go on to say that a CIBPS may be present in cancer patients who have no known residual tumor and who are apparently cured but develop a *cancerphobia*. This may present as difficult a problem for the significant others. In the presence of pain behaviors neither may be able to relinquish the fear of disease progression. An equally difficult situation may occur for the patient and his family if he finally gets pain control during the terminal phase of his disease. Even in situations where there have been seemingly good family relationships people may have come to acceptance of the death and said "goodbye." They, therefore, may find even the improved quality of the extended life less acceptable than the patient's death, because they are still confronted with another unknown. Now the question is "when?"

OTHER PAIN SYNDROMES

Labor Pain

In addition to our cultural value of stoicism by those experiencing pain, much emphasis has been placed on the psychological and physiological value to both the mother and fetus during a "natural childbirth" process. Bonica (1980, pp. 7–8) challenges these values. He documents his report that when uterine contraction pain is not relieved it will cause residual maternal emotional and psychological problems. Perhaps, more serious is his report that unmedicated primagravadas develop severe respiratory alkalosis due to the increased ventilation, increased cardiac output, increased blood pressure, decreased uterine blood flow and decreased uterine contractions due to the increased sympathetic activity. The latter may impair placental blood flow and compromise both the fetus and the mother, and increase fetal morbidity and mortality. It may cause the "high-risk" mother to be at further risk. According to Bonica well-documented studies. have shown that "parturients given no pain relief, or moderate pain relief with narcotics, developed progressive metabolic acidosis as did their fetuses, while those mothers managed with epidural analgesics did not develop metabolic acidosis nor did their fetuses" (p. 8). Pain assessment during the labor and delivery process needs to be carefully monitored especially in situations where the mother has little or no choice about medication and little or no preparation for her delivery.

The typist for this book, Turman (1982), suggests that we have omitted a very important pain syndrome from this chapter, phantom bedpan pain. She identified it during a recent hospitalization and suggests that it be classified as a pathological pain syndrome. Turman says it has the same characteristics as phantom limb pain, occurring specifically when the patient says "I'll only be a minute" and the nurse says "I'll be right back" but returns in half an hour. This is a pain syndrome that Turman believes is almost always preventable, and suggests that it is another case of the nurse not listening to the patient. With phantom bedpan pain, we will conclude this chapter on pain syndromes.

In the next chapter, Chapter 7, we will consider the effects of pain on the patient. Of concern are how the patient may respond and adjust physically, emotionally, and socially to his or her pain experience.

REFERENCES

Adams, R.D. Pain—General considerations. In K.J. Isselbacher, R.D. Adams, E. Braunwald, et al. (Eds.). Harrison's Principles of Internal Medicine (9th ed.). New York: McGraw-Hill, 1980, pp. 12–26.

Bond, M.R. Psychologic and emotional aspects of cancer pain. In J.J. Bonica & V. Ventafridda (Eds.), Advances in Pain Research and Therapy. Proceedings of the International Symposium on Pain of Advanced Cancer. New York: Raven Press, Vol. 2, pp. 81–88, 1979.

Bond, M.R., & Pearson, I.B. Psychological aspects of pain in women with advanced cancer of the cervix. J Psychosom Res 13: 13–19, 1969.

Bonica, J.J. Management of pain in general practice—Practical therapeutics. GP Jan.: 107–123, 1966.

Bonica, J.J. The relation of injury to pain (Letter to the Editor). Pain 6: 203–207, 1979.

Bonica, J.J. Pain research and therapy: Past and current status and future needs. In L.K. Ng & J.J. Bonica (Eds.), Pain Discomfort and Humanitarian Care. Proceedings of the National Conference, National Institutes of Health, Bethesda, MD, Feb. 15–16, 1979. New York: Elsevier/North Holland, 1980, pp. 1–46.

Brechner, T. Personal communication, January 22, 1982.

Craig, K.D. Social modeling influences on pain. In R.A. Sternbach (Ed.), The Psychology of Pain. New York: Raven Press, 1978.

Crue, B., Felsoory, A., Agnew, D., et al. The Team Concept in the Management of Pain in Patients with Cancer. Paper presented in part at Symposium on the Diagnosis and Management of the Complications of Cancer by the Scripps Clinic and Research Foundation, San Diego, CA, February 22, 1979.

Ferrer-Brechner, T., & Brechner, V.L. Evaluation of graduated multimodality pain management of outpatient cancer patients. Paper presented at the Third World Congress on Pain of the International Association for the Study of Pain, Edinburgh, Scotland, Sept. 4–11, 1981. (Abstract)

Ferrer-Brechner, T., & Gitelson, J. Treatment outcome of cancer pain: Correlation with physician-patient interaction. Paper presented at the Third World Congress on Pain of the International Association for the Study of Pain, Edinburgh, Scotland, Sept. 4–11, 1981. (Abstract)

Foley, K.M. The Management of Cancer Pain. Cancer Pain Syndrome, Vol. 1. Nutley, NJ: Roche Laboratories, 1981.

Foley, K.M., Rogers, A., & Houde, R. Pain in patients with cancer: A quantative reappraisal. Proc Amer Assoc Cancer Res 19, C–202: 357, 1978, (Abstract).

Frost, H.M. Musculoskeletal Pain. In Alling, C. C. (Ed.). Facial Pain. Philadelphia: Lea & Febiger, 1968.

Grummons, D.C. Personal communication. January 18, 1982.

Guyton, A. Textbook of Medical Physiology (6th ed.). Philadelphia: W. B. Saunders, 1981.

Harvey, A. M., Johns, R. J., McKusick, V.A., et al. The Principles and Practice of Medicine (12th ed.) New York: Appleton-Century Crofts, 1980.

Jensen, D. The principles of Physiology (2nd ed.) New York: Appleton-Century-Crofts, 1980.

Keegan, J.J. Variations of symptoms with herniation of intervertebral discs. Nebraska Medical Journal, 1958, *43*, 191.

Kraus, H. Clinical Treatment of Back and Neck Pain. New York: McGraw-Hill, 1970.

McKhann G.M. & Speed, W.G. III. Disorders of Sensation: Pain and Headache. In Harvey, A.M., Johns, R.J., McKusick, V.A., et al. The Principles and Practice of Medicine (12th ed.). New York: Appleton-Century-Crofts, 1980.

Melzack, R. The Puzzle of Pain. New York: Basic/Harper Torchbooks, 1973.

Melzack, R., & Loeser, J.D. Phantom body pain in paraplegics: Evidence for a central "pattern generating mechanism." Pain 4: 195–210, 1978.

Mountcastle, V.B. Medical Physiology. Vol. 1 (14th ed.) St. Louis: C.V. Mosby, 1980.

Plum, F. Headache. In P.B. Beeson, W. McDermott, & J.B. Wyngaarden (Eds.), Cecil Textbook of Medicine (15th ed.). Philadelphia: W.B. Saunders, 1979, pp. 728–733.

Posner, J.B. Pain. In P.B. Beeson, W. McDermott, & J.B. Wyngaarden (Eds.), Cecil, Textbook of Medicine (15th ed.). Philadelphia: W.B. Saunders, 1979, pp. 720–728.

Ruch, T.C. Pathophysiology of pain. In T. Rush & H. Patton (Eds.), Howell–Fulton —Physiology and Biophysics: The Brain and Neural Function (20th ed.). Philadelphia: W.B. Saunders, 1979, pp. 272–324.

Seiden, M.R. Practical Management of Chronic Neuralgic Problems. New York: Appleton-Century-Crofts, 1981.

Sternbach, R.A. Pain: A Psychophysiological Analysis. New York: Academic Press, 1968.

Turman, A. Personal communication. October 11, 1982.

Woodforde, J.M., & Fielding, J.L. Pain and Cancer. In M. Weisenburg (Ed.), Pain: Clinical and Experimental Perspectives. St. Louis: C.V. Mosby, 1975, pp. 332–336.

SUGGESTED READINGS

Appenzeller, O. Pathogenesis and Treatment of Headache. New York: Spectrum, 1976.

Bonica, J.J. (Ed.). Symposium on Pain. Arch Surg 112: 749-861, 1971.
Bonica, J.J. Management of Pain (2nd ed.). Philadelphia: Lea & Febiger, 1974.
Bonica, J.J. Basic principles in managing chronic pain. Arch Surg 112: 783-788, 1977.
Bonica, J.J. Cancer pain: A major national health problem. Can Nurse 1: 313–316, 1978.
Bouchard-Kurtz, R. Nursing Care of the Cancer Patient (4th ed.). St. Louis: C.V. Mosby, 1981.
Brewer, B.J. Low back pain. Amer Fam Phys 19: 114–118, 1979.
Caghan, S.B., McGrath, M.M., Morrow, M.G., et al. When adolescents complain of pain. Nurse Pract 3: 19–22, 1978.
Caillet, R. Soft Tissue Pain and Disability. Philadelphia: Davis, 1977.
Catalano, R.B. The medical approach to management of pain caused by cancer. Seminars Oncol 2: 379–392, 1975.
Davis, A.J. Pain q 3 hr. Amer J Nurs 80(5): 974, 1980.
Diamond, S., & Dalessio, D.J. The Practicing Physician's Approach to Headache (2nd ed.). Baltimore: Williams & Wilkins, 1978.
Friedman, A.P. Research and Clinical Studies in Headache. Baltimore: Williams & Wilkins, 1967.
Friedman, A.P. Clinical approach to the patient with headache. In A.P. Friedman (Ed.), Medical Clinics of North America: A Symposium on Headache and Related Pain Syndromes. Philadelphia: W.B. Saunders, Vol. 62, 1978.
Hanington, E. The Headache Bash. Westport, CT: Technomic, 1980.
Hoppenfeld, S. Physical Examination of the Spine and Extremities. New York: Appleton-Century-Crofts, 1976.
Jacox, A.K. (Ed.). Pain, A Sourcebook for Nurses and Other Health Professionals. Boston: Little, Brown, 1977.
Jacox, A.K., and Rogers, A.G. The nursing management of pain. In L.B. Marina (Ed.), Cancer Nursing. St. Louis: C.V. Mosby, 1981.
Johnson, M. Assessment of clinical pain. In A.K. Jacox (Ed.), Pain, A Sourcebook for Nurses and Other Health Professionals. Boston: Little, Brown, 1977.
Livingston, W.K. Pain Mechanisms: A Physiologic Interpretation of Causalgia and Its Related States. New York: Plenum Press, 1976.
McCaffery, M. The nurse's contribution to pain relief in labor. In S.R. Reeder, L., Mastroianni, Jr., L.L. Martin, et al. (Eds.), Maternity Nursing (14th ed.). Philadelphia: J.B. Lippincott, 1980, pp. 265–288.
McNeil, C., Danzig, W.M., Farrar, W.B., et al. Craniomandibular (TMJ) disorders —The state of the art. J Prosthet Dent 4: 434–437, 1980.
Merskey, H. On development of pain. Headache 10: 116–123, 1970.
Noyes, R. Treatment of Cancer Pain. Psychosomatic Medicine. 43 (1) Feb., 57–70, 1981.
Oster, J. Recurrent abdominal pain, headache, and limb pains in children and adolescents. Pediatrics 50: 429–436, 1972.
Rosse, C. The Musculoskeletal System in Health and Disease. Hagerstown, MD: Harper & Row, 1980.
Schochet, S.S., & McCormick, W.T. Essentials of Neuropathology. New York: Appleton-Century-Crofts, 1979.
Valentine, A.S., Steckel, S., Weintraub, M. Pain relief for cancer patients. Amer J Nurs 78: 2055–2056, 1978.

Vredevoe, D.L., Dirdiarian, A., Sarna, L.P., et al. Concepts of Oncology Nursing. Englewood Cliffs, NJ: Prentice-Hall, 1981.
Wiley, L. (Ed.). Caring for the cancer patient. Nurs 77 7: 30–33, 1977.
Wilkes, E. Some problems in Cancer Management, The Michael Williams Lecture. Practitioner, 213, July, 1273, 82–86, 1974.
Wolff, H.G. Headache and Other Head Pain (3rd ed.). New York: Oxford University Press, 1972.

7

Effects of Pain Upon The Patient

Knowing the effects of pain and assessing the patient's condition in light of the effects enables us to obtain at least two extremely important types of information:

1. *Clues that alert us to the existence and nature of the patient's pain.* If the patient denies pain or has difficulty communicating about his pain, these clues should alert us to examine further the possibility that the patient is, in fact, experiencing pain. Of course, as mentioned before, the absence of any effects of pain cannot be used to rule out the presence of pain.
2. *The potential or actual harm to the patient.* Pain is not a benign event that can be endured without exacting a price. Sometimes the cost may be minimal; at other times pain may pose a direct threat to the patient's life. As we explore the possible effects of pain upon the patient, in this chapter it will become clear, for example, that pain may impede physical recovery from acute illness by such things as decreasing one's natural defenses, causing sleep disturbances, nausea and vomiting, and reluctance to ambulate. Pain may constitute a disability, if the pain is chronic. In any event, pain, of both known and unknown etiology, may cause considerable emotional trauma including deterioration of relationships, both personal and with the health team, irritability, and decreased interest even in normally pleasurable activities. All of these factors serve to increase the patient's pain and suffering in a circular fashion.

Information such as this facilitates devising pain relief strategies with specific goals such as increasing sleep, improving nutrition, and decreasing anxiety and depression which may elevate the patient's pain tolerance, and general sense of well-being, thus decreasing or minimizing his suffering.

SUFFERING

It would seem that all pain results in suffering and when it does pain is of paramount concern to the patient and the practitioner. The problem of pain was described by Lewis (1962, p. 90; cited in Tu, 1980, p. 65).

> But the truth is that the word Pain has two senses which must now be distinguished. *a*. A particular kind of sensation, probably conveyed by specialized nerve fibers and, recognisable by the patient as that kind of sensation whether he dislikes it or not (e.g., the faint ache in my limbs would be recognised as an ache even if I didn't object to it). *b*. Any experience, whether physical or mental, which the patient dislikes. It will be noticed that all Pains in sense *a* become Pains in sense *b* if they are raised above a certain very low level of intensity, but that Pains in the *b* sense need not be Pains in the *a* sense. Pain in the *b* sense, in fact, is synonymous with "suffering," "anguish," "tribulation," "adversity," or "trouble," and it is about it that the problem of pain arises.

Suffering, like pain, defies definition and is entirely subjective. Copp (1974, p. 491) defines suffering as "the state of anguish of one who bears pain, injury, or loss." She notes that the phenomenon of suffering is almost an uncharted course. Krant (1978, p. 324) says suffering must "be understood in its broad perspective—humans struggling with their emotional and spiritual centers to make sense of their lives."

In one sense, suffering refers to the degree to which pain bothers or distresses the patient. Assessment of the degree of suffering in the patient with pain requires some understanding of the differences and intricate relationship between the intensity of the pain sensation, the patient's tolerance for pain and expressive style. All of these factors overlap to a certain extent and are described below. Other variables affecting the patient's suffering will be discussed in Chapter 8.

Pain tolerance, as described in Chapter 5, is that intensity or duration of pain that the person is willing to endure. Some patients may feel that it is senseless to experience even the mildest form of pain if something can be done about it. Other patients will not want anything done about severe pain. In the hospital setting, the fact that the patient calls for the nurse and tells her or him about pain usually implies that his tolerance level has been reached regardless of how the patient rates the severity of the pain. At that point the patient wants something done about pain and does not want to tolerate it any longer. At that point, it would ssem likely that suffering and anguish exist, if in fact they did not exist prior to that point.

Tolerance may also vary within the same person from one time to another. An interesting example of this in our culture currently has to do with the increasing number of women who want to go through labor and delivery without analgesia or anesthesia. The mother usually is motivated by desires to spare the infant the possible ill effects of medication and to be awake and aware at the time of delivery. This woman may be willing to endure pain that she would rate as severe, especially the pain intensity that she is likely to experience during the transition stage of labor. Yet in the postpartum period this same woman may request an oral narcotic for episiotomy pain that she rates as mild in intensity.

The patient who tolerates pain may nevertheless suffer. He or she may describe the pain as horrible and may fight back tears. The fact that such a patient is willing to tolerate pain should not be mistaken as meaning that he or she is masochistic, enjoys it, or does not suffer from it.

Some scales used to rate the intensity of pain also indicate the extent of suffering, or distress, such as the scale that uses the word "excruciating" to describe the highest intensity of pain. Other scales are aimed directly at assessing suffering. An example is: 0–normal, 2–bothered, 4–very bothered, 6–distressed, 8–very distressed, 10–extremely distressed (Scott & Barber, 1977). Scales used to rate distress usually are accompanied by a second scale that measures intensity of pain. (Pain scales are discussed in more detail in Chapter 5.)

In summary, many patients with pain will suffer. That is, pain will be more than an unpleasant event. Suffering is an ambiguous and individual matter. One patient may suffer with mild pain and not wish to tolerate it while another person will suffer and reach a maximum pain tolerance only when the pain becomes severe. Still another will tolerate severe pain, yet not admit to suffering with it. Further, each of these people may express or communicate his pain in very different ways.

There are important reasons why pain and suffering should be treated. When pain causes suffering or anguish, it reflects a high level of stress and a considerable emotional impact. Black (1980, p. 208) says that attempts to find the cause of suffering must be made because when patients do not respond to proven treatments "patients are often blamed for their bad response to good therapy." Fielding (1980, p. 707) says that "The sufferer who frustrates a keen doctor by failing to improve is in danger of meeting primitive human behavior, disguised as treatment." Referred to by Main (1957) as "therapeutic mania". The patient's ability to evoke a similar sadistic response in the nurse is discussed by Doherty (1979). The physician's response had been attributed, at least in part, as being due to failure during the assessment process to differentiate between pain caused by nociception and the pain behaviors that the suffering generates (Fordyce, 1980, p. 236). The nurse's behavior may be engendered by the powerlessness patients who do not improve or who continue to complain can invoke in us. As imprecise as it may be, the nurse needs to assess the degree to which pain results in suffering in the individual patient. She also needs to be introspective when experiencing negative feelings towards the patient in pain. As Fielding (p. 707) points out ". . . frustrations are often more apparent to the patient and our colleagues than to ourselves."

In addition to physiological manifestations of the patient's pain, observable behavioral responses must also be assessed. *Pain behaviors* are anything that a patient does or says in response to his pain, such as crying, and changes in posture or facial expression, or saying "it hurts." Pain behaviors in themselves are meaningful, purposeful, and understandable forms of communication. It is important to assess them both as a basis for treatment and to evaluate the success of treatment. We will first consider physiological manifestations of pain and then pain behaviors resulting from the effects of pain upon the patient.

PHYSIOLOGICAL MANIFESTATIONS

For many years, efforts have been made to correlate physiological parameters with the patient's rating of pain intensity. The results have been disappointing. As long ago as 1963, Barber noted that unfortunately there was no single physiological index and no combination of indices that unequivocally indicated the presence or absence of pain or suffering. Over ten years later it was again noted that attempts to relate pain to heart rate, galvanic skin response, and other correlates had been disappointing (Fetz, 1974). Hilgard (1969) succinctly asserts "that there is no physiological measure of pain which is either as discriminating of fine differences in stimulus conditions, as reliable upon repetition, and as lawfully related to changed conditions, as the subject's verbal report" (p. 109). In 1983, we believe this is still true.

An assessment of the physiological responses to pain, however, may alert us to the existence and nature of pain and its potential harm. For example, rapid heart rate, pallor, and perspiration may be excellent clues to the sudden onset of pain in a man who remains stoic. Acute pain that causes nausea and vomiting may endanger the electrolyte balance. Nausea accompanying chronic pain may cause weight loss and general physical deterioration.

Since anxiety, depression, and other emotions usually accompany pain, it is almost impossible to say whether the physiological manifestations reflect the emotions or the pain. But, this problem of uncertainty does not detract from the value of assessing the physiological manifestations of the patient's pain experience.

Physiological responses to pain are influenced by many factors, such as the individual's response style and the pain intensity. Therefore, it is impossible to state specific levels of physiological response, for example the exact change in heart rate or the specific amount of time that will elapse before the response will change. Here, physiological responses to pain will be presented in terms of the general duration of the pain, adhering to the basic sequence and principles suggested by Sternbach's (1968) review of the literature.

Activation

The first pattern of physiological responses to pain is referred to as *activation*, and usually takes place within the first second or so of a rather sudden and intense pain sensation. If the pain continues, the responses may be sustained for a few minutes up to about an hour. Activation is also characteristic of anger and fear and it has often been called the "fight or flight reaction." The original and classic description of these responses to a variety of conditions was done in 1929 by Cannon. The physiological changes appear to be directly serviceable to the individual. They prepare the individual for defense or escape, a reaction necessary for survival in a hostile environment.

During the period of activation, the sympathetic nervous system is dominant. What the nurse most often observes in the patient is an increase in pulse and respiratory rates, increase in diastolic and systolic blood pressure, pallor, dilated pupils, increase in muscle tension or various body movements, cold perspiration, and/or piloerection in some areas of the body. The patient may report nausea or a "hollow stomach." These observations reflect a tremendous amount of physiological activity. Blood moves from the viscera and superficial vessels, organs whose activities are deferable, to the organs immediately essential to muscular exertion such as the striated muscles, lungs, heart, and central nervous system. As a result, gastric secretions and contractions are inhibited. The bronchioles dilate to increase oxygenation of the blood and there is also an increase in the number of red blood cells. To combat fatigue, the circulating blood sugar increases through utilization of carbohydrate stored in the liver. The vigor of cardiac contraction increases, facilitating distribution of the enriched blood supply. The danger of bleeding is minimized by circulating adrenalin and a decreased coagulation time. These sympathetic nervous system activities are sustained by the secretion of adrenalin which mimics sympathetic activity. Some investigators noted that the responses to pain include not only an increase in respiratory rate but also an increase in alveolar ventilation and oxygen consumption and a decrease in alveolar carbon dioxide concentration (Masuda & Dudley, 1968).

Rebound

The next set of responses depends upon the duration and intensity of the pain sensation that initiated activation. If the original sensation was brief but intense, the phenomenon of *rebound* may occur. These responses are the opposite of activation: they are like parasympathetic responses and are usually of short duration. The nurse may observe rebound responses by noting that, in the aftermath phase of pain, the pulse rate is slower than it was before pain occurred or that the blood pressure is lower than it was prior to pain. The compensatory reflexes stimulated during activation outlast the sympathetic responses.

Adaptation

Adaptation occurs if the stimulus for activation is repetitive or of long duration. The extreme physiological activity of activation cannot continue indefinitely, but it may take some time, several hours, before the responses of adaptation can be observed. They are compensatory responses that are stimulated by the prolonged sympathetic responses. Adaptation is actually a decrease in the sympathetic responses and the nurse can observe that there is less of an increase in the pulse rate and the blood pressure. In other words, as time goes on there is a decrease in the magnitude of *response* to pain. As discussed in Chapter 2 the nociceptors themselves do not adapt. The exact mechanism underlying adaptation is not completely understood but may be related to antagonistic innervation, sympathetic inhibition and/or central inhibition at the spinal level.

Stress Reaction

The general *adaptation syndrome* or *stress reaction*, occurs when pain or another stressor persists for weeks, days, or many hours (Selye, 1946, 1956). While activation responses rely largely on autonomic innervation, the general adaptation syndrome depends upon hormonal reactions. These are more difficult responses for the nurse to observe, but she or he may note in the final stage of the stress reaction that tests reveal a greater production of 17-ketosteroids than 17-hydroxycorticosteroids and an increase in circulating eosinophiles, and that the physician's case history and physical analysis of the patient suggests various degenerative changes and an increased susceptibility to infections. Such findings probably are a result of the organism's inability to sustain a corticoid production sufficient to maintain resistance.

One woman, for example, was on medication for hypothyroidism prior to the onset of severe musculoskeletal pain. After several months of the severe pain, her medications for hypothyroidism needed to be increased. Another patient with a rheumatoid arthritis pain of about six months duration developed multiple skin lesions infected with staphylococci. The infection was resistant to antibiotic therapy and recurred several times over the next few months while the pain continued.

BEHAVIORAL RESPONSES

A thorough assessment of the patient's pain experience involves consideration of several main categories of behavioral response to pain: verbal, vocal, facial, body movement, and physical contact with others. The patient may express pain through some change in one or more of those behaviors. Observation of these behaviors is fairly easy and routine, indeed, almost unavoidable.

Verbal

A patient's verbal statements about his pain are of the utmost importance in pain assessment. The patient's ability to verbalize will also be considered in Chapter 9 in relation to the patient's communication about his pain experience. The nurse must interpret verbalizations about pain in light of the patient's cognitive ability. The focus here is on the patient's cognitive ability as an important limitation that may be placed on his ability to communicate verbally. For example the child's cognitive ability may be limited to his developmental age, whereas both the child's and the adult's cognitive ability may be limited by conditions such as brain damage or a lowering of the level of consciousness from anoxia. Sometimes pain distracts the patient and medications given for pain relief sedate the patient so that it becomes difficult for him to give an adequate description of his pain experience.

The child is sometimes unable to find the right words. He or she may have experienced the pain of a cut knee and said, "It hurts." But when he is faced with the new and strange experience of wound pain, he may not be able to understand that this is another form of pain to which the word "hurt" also applies (McCaffery, 1969). One four-year-old boy on the evening of his appendectomy was lying quietly in bed, perspiring, wide-eyed, and frowning. The nurse approached him and asked, "Do you hurt?" He shook his head to indicate "No," but the nurse stayed with him a while and repeated the question. He was silent for several seconds before he moved his hand toward his abdomen and looked up at her to say, "Hurt? Hurt. Yes." Sometimes the presence of pain in a younger child is indicated only by his calling for his mother or father.

When the adult's cognitive level is altered, the same lack of verbal ability may be exhibited as seen in the infant, or the language difficulties of the young child. The patient often is unable to find the right word to describe the pain. This may be seen especially if pain had not been a previous problem for this patient.

Vocalizations

Vocalizations refer to all emitted sounds that are not language, or at least cannot be understood as words by others. Patients who can verbalize may also use vocal behaviors to indicate the presence, severity, duration, or meaning of pain. Vocalizations include groaning, grunting, whimpering, whining, crying, sobbing, screaming, gasping, and many others. Some of these sounds are practically involuntary if pain is sudden, sharp, and unexpected. Such pain often elicits a gasp, a grunt, or even a scream.

Some adults, because of cultural expectations, will not have as many vocalizations as other adults or children. For children, however, who do not have great facility with language, vocalizations may be an important means of communication. This may be the child's only way to inform others that he or she is in pain and needs their assistance (McCaffery, 1969). A study of hospitalized patients with pain showed that crying because of the pain occurred in about half the patients studied (Marks & Sachar, 1973). However, both children and adults may hide their crying from others.

Although many people feel that they should, if possible, minimize vocalizations, such as crying and screaming, this belief certainly is not shared by all. A patient may view vocalizations as serving a purpose. Tanzer (1968) quoted one woman as saying that during labor "I was screaming purposely, because I was hoping one of the doctors would give me medication" (p. 69). The same attitude is described by Marie Edgeworth (1895), in *Ormond, a Tale*:

> In the middle of the night our hero was wakened by a loud bellowing. It was only King Corny in a paroxysm of gout. "Pray now," said he to Harry, who stood beside his bed,—"now that I've a moment's ease,—did you ever hear of the Stoics that the book-men talk of, and can you tell me what good any of them ever got by making a point to make no noise, when they'd be punished or racked with pains of body or mind? Why, I will tell you all they got—all they got was no pity;—and who would give them pity that did not require it? I could bleed to death in a bath as well as the rest of them, if I chose it; or chew a bullet, if I set my teeth to it, with any man in the regiment—but where's the use? Nature knows best, and she says, *roar*!" And he roared—for another twinge seized him.

Facial

The patient's facial expression may be the first or the only sign of pain, or facial expressions may accompany a variety of other behaviors. When a patient does not verbalize or vocalize, changes in facial expression may be an excellent indication of his pain experience. Some patients may have a rather normal, sober expression, such as opened eyes and no wrinkling of the skin in any part of the face. Others may have clenched teeth, tightly shut lips, spread lips, or be biting their lips, widely opened or tightly shut eyes, wrinkled forehead and tightened muscles in the jaw, or any number of other facial contortions.

As with vocalizations, facial expressions may indicate presence, severity, duration, and meaning of pain. They may be almost involuntary at times.

Body Movement

Restlessness may be an excellent indication of impending pain, as well as a sign of the presence of pain or its increasing intensity. Some patients find that restlessness warns them of pain before its onset (Copp, 1974). Practitioners, too, have found that restlessness can be used to predict that pain is imminent (Keats, 1974).

Other types of body movement may give clues about the presence, severity, duration, location, and meaning of pain. They include: immobilization, muscle tension or relaxation, purposeless or inaccurate body movements, protective movement, and rhythmic or rubbing actions.

Immobilization means that a patient sustains one particular position for either a part of the body or the total body. Patients often do this to minimize their pain. Young children tend to immobilize the total body down to the little finger following massive physical trauma. Small injuries to a portion of a limb often result in their failing to move the whole limb. Adults are particularly reluctant to move the first few hours after most major surgery. This reluctance to move may also occur after some accidental injuries that potentially involve many parts of the body or that may have resulted in life-threatening trauma. Patients may sustain whatever position they happen to be in or, they may purposely choose a position of maximum comfort such as a horizontal position for a spinal headache or a semi-Fowler's position after cholecystectomy. Apparently, even infants draw up their legs in response to abdominal cramping although they do not tend to remain in this position. Any patient who immobilizes only a small part of his body gives the nurse a fairly good indication of the location of his pain. For example following thoracic surgery, the patient may limit all movement to prevent the need to breathe deeply or rapidly because of the pain of moving the chest wall.

Visceral pain seems to exert an overall depressing effect upon behavioral responses (Wolff & Wolff, 1958). Thus, pain in the viscera may be associated with a generalized lack of movement.

During any type of voluntary immobilization the muscles may be relaxed or tense, and this is important to note. There is generally some amount of muscle tension, such as the easily observed clenched fist, but through experience some patients find that relaxation minimizes pain and they will attempt to relax. The patient trained in a method of childbirth, such as the Lamaze method, is an excellent example of using muscle relaxation to relieve pain. The patient's muscles may remain completely relaxed throughout labor.

The *purposeless* or *inaccurate body movements* that may accompany pain may be due to fear, the excess energy from the flight or fight response that usually occurs at the onset of severe pain, or the patient's inability to find any way to help himself. The patient may tremble, flail his arms, kick, or toss and turn in bed. Purposeful motions sometimes become inaccurate during pain. For example, the patient may reach for a glass and knock it over.

The patient's initial physiological responses to pain typically prepare him for the flight or fight reactions. The goal of protective movements associated with pain is to prevent the recurrence or increase of pain. These movements may take the form of consciously controlled flight reactions for which activation of the initial physiological processes so aptly prepares the person. Or, protective movements may be reflex responses, which are involuntary movements executed without conscious effort. Reflex responses, of course, are a type of flight reaction.

Voluntary flight reactions may range from literally running away from a threat of pain to careful shielding of the threatened part using the hands or objects. A child who is threatened with a venipuncture may get out of bed and try to leave the room or he may hug his arms to his body or lie down on them. An adult may splint his incision with a pillow before he turns from side to side.

Another way of fighting pain or the threat of pain is quite literally to attack the person who seems responsible for inflicting it. This *aggressive physical response* can be seen in the child who kicks, hits, pushes away, or bites the physician or nurse who approaches him with something he believes will induce pain. This occurs with less frequency and vigor in the adult, but an adult who has a tender liver, for example, may push away the physician's hand during palpation.

The patient's general level of physical activity is suggestive of the site of pain, in terms of whether it is cutaneous or visceral. It is also related to whether the cause of pain is perceived as internal or external. As we have noted, cutaneous pain tends to elicit fight or flight responses, whereas visceral pain tends to result in inactivity. The biological usefulness of these differences is apparent. Since external hostile assaults are most likely to pierce the skin first, the individual's tendency toward escape or combat is adaptive. Inactivity in response to visceral pain is equally appropriate since it is virtually impossible to run away from an attack from within.

Seven-year-old Charlie demonstrated these different responses. Several hours after a cystoscopy, he complained of a "hurt" as he pointed to his lower abdomen where his distended bladder could be easily observed. He remained motionless in bed with a wrinkled forehead and occasionally whined quietly. Earlier that day he had received a subcutaneous injection in preparation for the cystoscopy. During the injection he made repeated attempts to move away from the inserted needle. Throughout the injection of the medication he cried loudly. His distended bladder had a depressing effect upon his responses, the usual effect of visceral pain. However, when the nurse palpated Charlie's bladder, causing further visceral discomfort, he responded by attempting to move away from the nurse. Although the pain was visceral, the cause was external, and he responded in a manner similar to his response to cutaneous pain.

Patients with pain frequently utilize some type of *rhythmic* or *rubbing body movement*. A baby may rub an ear if otitis media is present. When teething, the baby is in effect rubbing swollen gums as he or she chews on an object. With a headache an adult or young child may rub the head. Rocking in a semifetal position is common with abdominal or uterine cramping. During labor a patient, because of her childbirth training lessons, may employ *effleurage*, a rhythmic massage of the abdomen with both hands. Rubbing or rhythmic movements may be excellent clues as to the location of pain.

GENERAL RESPONSE TO THE ENVIRONMENT

Pain tends to draw attention to itself, so much so that a focus on pain becomes involved in almost all the patient's responses. It seems that the patient with pain either succumbs to some extent and attends to the pain or fights doing so. In either case, the patient is reacting to the powerful force of the pain.

A patient admitted to the hospital with vascular headaches illustrates how pain may cause a person's interactions with environment, both objects and people, to drop to a minimum. This patient may fail to notice the flowers sent by a friend or not open cards. He or she may no longer initiate conversation, or may fail to respond when spoken to or give only short responses. He or she may focus only on the body and those things done that might affect the pain.

A patient with pain that lasts months and years may also markedly decrease his interactions with everyone and everything. His or her entire life may revolve around treating the pain, preventing it or relieving it. He or she may be not only uninterested in other things, but eventually be unable to converse about anything but the pain.

People who have learned to handle pain so that it does not appear to interfere with their lives, tell us that it is a constant, daily battle to win over the pain. Some people with pain are less successful in coping with it than others are. In the following discussion of the effects of pain on emotions, such as anxiety, anger and depression, and on daily activities, it is clear that much of the suffering and disability associated with pain is related to the magnetic demanding and unrelenting nature of the pain sensation.

Both brief acute pain and chronic pain often have profound effects upon the patient's daily activities and upon relationships with others. Chronic pain may be the most significant offender, but acute pain also poses serious problems. Whether the pain is acute or chronic, the patient may be emotionally distressed and may experience harmful alterations in many aspects of life.

Generally, the danger or harm that may result from acute pain is associated with recovery from the associated acute illness. Very simply, such pain may retard recovery. The harmful effects of chronic pain are associated, in general, with some degree of disability. Chronic pain may prevent successful rehabilitation or restoration to the patient's former life style.

The more severe the pain, generally, the greater its impact upon the patient's life (Timmermans & Sternbach, 1976). The harmful effects of pain upon daily activities and relationships also depend to some extent upon the pain's duration, that is, whether the pain is acute or chronic. But, pain, regardless of its duration, seems to interfere with the same areas of the patient's life, namely, sleep, concentration, eating, emotions (such as anxiety and depression), relationships with others, and physical activities at home and work.

When pain affects these areas of the patient's life, a spiraling process may ensue. In essence, the pain affects the patient's life in distressing and harmful ways; these effects increase the pain or make it more difficult for the patient to cope with the pain, which in turn, results in the pain having more harmful effects on the patient. Obviously the situation can easily worsen unless something is done. Hence, assessment must include determining not only the characteristic of the painful sensation, but also what it is doing to the patient's life.

Eating

Both acute and chronic severe pain often result in *weight loss* and decreased fluid and nutritional intake. In addition, both prolonged pain and pain due to inadequate analgesia may cause nausea and vomiting, loss of appetite and the refusal of food and fluid. With acute pain, this hampers recovery from illness since fluid and electrolyte balance are jeopardized and the general nutritional status is affected. Anderson & Krogh (1976) found that in postoperative patients who had undergone abdominal surgery when pain was relieved in patients who had both pain and nausea, the nausea usually was relieved too.

With chronic pain, weight loss, and failure to eat a balanced diet decreases the patient's resistance to additional disease. Thus, the pain problem may be complicated by other health problems.

Weight loss with chronic pain is not always due simply to decreased appetite. The patient with chronic pain often discovers that oral analgesics are more quickly and totally absorbed if they are taken on an empty stomach. Thus he may avoid eating prior to taking analgesics. Once the analgesic takes effect, the patient still may not eat if the analgesic causes sedation or nausea.

Weight gain, however, is by far the problem patients who have chronic pain of nonmalignant origin are faced with. Generalized decrease in physical activity probably contributes to the tendency toward weight gain. Also, chronic pain is associated with depression, and depression may be related to poor food choices and overeating. One patient with severe pain of six months' duration illustrates this problem. He had gained 40 pounds since the onset of pain. On rounds, he was found lying in bed eating a pint of ice cream by the spoonful directly from the carton. He explained that eating was almost the only thing he could do to bring pleasure and comfort to his body.

Since so many patients with chronic pain have muscle and joint problems, the tendency toward weight gain is especially important to keep in check. The more weight the patient carries around, the more likely they are to experience an increase in muscle and joint pain.

Sleep

"If I could only sleep" is a common lament of the patient with pain, acute or chronic. Pain, per se, is exhausting. Possibly people with pain have an increased need for sleep or rest but pain can prevent sleep. In a study of adult patients with pain hospitalized on a medical unit, specific questions about the effects of their acute pain showed that sleep was the most frequently reported area of disturbance (Marks & Sacher, 1973). For the patient with chronic pain, sleep tends to be such a constant problem that it has been said that a patient feels like he has eternal jet lag. Patients with pain are often treated with analgesics and sleep-deprived patients are often treated with hypnotics. However, it has been shown that short-acting analgesics on a PRN basis, as opposed to longer acting analgesics on a time-contingent basis and hypnotics on a regular basis, tend to compound the problem because they disrupt normal sleep patterns (Black, 1980, p. 211).

When pain interferes with sleep, the resulting fatigue may be very detrimental. In general, lack of sleep results in symptoms that are remarkably similar to those of sensory restrictions which are discussed in Chapter 8. Quite understandably, the feelings of tiredness and weariness cause the individual to begin to take the easy way out, choosing alternatives that demand the least of him physically and mentally. Since fatigue delays transmission of nerve impulses, reaction times may become uneven. As the mental processes slow down it becomes difficult to maintain a train of thought. Fantasies become more prevalent and hallucinations may occur. An excellent example of this is the experience of a disc jockey who stayed awake to broadcast for over eight days. On the last morning of this marathon, during one of the routine medical examinations, he decided the physician was an undertaker who had come to bury him, and immediately ran out of the building (Current Research on Sleep and Dreams, 1965).

Such effects of sleep deprivation suggest that fatigue will affect the patient's response to pain in several other ways. He or she will have less energy and mental ability to utilize usual strategies, such as distraction or imagination, for coping with pain. As a result he or she will tend to choose less demanding alternatives, such as analgesics. In addition the patient may indulge in horrible fantasies about the significance of the pain. This in turn may increase the subjective experience of the pain sensation. One example of some of these effects is a maternity patient who refused analgesics and anesthetics until she had labored for 24 hours and had been without sleep for 36 hours. At that point she began to say that the labor would never end and that her baby would die. A half hour later, she accepted an epidural block.

With acute pain, recovery from the accompanying acute illness depends to some extent upon rest. Considering that the illness itself may be fatiguing and that pain further exhausts the patient and prevents sleep, the accumulation of fatigue may seriously hamper recovery. In addition, the patient may simply be too tired to engage in activities that might speed his recovery and prevent complications. When the patient with acute pain and illness is deprived of a restful night's sleep, he or she is much less likely to ambulate, exercise his legs, turn in bed, breathe deeply, or cough. These activities require energy he may not have.

The significance of sleep difficulties is somewhat different for the patient with chronic pain. Day after day, month after month, the patient gets up tired in the morning. He or she is irritable with family, friends, and coworkers and eventually cannot even go to work. The perpetual fatigue causes a decrease in almost all activities. The patient is involved in fewer social activities and the general physical condition often deteriorates. He or she may fail to take care of himself or herself in some simple ways, such as brushing the teeth and bathing.

Sometimes it seems that sleeping problems are at the root of all the problems faced by the patient with pain. Certainly this is by no means entirely true, but lack of rest and sleep contribute to many of the effects discussed here.

To assess the effect of pain upon sleep, the nurse may ask specific questions such as the following: Does pain keep you from going to sleep at night? Does pain awaken you during the night or an afternoon nap? Does pain cause you to awaken earlier than your usual habit? How rested do you feel after sleeping?

Physical Activity

Many activities of daily living are affected by pain. Restlessness and various types of body movement, such as the protective or rubbing motions may result from pain. Here we are concerned with how pain interferes with the normal daily physical activities, such as walking. Generally the patient with pain decreases physical activities, often to the point of staying in bed.

Usually this is expected with acute pain. Because this pain is of brief duration, limited physical activity may be no more than a temporary inconvenience. With chronic pain, the problem is much more significant.

When the patient has prolonged or chronic pain, assessment involves asking specific questions about physical activities, such as the following: How often do you stop to rest and for how long? How far can you walk? Can you dress and undress yourself? Does pain interfere with physical activity associated with your job? What kinds of physical activities relieve your pain, cause it, or increase it? Are you able to walk up and down stairs? Have you had to give up your participation in any sports?

Sexual Activity

A decrease in sexual activity and interest often accompanies pain. Sometimes the physical movements involved in sexual activity cause the onset of pain or an increase in intensity. This is especially true for patients with pain in the back, arms, neck, head, or shoulders. For other patients it is a matter of decreased interest because the pain consumes their attention, and they also experience anxiety and depression.

If the pain is of brief duration, a temporary interruption in sexual activity may be tolerated well by the patient and sexual partner. However, with pain that lasts several weeks or longer, sexual inhibition may be a much greater problem. In one study of chronic pain patients two-thirds reported decreased quality and frequency of sexual activity and more than one-third reported deterioration in their marriages (Maruta & Osborne, 1978, p. 531).

It may be appropriate for the nurse to assess the effect of pain upon the patient's sexual activity. Early detection of a problem can result in counseling to help improve or restore the patient's level of sexual functioning. Otherwise, some authors feel that sexual dysfunction with prolonged pain can become irreversible. They also say that return of sexual interest and activity exerts a positive therapeutic effect by relieving anxiety, distracting attention from pain, and providing affectionate and warm relationships (Naughton & Chiu, 1975). Even the patient with chronic back and neck problems can be helped to find alternatives that allow sexual function (Rubin, 1970).

Social Interactions

Both casual and intimate relationships with others tend to deteriorate when the patient has pain. The longer the pain lasts, the more isolated the patient usually becomes. Again, the problem occurs with both acute and chronic pain but is of more significance for the chronic pain patient.

The patient with acute pain may use visitors to distract from the pain or he or she may prefer to be alone with pain. As the pain subsides, relationships with others usually resume.

When pain continues month after month, maintaining relationships with others can become an almost insurmountable problem for the chronic pain patient. The patient may suffer from a combination of several effects of pain such as those previously mentioned, plus body disfigurement associated with the pain problem, time consumed in regimens to control the pain, and other feelings such as anxiety, depression, irritability, anger, and confusion. The patient may become extremely self-centered and "pull-out" of all normal activities and relationship with others. The patient may elect to spend time only with people who have a similar problem feeling he or she can no longer continue to burden his or her significant others with the ongoing pain and depression. The patient may even hope or plead for a premature death.

Not only may the patient have a decreased investment in his relationship with others but family and friends may find that the patient is quite unpleasant to be around. Maltbie, et al. (1978, p. 359) say that "When the source of pain is physically apparent, empathy is more readily maintained." The *empathy* may be directly proportional to the patient's *perceived pain* and *suffering*. Once all efforts to relieve the suffering have failed there is usually a deterioration in the patient's relationship with significant others and the health care professionals. Marital relationships are often adversely affected. It is estimated that 40–50 percent of chronic pain sufferers have been divorced (Gaumer, 1974). Significant others often feel angry both because of their helplessness and because of the disruptions to their own life. The more essential parts of one's life that have been effected such as social interactions or financial security, the more anger and guilt the significant others may feel. Even though nurses and physicians may be aware that it is through no fault of theirs that the patient experiences pain, irrational anger at the patient is not uncommonly expressed as was previously discussed.

In working with cancer patients, Sutherland (1981, p. 166) reports that even with advanced cancer where a patient has marked physical deterioration, when the relationship was based on mutual trust and affection and there were no conflicts in the economic or sexual spheres, the patient can expect the same warmth, caring, and even suppression of the spouse's grief to further support him or her. In "facade marriages" (marriages which have endured primarily for some social or economic reason) and "hostile marriages" the patient may well be abandoned emotionally, physically, and economically.

To assess the effect of pain upon the patient's social interactions, the nurse must ask about the patient's relationships at home and at work. With whom does the patient spend time and what do they do together? How have others reacted to pain? How do relationships now compare with those before the onset of pain? Information more specifically related to the presence, attitudes, and feelings of others toward the patient with pain is discussed in Chapter 8.

FEELINGS, THOUGHTS—EMOTIONAL RESPONSES TO PAIN

A myriad of thoughts and feelings occur in the patient with pain. All at the same time the patient can feel anxious, depressed, lonely, confused, angry, irritable, resentful, and guilty. The nurse's assessment of these feelings is facilitated by understanding some of their variations and by appreciating just how difficult it may be for some patients with pain.

No matter how much we try to understand, it is very hard to know what pain does to another person. The practitioner's personal experience with pain is significant. If you have never experienced either severe or chronic pain, it is almost impossible to know how intense pain can become or what prolonged pain can do to your life. On the other hand, if you have experienced severe pain or chronic pain, there is always the risk that you may, like many others, feel that this increases your expertise on the subject. In a sense it does, but pain is a highly individualized experience. Our personal experiences with pain shed some light on what others endure, but they can never be used as *the* standard against which to judge another's pain experience. It is, of course, impossible that the practitioner have personal experience with every type of pain, but the practitioner's experience with pain seems to make a difference. Unfortunately the effects are not always in the direction of concern, sympathy or empathy for the patient as are discussed in Chapter 3.

There do not appear to be any systematic studies about the stages of emotional adjustment and responses patients go through as they experience pain over a period of time. However, Pinsky (1979, pp. 312–313) describes the grief response for the patient with pain. He identifies "somatic distress, preoccupation with the premorbid self, anger, and bitterness about medical and surgical treatment outcomes and changes in conduct patterns such as restlessness, inactivity, insomnia, and diminished psychosocial activity" as components. These changes are similar to those of individuals undergoing other major losses. The striking possibility, however, for the patient with chronic pain is that these losses occur in addition to major changes in body image and roles, and all at almost the same time. Thus the grief process may be significantly intensified as would the possibility for incomplete or pathological grief.

Both denial of emotions accompanying pain and loss and the meaning the patient ascribes to his pain may lead to an overreaction to it (Fielding, 1980, p. 705). Therefore, thinking of the person as going through certain stages of emotional adjustment and response during the pain experience is useful for the nurse when assessing the patient with pain. Identifying the present characteristics of a patient's response, attitude, and adjustment to pain helps anticipate more accurately the effects of the pain upon the patient and the types of relief that the patient may accept, both for pain and the emotional response to it.

Anxiety

Anxiety is the emotion most often associated with acute pain, is recognized as increasing pain perception and is experienced in several ways. It is related to the severity of the pain and possible meanings pain has for the patient. In general, the more severe the anxiety, the greater the reaction to pain stimulation (Bronzo & Powers, 1967; Jones, et al. 1966; Katz, 1979; 1982; Katz, et al., 1980, 1982 a; b; Malmo & Shagass, 1949; Merskey, 1978; Pinsky & Malyon, 1979 a; b).

Here we are concerned with the nature of the feeling of anxiety. The patient simply may be fearful of something that he can easily identify. This is illustrated by a woman who had surgical removal of an abdominal malignancy four years ago. Now she has been experiencing abdominal pain of several days' duration and awaiting hospitalization for diagnostic tests. She said, "I'm in a panic. The only thing I can think of is cancer. I wake up in the middle of the night with a pain but all I think about is cancer. But I just try not to think about it. What else can I do until I know?" This interfered considerably with her ability to work. She experienced marked confusion and difficulty concentrating. She said she was able to do only routine activities, nothing that demanded creativity.

Black (1980, p. 215) discusses the relationship of pain and anxiety in the patient with *cancer*, which he calls the "most unfortunate diagnosis." He says that cancer becomes an explanation for every ache and discomfort when these really represent the patient's anxiety, fear, and depression about the diagnosis. Even after the cancer pain has been successfully treated, unrelieved anxiety can intensify pain and lead to the use of strong analgesics when a more helpful approach might be an exploration of the meaning of the pain and other treatments more specifically directed toward the anxiety. It seems likely that *patients* with any *condition* which they *believe* has an *ominous prognosis* and which is accompanied by pain may experience similar anxiety reactions. They too may benefit from the above suggested approach and treatment of their anxiety.

Other patients may be anxious, but may not be able to identify exactly why. This is illustrated by a man who was hospitalized with ureteral colic. Even when he was not in pain, he said he was unable to do any of the paper work he had brought with him to the hospital. He said, "I don't know what is bothering me. They [the physicians] seem to know what causes it [the pain]. But they don't seem to know what to do about it. I just don't know what's going to happen." He seemed to be expressing anxiety over the *uncertainty* of all aspects of his situation—prognosis, future pain, treatment, ability to work. He, too, had difficulty concentrating and thinking in his usual fashion.

Katz et al. (1980, p. 363) studying anxiety in children with leukemia undergoing repeated painful procedures found that young children consistently exhibit higher levels of behavioral distress (anxiety, fear, and pain), and a greater variety of anxious responses occurring over a longer period of time than do older children. They explain these findings based on the work of Mussen et al. (1974), who indicate that younger children have a greater tendency for stimulus generalization and are less inhibited in their behavioral expression. Kauffman (1980, p. 283) says that infants and young children may respond to a lesser degree and for a shorter period of time in relation to pain or the threat of pain. Exemplifying this, he says the seven- to eight-month-old baby exhibits pain behaviors only while the painful stimuli is occurring in contrast to the child of one year who demonstrates anxiety and fear by crying when he sees someone enter the room with a syringe. Levy (1960) reports that this recognition of signals that may indicate pain is noted after six-months of age. Izard et al. (1980) report that by the seventh or eighth month children recognize, anticipate, and respond with specific emotional expressions to the potentially painful stimuli.

Unfortunately for children who have repeated painful experiences, this anxiety and associated behavioral responses do not decrease. Further acute painful experiences are significantly influenced by preceeding emotional factors (Katz et al. 1981). Therefore, if the anxiety is not treated, children who are highly anxious and experience more pain will have their fear and avoidance reinforced in a circular manner (Katz, 1982). In one study of leukemic children, Spinetta & Maloney (1975) reported that as the duration of their illness increased and repeated outpatient visits were necessary, the children became significantly more anxious. Further, the anxiety and pain may seriously disrupt the continuation of normal life activities of children (Katz, 1982). Katz et al. (1980, p. 364) found that children who were inquisitive about procedures exhibited fewer anxious behaviors than children who did not question. This lead them to speculate that children were asking questions in an attempt to enable themselves to cope more effectively.

In addition to increasing the perceived intensity of their pain experience patients with relatively high anxiety levels may suffer from distorted communication about their pain. Because such patients may be less able to articulate clearly or may not verbalize at all, health care professionals may be more likely to ignore, minimize, or dismiss their pain complaints. Thus, these patients may receive less than optimum assessment and treatment for their pain problem.

Treating either pain or anxiety has been shown to be mutually beneficial because decreasing one decreases the other. Capka, et al. (1979, p. 383) report that one benefit of relieving the patient's pain is that it desensitizes him to the anxiety associated with the pain. Chapman (1978, p. 179), Sternbach (1978, p. 243), and Sutherland (1981, p. 170) report different positive effects of decreasing the patient's anxiety. Chapman (1979) reports that decreasing the patient's anxiety with appropriate information helps maximize the patient's coping skills. Sternbach (1978) says that when anxiolytic agents, explanations, and reassurance are appropriately used, patients report less pain, and Sutherland (1981) has found that there is an overall benefit of decreasing the patient's anxiety. It fosters hope and resumption of adaptive coping. He suggests this can be accomplished by encouraging the patient to verbalize without the fear of rejection and helping the patient feel confident that the advice and treatment he has received is appropriate and well motivated.

These techniques may not benefit all patients. It has been found that even when preparatory messages are used for the purpose of decreasing the distress associated with pain, they are not consistently effective. In one study such information prior to a painful procedure reduced distress for low-fear women but exacerbated anxiety and stress for high-fear women, especially during the early parts of the test (McCaul, 1980, pp. 502–503). The most beneficial intervention for the patient with anxiety accompanying pain may come from the patient. Thus, the nurse should ask him what he has found effective in the past.

Depression

Depression is almost invariably associated with chronic or prolonged pain. This is a *reactive* or *neurotic* type of *depression*, as opposed to *endogenous depression*. In other words, the depression is in general a reaction to an event that involves loss, in this case, the loss is imposed by the pain. All of the previously mentioned effects of pain on the patient in this chapter also occur in response to depression due to habituation of the autonomic nervous system (Sternbach, 1978, p. 243). Obviously, then, pain and depression are capable of reinforcing each other. Feelings of depression in the patient with pain takes many forms. The patient feels *lonely, discouraged, helpless, hopeless, abandoned, disinterested, agitated, angry,* and *irritable*. These feelings tend to increase during the day, becoming worse at night (Sternbach, 1974 a).

It is generally accepted that reactive depression occurs with chronic pain and that it makes the pain experience more difficult for the patient. The patient's lack of interest in surroundings and lack of motivation decrease the chances of doing what is necessary to relieve the pain or of living a productive satisfying life in spite of the pain. The depression, accompanied as it is with a focus on the self, serves to increase the perceived intensity of pain. Sternbach (1974 a) says that focusing on the pain, somatization, may be adaptive for the patient's depression because it may help him avoid an awareness of the depressed feelings.

What is not fully understood is the cause and effect relationship between chronic pain and depression. One view is that the depressive mood is characteristic of chronic pain patients whether the cause of pain is environmental (psychogenic) or organic, that most functioned quite normally or adequately prior to the onset of pain, and that relief of the pain reduces or eliminates the depression (Sternbach, 1974a; Sternbach & Timmermans, 1975). Pinsky (1979, p. 311) is in agreement. He believes that the depressive demeanor is the result of multiple treatment failures including antidepressant medications. Further, he and his associates have found that no matter how longstanding the disturbance, and in spite of its depth, it responds very positively and rapidly to a caring and hopeful treatment situation. Thus he recommends the use of the word *demoralizing* instead of *depression*. From these workers in the field of pain it would appear that depression is the result, not the cause of chronic pain. However, other researchers disagree to the extent that they find that many patients with pain retain abnormal personality profiles despite the alleviation of pain. Thus, it is possible that the higher incidence of depression and somatic concern in patients with chronic pain may constitute a preexisting personality pattern that facilitates the continuation of the pain (Pilowsky & Spence, 1976). Patients with postoperative cancer pain and reactive depression may be at especially high risk for unrelenting reactive depression. Sutherland (1981, p. 164) reports that if a basic pattern is disrupted, the reactive depression may persist indefinitely throughout the individual's entire life.

While the question of cause and effect remains unanswered, the frequency of depression makes it a highly significant aspect of assessment of the patient with pain. One reason that the relationship between depression and pain is addressed here is because of the harm that can be done if depression is assessed with the attitude that the pain is due to the patient's depression. This impression is easily conveyed if, for example, the nurse tries to identify some depressing event in the patient's past that occurred prior to or at the same time as the onset of pain. This may or may not be relevant. The important point is that it can increase the patient's depression if it is felt that the nurse is attempting to ascribe the pain to psychological rather than organic causes. Patients and some health professionals tend to discount pain that has an unidentifiable emotional component. The nurse *must* make it very clear to the patient that it would be unusual if pain, regardless of its cause, did not result in some feelings of depression. Another point that needs to be communicated to the patient is that treatment of depression has been found to significantly decrease pain and treatment of the pain significantly decreases the depression (Sternbach, 1978, p. 243). Informing the patient of this may make him more receptive both to discussing his depression and becoming more amenable to possible treatment of it.

If you have never experienced chronic pain, the effects of the pain and the nature of the depression may be more easily understood if you participate in a mental exercise: Remember the last time you experienced pain. Regardless of its location and quality, it probably represents chronic pain for someone. Now slowly and seriously try to imagine that the pain never went away. You thought it would subside, but it did not. You tried a few simple remedies and finally consulted your physician, who suggested a few methods of treatment. These were not successful, the pain continued, and you saw another physician. By now you have consulted several people, and not necessarily all of them were members of the health team. Months have passed and the pain remains. Try to imagine what this would have done to your life. How much money would it have cost? How much time would be devoted to the care of the pain? How would it affect your normal day? Think of getting up in the morning (could you get out of bed?) and going through each activity of your usual day. Remember, the pain is with you always, not only occasionally, changing in intensity or quality. With these thoughts, consider the following descriptions of living with chronic pain.

The similarities between chronic pain and a nightmare are enumerated in a sensitive account by LeShan (1964). First, in both instances, terrible things are being done to the person. Things may become worse. Second, the person is not in control of what is happening. He or she feels helpless. Third, there is no limit to the experience. He cannot predict when it will be over, if ever. In addition to this, the experience becomes meaningless. Acute pain can be thought of as serving a purpose because it may warn of bodily harm and of the need to do something to help ourselves. Chronic pain may seem to serve no purpose; it may be utterly senseless.

The loneliness and nightmare quality of chronic pain is succinctly expressed by a patient, quoted by Sternbach (1974a, p. 7) as saying, "It's always 3 o'clock in the morning." That is indeed a lonely time.

Another patient described pain as being a prison. He told us his painful body formed a prison around the person he really was. He said he was still the same person he was before the onset of pain. He still wanted to laugh, enjoy life, and engage in all the activities that constituted his previous daily life. Yet he said his pain acted like the walls of a prison, keeping him from stepping out into his former life. One of his fantasies was to walk away from his painful body, leaving it behind even if it were in the prison.

Still another patient said that his chronic pain made him feel like an old man. He specifically said he did not wish to discuss his pain unless it was absolutely necessary. He said conversations about his pain made him feel very old. In particular, he said that focusing on his pain made him feel dependent upon others and unable to do the things that adults his age could do. He was 31 years old and had suffered low back pain for 18 months. Until the onset of his pain he was very active in a variety of sports, such a snow skiing and weight lifting. As he reluctantly continued, upon our request, to describe his feelings, he said that being an old man was something like being a child. Again, he focused on being deprived of adult activities and independence.

Thus the depression associated with pain, especially chronic pain, is felt in many ways. It is *loneliness*, a *nightmare*, a *prison*, or *being an old man*. Doubtless many other patients with pain have equally descriptive ways to explain their feelings about the affect their pain has had on them.

Suicidal attempts and thoughts may occur in patients with pain, especially severe, uncontrolled pain. The pain need not be chronic. It may be of only several weeks' duration. Comedian Jerry Lewis (1982) openly discussed how close he has come to committing suicide because of the constant pain he suffers from a spinal injury incurred from a stage fall. At one point, he actually had the barrel of a loaded gun in his mouth.

Statistics on successful suicide to escape pain are essentially nonexistent as far as we have been able to determine. However, suicide is mentioned in the literature on pain, but there is a remarkable lack of discussion. The extreme and finite end of the pain intensity scale devised by Sternbach (1974a) is labeled suicide. Marks & Sacher (1973) describe briefly one patient with sickle-cell crisis who threatened suicide as a desperate attempt to get more medication for her severe pain. Pasnau (1975), a practicing psychiatrist, says that when a patient with chronic pain is referred to him he quickly assesses the degree of depression since the patient could be suicidal. Occasionally one hears that a high incidence of suicide is associated with a certain type of pain, such as cluster headache or trigeminal neuralgia.

The occurrence of attempted suicide is illustrated by a woman who was hospitalized with a low back pain of undiagnosed origin and of several weeks' duration. She described it as unbearable. Although she was receiving medication for the pain, morphine 5 mg IM, the degree of relief was not satisfactory to her. She was described by the nursing staff as very depressed. On several occasions she asked her physician to consider a cordotomy. Once she initiated a lengthy conversation with him about the possibility of increasing her medication for pain. The physician refused both suggestions, and he and the staff began to avoid contact with the patient. After being hospitalized for about three weeks, she attempted suicide. The result was a reversal of action on the part of the health team. The dosage of morphine was tripled and she was transferred to another hospital for evaluation of a possible cordotomy. This is a truly unfortunate situation. It is quite likely that more satisfactory pain relief could have been achieved with fewer oppressive side effects for this patient. An example of a successful suicide by a patient with prolonged pain was reported by Jones (1981). A 59-year-old man with neck pain of several years' duration had gone to many physicians seeking relief for his pain. The last physician he had seen had x-rayed his neck, found no cause for the neck pain, and told the patient he would have to "learn to live with it." That night the patient shot himself.

The severely depressed patient with pain may not attempt suicide, but may lose what we so often refer to as the will to live. This happened in a teenage girl who had suffered about two months with pain from osteomyelitis of the femur. Eventually she had an open, draining wound that was surgically debrided and packed once a week. From the beginning, her pain rarely was well controlled. Finally she began refusing all medication for pain, since she said it did not help anyway. For several days she cried all day and almost all night. She hardly talked with anyone and did not call the nurses for assistance with toileting. Consequently, she would simply lay in her own feces and urine until it was discovered on a routine check. Naturally, she refused all rehabilitative measures such as physical therapy. The staff felt it was increasingly likely that her leg would have to be amputated. However, when her medication for pain was adjusted to provide pain relief, her depression lifted almost immediately. Once again she cooperated with the health team and took part in her own recovery. Amputation was not necessary and several weeks later she was discharged.

Anger

Pain results in other feelings we may find more difficult to accept. Pain makes some people *angry, hostile, resentful, aggressive,* and *irritable.* Patients with pain not only scream, they also curse. This is a common sight when a person accidentally, for example, hits her thumb with a hammer or bangs his head on a cabinet door. When pain persists for weeks, the patient may also at times have an overwhelming desire to use obscenities. On several occasions, we have closed the door to a patient's room while he or she uttered a string of curse words and profanities that other patients and visitors might find offensive.

If a man told you that five or six times a day another person hit him in the back with a lead pipe, it would not be very surprising if he also said this made him extremely angry. Yet sometimes we fail to appreciate that pain, regardless of its origin, is likely to cause anger. Thus, the man with chronic low back pain of unknown cause may very well exhibit periods of anger.

Reviews of the literature reveal much evidence that pain elicits aggressive behavior and irritability. When pain is felt on the skin, as opposed to internally, aggression may be especially likely. Also, resentment seems to be aroused fairly easily in patients with pain. It may be expressed towards physicians or others (Merskey, 1976; Sternbach, 1968).

Anger turned inward is traditionally thought of as depression. Some depressed patients may have difficulty expressing hostility, but others may manifest angry outbursts. *Repressed hostility* may also be related to anxiety (Pilowsky & Spence, 1976). Anger turned outward may take the form of aggression, resentment, irritability, and *manipulativeness.* This occurs with both acute and chronic pain.

In one study, about half of a group of patients hospitalized with acute pain reported that they had significant difficulty with *irritability* (Marks &

Sacher, 1973). The effect this has upon relationships with others can be devastating. One patient who had occasional headaches lasting several days told us she went to bed each night deeply ashamed of how irritable the headaches caused her to be with her husband and child. Another person told us he knew his pain was not his physician's fault, but he could not help *blaming* the physician for the pain. No doubt this man expected, as do most patients, that the physician will heal whatever malady they may have. The physician and nurse often are blamed if they fail, perhaps sometimes only because the patient needs to place blame somewhere.

The presence of irritability in children who have pain may be the major presenting behavior of an illness. We have often seen children described as becoming spoiled and demanding only to discover some days later that this child has had a severe ear infection or tonsillitis. We have come to regard irritability in a child as an excellent clue to the possibility of pain.

There are somewhat conflicting reports about anger in patients with chronic pain. One study compared patients with chronic intractable pain who were referred to a pain clinic with outpatients with chronic pain responsive to conventional management. Those with intractable pain reported greater inhibition of angry feelings (Pilowsky & Spence, 1976). Others have reported that these patients are also more liable to frequent anger (Engel, 1959). In another study, patients with chronic low back pain showed more agitation, and those who had litigation pending showed higher anger, *resentment* against authority figures, and rebelliousness (Sternbach et al. 1973).

Certainly there is reason to suspect the presence of some form of anger in the patient with pain. Assessment needs to include questions about anger and its variations such as feelings of hostility, resentment, irritability, blame, bitterness, and actions such as *striking out* against others or breaking or smashing things.

Guilt

The relationship of guilt is not as frequently or clearly dealt with in relationship to pain in the literature. When mentioned it usually is in relationship to pain being used to expiate guilt or guilt over dependency needs and/or secondary gains associated with the pain and unacceptable anger. The anger may be in relation to the individual not getting what he wants from other people or situations. However, it seems likely that there are at least two instances in which the patient with pain may experience guilt which may also intensify his pain experience. First, if the patient has knowingly done anything which has caused or increased his pain, and second, when the patient is confronted with the fact that his pain may be providing secondary gains. That is the patient may need and perpetuate his pain either consciously or unconsciously. Secondary gains related to pain will be discussed in Chapter 8. At the time of confrontation it is likely that the patient will experience guilt and increasing anxiety, depression and, possibly denial, at least initially. Crue (1979, pp. 406–407) in working with patients with CIBPS says that presenting the information to patients "that they have a subconscious need to continue to hurt" results in "considerable heated discussion." In presenting this information to patients Crue says that he attempts to empathize while pointing out to patients that the " 'unconscious' thoughts, feelings or conflicts may be 'more painful' to confront than the painful syndromes from which they are suffering." It seems possible that the patient's "heated discussions" may be due to guilt. As mentioned in Chapter 5, another time patients with pain sometimes experience guilt is when they have "failed" to respond to a treatment plan.

Thought Disturbances

Thought disturbances appear frequently in patients with pain. In a study of adults with pain who were hospitalized on a medical unit, it was found that *difficulty with concentration* was the second most frequently reported disturbance of function, sleep being the most frequent (Marks & Sacher, 1973). No doubt the sleeping difficulties contributed to the problems with concentration. In elderly patients with brain impairment, the onset of *confusion* may signal the onset of pain (Hunt, 1976). Patients with pain not uncommonly say that they feel they are losing their minds.

Thought disturbances may become extreme. In a study of patients who had cardiac surgery, over half the patients reported hallucinatory-type experiences, defined as perceptions for which there were no apparent appropriate stimuli within the patient's environment. The patients described experiences of varying specificity. One patient's experience included a "bared-fang menacing black bear" and copper rods that exuded a vile smell. Another patient reported "half dreams" of "hazy unpleasantness." A significant number of patients associated their thought disturbances with uncontrolled pain (Ellis, 1972).

Body Image

Body image refers to one's concept of what constitutes the self. The neonate's first experiences are through body experiences. Body organs or parts are vested with certain individually specific meanings and are usually intimately connected with one's patterns of adjustment, relationship with others, and styles of communications. Sutherland (1981, p. 161) says "The loss of a body part has a much wider context than its impact upon the individual's 'body image'." This is so to a large degree due to its significance in determining the types of disruptions the patient expects in his entire life. Because valued life activities are intimately related to basic character defenses, patterns of adaptation and maintenance of self-respect, even a temporary disruption can produce significant problems for a patient. Robinson (1976, p. 8) says that the patient may treat the involved body part "as an anxious parent treats a sick child."

Engel (1959) extends the idea of body image to a "*body pain image*." By this he means both areas of the body in which pain was previously experienced and memories of past experiences with pain. Szasz (1957) says that individuals may project their feelings on to their body in the same way that they do to other people. Pilowsky (1978, p. 207) exemplifies this in relation to the pain experience saying that an individual may perceive his pain as an attack from his own body.

It is not uncommon to hear a patient with pain say "I feel like I no longer know who I am" or "I no longer am who I was." Some patients may not be able to conceal their pain behaviors such as limping, therefore are unable to project the self-image they desire and may be fearful of alienating others. In one study, impairment and disability were positively correlated with pain behaviors (Brena, et al. 1979, p. 387). Thus, role changes may either cause or result in further body image and role changes. Even patients who have no visible changes in their body may suffer from changes in their body image. For these individuals the change may be equally traumatic and at times more so. Patients who suffer from very painful or discomforting diseases which are not visible to others stand a considerable chance of not being able to legitimatize their pain behaviors to others. Strauss & Glasser (1975, p. 50) see this as a great disadvantage to the patient because others are likely to believe the patient is "malingering, somewhat sick but not *that* sick or even pretty neurotic."

Especially with prolonged pain, one's loss of self-esteem and one's thoughts and feelings about pain and body image may significantly influence feelings of future competency, ability to participate in life as one formerly enjoyed it and one's potential for rehabilitation. Even the patient who restructures his or her life and is considered successfully rehabilitated is constantly confronted by the changes in identity, with anxiety about continued abilities, sustaining relationships and desired activities. Moreover, when patients have diseases which are disfiguring or stigmatizing *even* if they are successful in not having a negative self-image they must develop adaptive processes to avoid such feelings (p. 52).

ADJUSTMENT TO PROLONGED PAIN

The patient with prolonged pain is a very vulnerable individual being exposed to innumerable crises and losses. These very realities may force the patient to focus on his pain as a necessity for self-protection and self-preservation. Indeed, the patient often will have been instructed that he or she *must focus* on his or her body and become intensely aware of any biological changes as they may herald an impending condition that carries with it the potential of intensifying their pain. Strauss & Glaser (1975, p. 18) say that "when the patient is his own protective agent, he carries a heavy burden." One thing the patient cannot delegate is the responsibility for body and mind.

Vigilance by the patient with prolonged pain will involve being aware of early signs and symptoms and attempting to identify their possible significance in relation to the pain experience. The patient must know the quality, the duration, and anything that may or may not be done that will influence the pain. For example, a patient may have a dull ache in a calf that lasts for 20 minutes and remits by itself requiring no intervention. On the other hand, if the pain persists beyond that point it may signal the need for protective or therapeutic modalities. The patient must also know the impact of some types of pain or other symptoms and their relationship to his tolerance. Does the dull ache, in the above example, result in severe burning pain after 20 minutes which the patient finds intolerable? The patient must also become aware under what circumstances he can tolerate pain. Does work or play increase his tolerance to his pain? How a patient manages his routine is intimately involved in his value system. For example, a man with low back pain may elect to lift an object knowing this may increase his pain rather than suffer the embarrassment of asking a woman for assistance.

Attempts at Normalizing

Strauss & Glasser (1975, pp. 74–80) discuss the arduous and endless tasks and maneuvers which are involved for a patient with a chronic illness who is attempting to regain and maintain some semblance of his or her former life. This information will be applied to the patient with chronic pain. For the patient with chronic pain "adjusting" involves keeping pain behaviors to a minimum and appearing as normal as possible. Maneuvers to accomplish this include covering-up, keeping-up, justifying inaction, pacing, reducing activity, eliciting help, and balancing options. *Both success* and *failure* at any of these activities is likely to result in increased pain, fatigue and stress, thus *exacerbating* the very pain that the patient is attempting to prevent or cope with.

Covering up or *concealing pain* and *disability* differs from denial in that the patient is consciously attempting to separate his or her total social and interactional self from the pain problem. *Keeping up* involves trying to maintain what the individual sees as normal for him or her. When both children and adults have minimal pain or have pain-free periods they often indulge in a type of *super-normalizing* in an attempt to make up for lost time, "proving their capacity or denying their incapacity or recapturing a former identity" (p. 75). This "super-normalizing" may temporarily distract the patient from the pain but usually there is a high price for his temporary freedom. He or she loses more time and self-esteem through the subsequent increased pain, disability, and oscillating periods of better and worse.

Some patients with pain have difficulty in *justifying* their *inactivity* to others. Although many individuals pride themselves on concealing their pain, they usually have an intense desire for someone to "just understand" and minimize the social isolation. One patient described the feelings as "Pain is essentially private. Sometimes you wish for someone to understand and be patient with your pain. To allow you to have it!! I do not mean sympathy or pity" (p. 76).

Pacing involves the patient becoming very attuned to the body and making constant decisions, sometimes by the minute or hour, relative to activities he or she is capable of doing, their frequency, and under what circumstances. Both pacing oneself and failure to pace oneself may result in increased pain problems, fatigue, and stress for the patient. When it becomes necessary for the patient to *elicit help* with certain activities to better pace himself it becomes impossible for the patient to cover up. Further, his inability to keep-up and feelings of a lack of competency and dependency are likely to escalate. The patient's increased dependency needs due to the escalating pain and disability may cause the patient to fear that others may not or will not help, and may also result in undesired role reversal.

The life of the patient with prolonged pain becomes one of *balancing options*. Only the person who is experiencing the pain can know what price his choices may exact. When there is a *lack of predictability* as to their effect on his pain the patient can be expected to experience *increased vulnerability* to pain and disability and the anticipatory anxiety related to their potential consequences.

The Pain Regimen

To mitigate against potential pain crises, the patient must ingeniously devise singlely or in collaboration with the physician, other health professionals, or significant others, a routine that will afford the greatest protection yet the greatest flexibility and freedom. Strauss & Glasser (1975, p. 27) have identified the many considerations that the patient must make in deciding the merits of and his willingness to adhere to such a routine. These include:

1. Is it difficult or easy to learn and to carry out.
2. Takes much or little time [limits flexibility or fragments one's time].
3. Causes much or little discomfort or pain.
4. Does or does not cause side effects, especially if they are actually or seemingly risky ones.
5. Needs much or little effort or energy to carry out.
6. Is or is not visible to others.

7. If known, might or might not cause others to stigmatize the person.
8. Does or does not seem efficient.
9. Is or is not expensive.
10. Does or does not lead to increasing social isolation

About the imposition of routines either by self or others, Strauss & Glasser (p. 27) address health care professionals. They say that listing the considerations of a regimen is done

> in order to emphasize, as if underlined in red, that the view of a patient's breaking the regimen (foolish, ignorant, obstinate) that is often held by health personnel [and the patient's significant others] is just too simplistic, too stereotyped. Just scanning the list is likely to make one wonder at how anyone (including himself) manages to stay with his regimen, even in modified form.

We could not be more in agreement with this attitude toward the patient with pain. Indeed the "attacks" on patients by physician and nurses that were discussed earlier may be minimized if we could only keep the patient's realities in mind. Clarifying goals—the patient's versus ours—may also help.

As the pain comes under better and better control, for understandable reasons, the patient is likely to relax the defensive routine. This may include something seemingly as simple as not taking an analgesic, not wearing a brace, not doing exercises, or not sleeping in the prescribed position. The desire for regaining control of one's body and life is usually strong. One patient so resented the necessity of constantly focusing and being vigilant that her explanation for not adhering to her regimen was that it made her feel like a "neurotic" and "hypochondriac." Attempting to elicit compliance, her nurse explained that it was potentially "more neurotic" and "hypochrondriacal" to relax her guard and reexperience or intensify her pain and concomitant disability.

Indeed, patients who are under the supervision of more than one health care professional may be subject to even more labeling when there is inadequate communication among their health care team. For example, the patient with low back pain and angina has two conditions which may result in different types of pain and potentially conflicting regimens just in relation to position for sleep.

Balancing one's life with routines may be such a delicate matter that the patient may find that the constant juggling is just not worth it. The effect of the patient's pain on communication and relationships with significant others will be discussed in Chapters 8 and 9.

POSSIBLE ADAPTIVE STRATEGIES FOR PROLONGED PAIN

The components of the grieving process usually include the feelings and ideas previously discussed such as denial, anger, grief, depression, and bargaining (Kubler-Ross, 1969; Lazarus, 1975).

Usually when one discusses loss the notion that is conveyed is that of an isolated event such as the loss of an object. Further, Lazarus (1975, p. 50) says that the individual who goes through a loss is "expected to experience and display grief appropriately, that is in the proper degree, in the appropriate circumstances, and in the appropriate form."

When one considers the reverberatory losses involved for a patient described by McCaffery (1979, p. 275), who experienced a prolonged uncontrolled pain problem one wonders just what would constitute appropriate grieving. McCaffery says this

> A 43-year-old woman had severe muscle spasms of the neck and shoulders for approximately nine months before they were controlled sufficiently for the patient to be allowed to return to work. In the meantime, her losses included a $25,000 a year job; the need to live on workman's compensation; sell her new sports car, and buy an older car with power steering and automatic shift; move to a less expensive apartment; and only have enough money to buy used furniture. She gained 35 pounds and none of her clothes fit. Her boyfriend broke their engagement. In order for her to return to work it was necessary for her to take a job paying significantly less. In addition, to prevent recurrences and muscle strain, her life revolved around many daily exercises, watching her diet, getting enough rest, and numerous alterations in her environment. Some of these included the aggravation of having to water her houseplants with a garden hose, installing sliding shelves in the kitchen, finding someone to push her cart at the grocery store, and purchasing a desk with ball bearing drawers, an adjustable bed, a lightweight vacuum cleaner, and a lightweight iron. The summer before she was a busy, spontaneous woman, playing tennis several times a week, swimming in a bikini at the pool in her apartment building, dating a man she planned to marry, and enjoying considerable professional success.

This patient was interviewed three years later. In the interim she had experienced serious suicidal ideation and her weight gain increased to 55 pounds. Many additional adaptations in her activities of daily living were necessary. She had been sent to a psychologist to help her "learn to live with her pain." Her response to biofeedback was not typical of the chronic benign pain patient so she was referred back for further diagnostic workup. [Biofeedback is not considered to be effective in the treatment of acute pain (Orne, 1980, p. 269).] Her disability carrier refused to allow payment either for the studies or the recommended treatment based on these, creating further economic and psychological burdens. In desperation and with the hope of recapturing some semblance of her former life this patient elected to use all of her savings and private insurance to pay for the diagnostic studies and recommended extensive orthopedic and neurosurgery. Her pain was significantly improved; the functional ability in her arms was not. When she was ready to return to work, her employer refused to take her back in spite of the fact that she previously had been hired with the same functional limitations.

Understanding the stages of grief, she discussed the magnitude of the losses associated with her pain problem. She said that she felt for *each loss,* in varying degrees and for varying periods of time, she had gone through all of the stages of the grieving process. Adding that during periods of recurrent acute pain and on significant anniversaries she reexperienced many of the associated feelings in modified form. She commented that after 4½ years that she was finally just getting around to dealing with the losses which provided her the most satisfaction and pleasure including such things as participating in new recreational activities, reentering a relationship, and losing weight.

This patient's depression is not atypical of individuals who believe or have had to accept that their pain will persist indefinitely and that there is no good solution to their pain problem. Merskey (1978, p. 120) discusses the effects of chronic pain on personality which may further compound the patient's pain experience. He says that many individuals are aware of the damage to their personality from a prolonged pain experience citing increased vulnerability to anxiety and depression as significant symptoms. Consider the above patient's earlier experiences of being informed that the cause of her pain could not be found and the duration was unknown, how this patient adapts is likely to be quite different from another person who has possessed the same knowledge about himself for years. At first, and sometimes for years, the patient will avoid and deny the notion that the cause of his pain cannot be diagnosed. Each time the patient is confronted with this conclusion, he may insist upon being referred to another physician. The patient may be unwilling to accept anything less than definitive diagnosis and cure except perhaps the elimination of the pain without learning the cause.

Failure to appreciate the patient's orientation toward diagnosis and cure can cause us to repeat unsuccessful diagnostic procedures and treatments, increase the patient's frustration, and *increase* the patient's *resistance* to *other modalities.* This is illustrated by a 35-year-old man with chest pain of one year's duration. He had been admitted to the hospital for repeated diagnostic procedures, but the cause of his pain could not be found. The nurses suggested numerous palliative pain relief methods, such as relaxation techniques and transcutaneous electric nerve stimulation (TENS). Each suggestion infuriated the patient, and he continued to demand medication for his pain. He told the staff "I expect you to find out what causes this pain. When you do, you'll fix it and this time I'll walk out of here without pain." With this *denial* and belief system, naturally, it was difficult for this man to see any sense in spending time and perhaps money to learn palliative pain relief methods. We told him that we hoped a cure for his pain could be found. In addition because readiness and motivation are the crux of learning, we told him that if this did not happen other options for pain relief were available including a referral to a pain clinic.

Another patient may respond to chronic pain simply by *"giving up and going to bed."* The patient lives, but is disabled. In a way, he or she makes the best of the situation, but does so by being dependent upon others. The patient may feel perfectly justified in making demands upon others who do not have pain and in collecting money available through litigation or insurance. This patient may be very resistant to taking an active part in his pain relief. At least initially, he or she may be willing to try only those pain relief measures that allow passivity. For example, if massage of the painful area seems indicated, the patient may allow someone else to massage him or her, but will not do so by themself.

Defiance of the pain is another type of adjustment to the realization that pain may not end. This patient may be willing to try anything to achieve pain relief, but tries desperately not to change his or her life because of the pain. This often results in "peaks and valleys" in the patient's pain experience. A distinguishing feature may be that the patient does something that may initially seem totally illogical—causes the pain to occur or to increase. Usually he or she does so by engaging in an activity he enjoys. To the patient, the whole point of pain relief may be to enable him to be "normal" again. This is illustrated by a man with an arthritic spine. He enjoyed mowing his lawn but it caused extreme back pain. He would comply with the physician's orders to take medication, apply ice, and stay in bed. However, as soon as the pain began to subside he was out mowing his lawn again. He has continued this type of behavior for about ten years. Occasionally he will resist harmful physical activity for a matter of months, but then the *cycle* of *activity–pain–relief–activity* starts again. In discussing this patient's pain with him, he says that thinking that he cannot do something that pleases him is less tolerable than the subsequent pain he experiences from doing it and "paying the price." He further said that he still holds onto the hope that some day his pain will completely go away and every now and then he tests it fully knowing that he most likely will again increase the pain.

A variation of this adjustment is the patient who also is *willing to try almost any method of pain relief* but at the same time *adjusts* his or her *life style* to the fact that pain exists. This patient, for example, would not mow the lawn if he or she had an arthritic spine, and would try to prevent pain by limiting his physical activities. This type of patient *compliance* is less common. In addition to minimizing the patient's pain it is likely to endear him to the health team.

Still another type of adjustment may occur when the patient expects the pain to persist. This is the patient who *refuses most forms* of *pain relief* and makes every effort to keep pain from changing his or her daily life. This patient is seldom seen by health team members so information on this type of adjustment is not as clearly documented.

The patient may, of course, pass from one stage of adjustment to another in either the direction of progression or regression. As previously described, at first the patient may refuse to believe that the cause of the pain cannot be diagnosed and cured. Then the patient may become angry, depressed and withdrawn, giving up for a time. He may limit his activities severely and accept only those pain relief measures that allow him to remain passive and dependent. He may move from this stage to a more active one in which he resumes activities that do not adversely affect his pain, and he may be willing to assume some responsibility for his pain relief. As a result he may begin to learn how to use some palliative noninvasive measures such as guided imagery.

One young woman experienced the loss of her pain-free self and the loss of her husband, both abruptly. Her husband died mountain climbing and she had a traumatic amputation of her dominant right hand resulting in phantom limb pain. In comparing these two major losses the woman said that in the marriage she saw herself as part of a partnership and incomplete without her spouse. With the amputation, she also viewed herself as incomplete. She described feelings commonly associated with loss in both situations, commenting that they were like falling off the top of a mountain and having to begin all over again. She believed that the feelings of loss associated with her chronic pain were more difficult to cope with. Explaining this, she said that with the loss of her husband the finality was immediate and undeniable. She said,

> Although no two individuals are alike at least I was able to reestablish another relationship with a comparable life style. Although I felt that a part of me had died in reality I knew that this was not true. With the chronic pain even though I feel that I have been successfully rehabilitated [returned to gainful employment and remarried] I am constantly reminded that I am incomplete. When the pain is intense I am unable to deny my lost hand. Sometimes it makes me feel angry, other times very sad and depressed.

Some other possible adjustments or maladjustments to pain include the patient becoming resigned, stoic, empathetic to others with pain, indifferent, vindictive, and perhaps sadistic especially if those at whom it is directed have had any part in his pain.

No doubt there are other types or progressions of adjustment to pain. This discussion was meant to be suggestive of some of the possible effects of pain upon the patient. It is not comprehensive and certainly not final.

Sternbach & Timmermans (1975) have documented their finding that when there is relief of the chronic pain there is also some reversal of the personality changes. Unfortunately, for a great many patients the pain experience is not interrupted or minimized. It becomes more and more difficult for them. Although the pain may not actually increase in intensity, the pain may become increasingly bothersome or intolerable. As time passes the patient's adjustment may worsen considerably with respect to attitude and activities. When months pass with unrelenting pain, he or she may feel progressively more helpless and hopeless. The pain may deplete emotional and physical energy, leaving him or her less able to interact with family or to go to work. The patient's world shrinks and his life is dominated by pain. In effect, the longer the pain exists, the more the patient tends to suffer.

Nursing care of the patient with pain is to first acknowledge that all behavior is meaningful, purposeful, and can be understood; the nurse can then recognize and respond to the stage of adjustment that the patient is in. Also important to recognize is that it may take time to move from one step to another and that regression is not uncommon especially if there is an exacerbation of the pain problem.

Situational factors which affect the patient's pain experiences in some ways may be very closely related to the effects of pain on the patient and results in some overlapping of content. They will be discussed in the next chapter, Chapter 8.

REFERENCES

Anderson, R., & Krogh, K. Pain as a major cause of postoperative nausea. Can Anesth Soc J 23: 363–369, 1976.

Barber, T.X. The effects of "hypnosis" on pain: A critical review of experimental and clinical findings. Psychosom Med 25: 303–333, 1963.

Black, R.G. The clinical syndrome of chronic pain. In L.K.Y. Ng & J.J. Bonica, (Eds.) Pain, Discomfort and Humanitarian Care, Proceedings of the National Conference Held at the National Institutes of Health, Bethesda, MD, Feb. 15–16, 1979. New York: Elsevier/North-Holland, 1980, pp. 207–219.

Brena, S.F., Chapman, S.L., Stegall, P.G., et al.: Chronic pain states: Their relationship to impairment and disability. Arch Phys Med Rehab 60: 387, 1979.

Bronzo, A., Jr., & Powers, G. Relationship of anxiety with pain threshold. J Psychol 66: 181–183, 1967.

Cannon, W.B. Bodily Changes in Pain, Hunger, Fear and Rage. (2nd ed.) New York: Appleton-Century Co., 1929.

Capka, D., Griffin, S., Harris, G., et al.: Selected psychometric evaluations before and after treatment on a pain unit. In B.L. Crue (Ed.), Chronic Pain: Further Observations from the City of Hope National Medical Center. New York: SP Medical and Scientific Books, 1979, pp. 373–384.

Chapman, C.R. The perception of noxious events. In R.A. Sternbach (Ed.), The Psychology of Pain. New York: Raven Press, 1978, pp. 169–202.

Copp, L.A. The spectrum of suffering. Amer J Nurs 74: 491–495, 1974.

Craig, K.D. Social modelling influences on pain. In R.A. Sternbach (Ed.), The Psychology of Pain. New York: Raven Press, 1978, pp. 73–109.

Crue, B.L., Jr. A role for a neurosurgeon on the pain unit. In B.L. Crue, Jr. (Ed.), Chronic Pain: Further Observations from the City of Hope National Medical Center. New York: SP Medical and Scientific Books, 1979, pp. 397–412.

Current Research on Sleep and Dreams. Public Health Service Publication, No. 1389. Washington, D.C.: U.S. Government Printing Office, 1965.

Davitz, L.J., & Davitz, J.R. How nurses view patient suffering. RN 38: 69–72, 1975.

Doherty, XX. The patient in pain: Handling the guilt feelings. Can Nurse (Feb.): 31, 1979.

Edgeworth, M. Ormond, A Tale. London: Macmillan, 1895.

Ellis, R. Unusual sensory and thought disturbances after cardiac surgery. Amer J Nurs 72: 2021–2025, 1972.

Engel, G.L. Psychogenic pain and the pain-prone patient. Amer J Med 26: 899–918, 1959.

Fetz, E.E. Floor discussion: Psychologic aspects. In J.J. Bonica (Ed.), Advances in Neurology, Vol. 4. New York: Raven Press, 1974, pp. 297–300.

Fielding, J.M. Psychiatric aspects of pain. Med J Austral 2: 705–707, 1980.

Fordyce, W.E. A behavioral perspective on chronic pain. In L.K.Y. Ng & J.J. Bonica (Eds.), Pain, Discomfort and Humanitarian Care, Proceedings of the National Conference held at the National Institutes of Health, Bethesda, MD, Feb. 15–16, 1979. New York: Elsevier/North-Holland, 1980, pp. 233–252.

Gaumer, W.C. Psychological potentials of chronic pain. J Psychiatr Nurs 12(5): 23–24, 1974.

Hilgard, E.R. Pain as a puzzle for psychology and physiology. Amer Psychol 24: 103–113, 1969.

Izard, C.E., Huebner, R.R., Rissner, D., et al.: The young infant's ability to produce discrete emotional expressions. Devel Psychol 16: 132–140, 1980.

Jones, A., Bentler, P.M., & Petry, G. The reduction of uncertainty concerning future pain. J Abnormal Psychol 71: 87–94, 1966.

Jones, J. Personal communication, Lexington, Kentucky, Sept. 21, 1981.

Katz, E.R. Distress Behavior in Children with Leukemia Undergoing Medical Procedures. Paper presented at the Meeting of the American Psychological Assoc. Convention, New York City, Sept. 1979.

Katz, E.R. Behavioral Approaches to Pain and Distress in Children with Cancer. Paper presented at the Meeting of the Western States Conference on Cancer Rehabilitation, San Francisco, March, 1982.

Katz, E.R., Kellerman, J., & Siegel, S.E. Behavioral distress in children with cancer undergoing medical procedures: Developmental considerations. J Consult Clin Psychol 48(3): 356–365, 1980.

Katz, E.R., Kellerman, J., & Siegel, S.E. Anxiety as an affective focus in the clinical study of acute behavioral distress: A reply to Shacham and Daut. J Consult Clin Psychol 49(3): 470–471, 1981.

Katz, E.R., Kellerman, J., & Siegel, S.E. Self-Report and Observational Measurement of Acute Pain, Fear and Behavioral Distress in Children with Leukemia. Paper presented at the Annual Meeting of the Soc. of Behavioral Medicine, Chicago, IL, 1982a.

Katz, E.R., Kellerman, J., & Siegel, S.E. Direct Self-report of acute pain and fear in children with leukemia undergoing medical procedures. Manuscript submitted for publication, 1982b.

Kaufman, R.E. Pain. In H.C. Shirkey (Ed.), Pediatric Therapy. 6th ed. St. Louis: C.V. Mosby, 1980, Chap. 23, pp. 283–287.

Keats, A.S. Floor discussion: Other drugs. In J.J. Bonica (Ed.), Advances in Neurology, Vol. 4. New York: Raven Press, 1974, pp. 557–558.

Krant, M.J. Oh death—Where is thy sting? In L.K.Y. Ng & J.J. Bonica (Eds.), Pain, Discomfort and Humanitarian Care, Proceedings of the National Conference Held at the National Institutes of Health, Bethesda, MD, Feb. 15–16, 1978. New York: Elsevier/North-Holland, 1980, pp. 313–328.

Kubler-Ross, E. On Death and Dying. New York: The Macmillan Co., 1969.

Lazarus, R.S. The self-regulation of emotions. In L. Levi (Ed.), Emotions—Their Parameters and Measurement. New York: Raven Press, 1975.

LeShan, L. The world of the patient in severe pain of long duration. J Chron Dis 17: 119–126, 1964.

Levy, D.M. The infant's earliest memory of innoculation. J Gen Psychol 96: 3–46, 1960.

Lewis, C.S. The Problem of Pain. New York: Macmillan, 1962.

Lewis, J. Television interview. On Tom Cottle: Up close. Death: Jerry Lewis, Part II. Los Angeles, Channel 5, November 30, 1982.

Main, T.F. The ailment. The Brit J Med Psychol, 30:129, 1957.

Malmo, R., & Shagass, C. Physiologic studies to reaction to stress in anxiety and early schizophrenia. Psychosom Med 11: 9–24, 1949.

Maltbie, A.A., Cavenar, J.O., Hammett, E.B., et al.: A diagnostic approach to pain. Psychosomatics 19(6): 359–366, 1978.

Marks, R.M., & Sachar, E.J. Undertreatment of medical inpatients with narcotic analgesics. Ann Intern Med 78: 173–181, 1973.

Maruta, T., & Osborne, D. Sexual activity in chronic pain patients. Psychosomatics 19(9): 531–537, 1978.

Masuda, M., & Dudley, D.L. Physiologic responses to noxious head stimuli. J Psychosom Res 12: 205–214, 1968.

McCaffery, M. Brief episodes of pain in children. In B.S. Bergersen, E.H. Anderson, M. Duffey, et al. (Eds.), Current Concepts in Clinical Nursing, Vol 2. St. Louis: C.V. Mosby, 1969, pp. 178–191.

McCaffery, M. Nursing Management of the Patient with Pain. Philadelphia: J.B. Lippincott, 1979.

McCaul, K.D. Sensory information, fear level, and reactions to pain. J Personality 48(4): 494–504, 1980.

Merskey, H. Psychiatric aspect of the control of pain. In J.J. Bonica & D. Albe-

Fessard (Eds.), Advances in Pain Research and Therapy, Vol. 1. New York: Raven Press, 1976, pp. 711–716.

Merskey, H. Pain and personality. In R.A. Sternbach (Ed.), The Psychology of Pain. New York: Raven Press, 1978, pp. 111–127.

Mussen, P.H., Conger, J.J., & Kagan, J. Child Development and Personality, 4th Ed. New York: Harper & Row, 1974.

Naughton, J., & Chiu, W.S. The inhibitory effect of pain on sexual performance. Curr Concepts Pain Analgesia 3: 1–3; 9, 1975.

Orne, M.T. Nonpharmacological approaches to pain relief: Hypnosis, biofeedback, placebo effects. In L.K.Y. Ng, & J.J. Bonica (Eds.), Pain, Discomfort and Humanitarian Care, Proceedings of the National Conference held at the National Institutes of Health, Bethesda, MD, Feb. 15–16, 1979. New York: Elsevier/North-Holland, 1980, pp. 253–274.

Pasnau, R.O. The interdisciplinary pain clinic—A panel discussion. Panel participant, First Annual Meeting of the Western Chapter of the International Association for the Study of Pain, University of California at Los Angeles, Los Angeles, CA, May 10, 1975.

Pilowsky, I. Psychodynamic aspects of the pain experience. In R.A. Sternbach (Ed.), The Psychology of Pain. New York: Raven Press, 1978, pp. 203–217.

Pilowsky, I., & Spence, N.D. Pain, anger and illness behavior. J Psychosom Res 20: 411–416, 1976.

Pinsky, J.J. Aspects of the psychology of pain. In B.L. Crue, Jr. (Ed.), Chronic Pain: Further Observations from the City of Hope National Medical Center. New York: SP Medical and Scientific Publications, 1979, pp. 301–314.

Pinsky, J.J., & Malyon, A.K. The intractable pain and suffering process—Facilitating change. In B.L. Crue, Jr. (Ed.), Chronic Pain—Further Observations from the City of Hope National Medical Center. New York: SP Medical and Scientific Publications, 1979, pp. 315–320a.

Pinsky, J.J., & Malyon, A.K. The eclectic nature of psychotherapy in the treatment of chronic pain syndromes. In B.L. Crue, Jr. (Ed.), Chronic Pain—Further Observations from the City of Hope National Medical Center. New York: SP Medical and Scientific Publications, 1979, pp. 324–327b.

Robinson, L. Psychological Aspects of the Care of Hospitalized Patients. Philadelphia: F.A. Davis, 1976.

Rubin, D. The no!—or the yes and how of sex for patients with neck, back and radicular pain syndromes. Calif Med 113: 12–15, 1970.

Scott, D.S., & Barber, T.X. Cognitive control of pain: Four serendipitious results. Percept Motor Skills 44: 569–570, 1977.

Selye, H. The general adaptation syndrome and diseases of adaptation. J Clin Endocrinol, 6: 217–230, 1946.

Selye, H. The Stress of Life. New York: McGraw-Hill, 1956.

Spinetta, J.J., & Maloney, L.J. Death anxiety in the outpatient leukemic child. Pediatrics 56: 1034–1037, 1975.

Sternbach, R.A. A Psychophysiological Analysis. New York: Academic Press, 1968.

Sternbach, R.A. Pain Patients: Traits and Treatment. New York: Academic Press, 1974a.

Sternbach, R.A., & Timmermans, G. Personality changes associated with the reduction of pain. Pain 1: 177–181, 1975.

Sternbach, R.A., Wolf, S.R., Murphy, R.W., et al.: Traits of pain patients. The low-back loser. Psychosomatics 14: 226–229, 1973.

Strauss, A.L., & Glasser, B.G. Chronic Illness and the Quality of Life. St. Louis: C.V. Mosby, 1975.

Sutherland, A.M. Psychological impact of cancer and its treatment. Med Clin North Amer 40: 705–720, 1956; rpt. in CA—Cancer J Clinicians 31(3): 159–170, 1981.

Szasz, T. Pain and Pleasure. London: Tavistock Press, 1957.

Tanzer, D. Natural childbirth: Pain or peak experience. Psychol Today 2: 17–21, 69, 1968.

Timmermans, G., & Sternbach, R.A. Human chronic pain and personality: A canonical correlation analysis. In J.J. Bonica & D. Albe-Fessard (Eds.), Advances in Pain Research and Therapy, Vol. 1. New York: Raven Press, 1976, pp. 307–310.

Tu, W. A religiophilosophical perspective on pain. In H.W. Kosterlitz & L.Y. Terenius (Eds.), Pain and Society, Report of the Dahlem Workshop on Pain and Society, Berlin, Nov. 26–30, 1979. Weinheim: Verlag Chemie, 1980, pp. 63–67.

Wolff, H., & Wolff, S. Pain. 2nd ed. Springfield, IL: Charles C. Thomas, 1958.

SUGGESTED READINGS

Apley, J., & MacLeith, R. The Child and his Symptoms. Oxford: Blackwell, 1968.

Baker, J.W., & Merskey, H. Pain in general practice. J Psychosom Res 10: 383–387, 1967.

Barber, T.X. Effects of Hypnotic Induction, Suggestions of Anesthesia and Distraction on Subjective and Physiological Responses to Pain. Paper presented at the Annual Meeting of the Eastern Psychological Association, Philadelphia, Apr. 10, 1969.

Barber, T.X., & Cooper, B.J. The effects of pain of experimentally induced and spontaneous distraction. Psychol Rep 31: 647–651, 1972.

Beecher, H.K. Limiting factors in experimental pain. J Chron Dis 4: 1121, 1956.

Beecher, H.K. Relationship of significance of wound to pain. J Amer Med Assoc 161: 1609–1613, 1956.

Beecher, H.K. The subjective response and reaction to sensation. Amer J Med 20: 107–113, 1956.

Beecher, H.K. Generalization from pain of various types and diverse origins. Science 130: 267–268, 1959.

Beecher, H.K. Pain: One mystery solved. Science 151: 840–841, 1966.

Blinchik, E.R., & Grzesiak, R.C. Reinterpretative cognitive strategies in chronic pain management. Arch Phys Med Rehab 60: 609–612, 1979.

Blumer, D. Psychiatric and psychological aspects of chronic pain. Clinical Neurosurgery. Proceedings of the Congress of the Neurological Surgeons, San Francisco, CA, 1977. Baltimore: Williams & Wilkins, 1978.

Bonica, J.J. The relation of injury to pain (Letter to the editor). Pain 7: 203–207, 1979.

Booker, J.E. Pain: It's all in your patient's head (or is it?) Nursing 82, 12: (Mar.) 47–52, 1982.

Boyle, P., & Parbrook, G.D. The interrelation of personality and postoperative factors. Brit J Anaesth 49(31): 259–264, 1977.

Chapman, C.R. Psychological aspects of pain patient treatments. Arch Surg 112: 767–772, 1977.

Chapman, C.R., Sola, A.E., & Bonica, J.J. Illness behavior and depression compared in pain center and private practice patients. Pain 6: 1–7, 1979.

Cousins, N. Anatomy of an illness (as perceived by the patient). N Engl J Med 295: 1458–1463, 1976.

Cramer, B., Gershberg, M.R., & Stern, M. Munchausen Syndrome. Its relation to malingering, hysteria, and the physician-patient relationship. Arch Gen Psychiatr 24: 573–578, 1971.

Davenport-Slack, B., & Boylan, C.H. Psychological correlates of childbirth pain. Psychosom Med 36: 215–223, 1974.

Davitz, L.J., & Davitz, J.R. Inferences of Patients' Pain and Psychological Distress. New York: Springer, 1980.

Davitz, L.J., Sameshima, Y., & Davitz, J.R. Suffering as viewed in six different cultures. Amer J Nurs 76: 1296–1297, 1976.

Driscoll, D.J., Glicklich, L.B., & Galkin, W.J. Chest pain in children: A prospective study. Pediatrics 57: 648–651, 1976.

Egbert, L.D., Battit, G.E., Welch, C.E., et al. Reduction of postoperative pain by encouragement and instruction of patients. N Engl J Med 270: 825–827, 1964.

Eland, J.M. Living with pain. Nurs Outlook 7: 430–431, 1978.

Elton, D., Stanley, G.V., & Burrows, G.D. Self-esteem and chronic pain. J Psychosom Res 22: 25–30, 1978.

Eysenck, S.B.G. Personality, and pain assessment in childbirth of married and unmarried mothers. J Mental Sci 107: 417–430, 1961.

Gildea, J.H., & Quirk, T.R. Assessing the pain experience in children. Nurs Clin North Amer 12: 631–637, 1977.

Glennon, B., & Weisz, J.R. An observational approach to the assessment of anxiety in young children. J Consult Clin Psychol 46: 1246–1257, 1978.

Gomez, J., & Dally, P. Psychologically mediated abdominal pain in surgical and medical outpatient clinics. Brit Med J 1(6074): 1451–1453, 1977.

von Graffenried, B. The influence of anxiety and pain sensitivity on experimental pain in man. Pain 4: 253–263, 1978.

Hart, H. Displacement guilt and pain. Psychoanal Rev 34: 259–272, 1947.

Haltzerbuehler, L.C., & Schroder, H.E. Desensitization procedures in the treatment of childhood disorders. Psychol Bull 85: 831–844, 1978.

Hayter, J. The rhythm of sleep. Amer J Nurs 80: 457–461, 1980.

Hunt, T.E. Management of chronic pain in the elderly. J Am Ger Soc, 1976, 24, Sept., 402–426.

Jacox, A.K. Sociocultural and psychological aspects of pain. In A.K. Jacox (Ed.), Pain: A Source Book for Nurses and Other Allied Health Professionals. Boston: Little, Brown, 1977.

Janis, I.L. Psychol Stress. New York: John Wiley & Sons, 1958, pp. 374–394.

Johnson, J.E., Kirchoff, K.T., & Endress, M.P. Altering children's distress behavior during orthopedic cast removal. Nurs Res 24: 404–410, 1975.

de Jong, R.H. Occasional notes—Prof. Wall's three phases of pain. N Engl J Med 301: 1129–1130, 1979.

Katz, E.R. Beta-endorphin and Acute Behavioral Distress in Children with Leukemia. Unpublished doctoral dissertation, University of Southern California, 1980.
Knox, V.J., Morgan, A.H., & Hilgard, E.R. Pain and suffering in ischemia. Arch Gen Psychiatr 30: 840–847, 1974.
Lazarus, A.A. "Has behavior therapy outlived its usefulness?" Amer Psychol 32(7): 53, 1977.
Leventhal, H., & Everhart, D. Emotion, pain, and physical illness. In C.E. Izard (Ed.), Emotions and Psychopathology. New York: Plenum Press, 1979.
Lewis, N. The needle is like an animal. Child Today 7: 18–21, 1978.
Liebskind, J., & Paul, L. Psychological and mechanisms of pain. Ann Rev Psychol 28: 41–60, 1977.
Martinez-Urrutia, A. Anxiety and pain in surgical patients. J Consult Clin Psychol 43: 437–442, 1975.
McCaffery, M. Cognition, Bodily Pain, and Man—Environment Interactions. Los Angeles: University of California Student Store, 1968.
McKee, K. Neurotic bodily pain in children. Amer J Nurs 70: 130–131, 1970.
Melzack, R. Psychologic aspects of pain. In J.J. Bonica (Ed.), Pain, Research Publications: Association for Research in Nervous and Mental Disease, Vol. 58. New York: Raven Press, 1980, pp. 143–154.
Merskey, H. Pain, learning and memory. J Psychosom Res 19: 319–324, 1975.
Merskey, H. & Spear, F.G. Pain: Psychological and Psychiatric Aspects. Baltimore: Williams & Wilkins, 1967.
Petrie, A. Individuality in Pain and Suffering. Chicago: University of Chicago Press, 1967.
Pilling, L.F., Brannick, T.L., & Swenson, W.M. Psychologic characteristics of psychiatric patients having pain as a presenting symptom. Can Med Assoc J 97: 387–394, 1967.
Pilowsky, I. Psychiatrist and the pain clinic. Amer J Psychiatr 133: 752, 1977.
Pinsky, J.J. Psychodynamics and psychotherapy in the treatment of patients with chronic intractable pain. In B.L. Crue, Jr. (Ed.), Pain, Research and Treatment. New York: Academic Press, 1975, Chap. 34.
Pozanski, E.O. Children's reactions to pain: A psychiatrist's perspective. Clin Pediatr 15: 1114–1119, 1976.
Price, D.D., Barrell, J.J., & Gracely, R.H. A psychophysical analysis of experimental factors that selectively influence the affective dimension of pain. Pain 8: 137–149, 1980.
Raney, J.O. Pain, emotion and a rationale for therapy. Northwest Med 69: 659–661, 1970.
Richards, J.S., Meredith, R.L., Nepomuceno, C., et al. Psycho-social aspects of chronic pain in spinal cord injury. Pain 8: 355–366, 1980.
Rook, J.C., Pesch, R.N., & Keeler, E.C. Chronic pain and the questionable use of the Minnesota Multiphasic Personality Inventory. Arch Phys Med Rehab 62(8): 373–376, 1981.
Schmeck, H.M. Pain and why it hurts so much. New York Times, Feb. 26, 1978.
Schmitt, M. The nature of pain with some personal notes. Nurs Clin North Amer 12(4): 621–629, 1977.
Scott, D.S., & Barber, T.X. Cognitive control of pain: Effects of multiple cognitive strategies. Psychol Rec 2: 373–383, 1977.

Seligman, M.E.P. Helpless: On Depression, Development, and Death. San Francisco: W.H. Freeman, 1975.
Shacham, S., & Daut, R. Anxiety on pain: What does the scale measure? J Consult Clin Psychol 49: 468–469, 1981.
Shapiro, A.K. The placebo effect: The physician's role as healer, priest and scientist. Pain 4: 1–2, 1976.
Spear, F.G. Pain in psychiatric patients. J Psychosom Res 11: 187–193, 1967.
Sternbach, R.A. Psychological factors in pain. In J.J. Bonica & D. Albe-Fessard (Eds.), Adv Pain Res Ther Vol. 1. New York: Raven Press, 1976, pp. 293–299.
Swanson, D.W., & Maruta, T. Patients complaining of extreme pain. Mayo Clin Proc 55: 563–566, 1980.
Szasz, T.S. Pain and Pleasure: A Study of Bodily Feelings. New York: Basic Books, 1957.
Terenius, L. Endorphins and pain. In L.H. Rees & T.B. van Wimersma Greidanus, (Eds.) Front Hormone Res 8: 162–177, 1981.
Veilleux, S., & Melzack, R. Pain in psychotic patients. Exp Neurol 52: 535–543, 1976.
Webb, W.L. The therapy of psychosomatic pain. In J.H. Masserman (Ed.), Current Psychiatric Therapies, Vol. 18. New York: Grune & Stratton, 1978, pp. 73–84.
Wilson, W.L., Blazer, D.G., & Nashold, B.S. Observations on pain and suffering. Psychosomatics 17: 73–76, 1976.
Zelter, L., Kellerman, J., Ellenberg, L., et al. The psychologic effects of illness in adolescence: Crucial issues and coping styles. J Pediatr. In press, 1982.

8

Situational Factors that Influence the Patient's Pain Experience

The patient's experience of pain is affected by an almost infinite variety of factors, known or unknown. Those fairly stable and unalterable forces that preexist in an individual such as neurophysiological, cultural, psychological, and pain syndromes that help to explain his particular response to a pain experience were discussed in previous chapters. Here we are concerned with those factors that influence the patient's pain experience, but are more or less situational, that is, they arise out of the present circumstance. These factors may change over time, or it may be possible for the patient or health team member to alter them in some way, thereby altering the contribution they make to the patient's experience of pain. Because they are subject to change or can be changed deliberately, it is especially important that they be assessed. To facilitate analysis and discussion here, the situational factors are divided into several categories, however, these categories overlap considerably.

MEANING AND VALUE OF PAIN

Most of the other factors that influence the pain sensation and response culminate to produce what many people feel is the most significant influence on the patient's pain experience—the meaning of the pain to the patient. Beecher's (1956) now classic and much-quoted study gives dramatic support to the notion that the perceived intensity of pain and the behavioral responses to pain are largely determined by what the pain means to the patient. He compared a group of men who had wartime casualties with a group of male civilian patients who had comparable wounds. The soldiers had extensive injuries, were mentally alert and were not in shock. When they were questioned, only 32 percent of them said they had enough pain to want anything done about it. By contrast, 85 percent of the civilian patients desired narcotics for their pain. This study found no significant *relationship between* the *extent* of *injury* and the *pain* experienced, nor were there differences between sudden injury and chronic illness. These results have been interpreted to mean that the soldier's pain was associated with an improvement in his life situation; that is, he was removed from combat and safely returned to a hospital. On the other hand, the civilian's pain was associated with an unfavorable change in his situation and threatened his life-style. To the civilian, pain implied death or serious illness, but to the soldier, pain meant escape from a greater threat and this decreased his complaints of pain and perhaps also the perceived intensity of pain. Therefore, when pain threatens the patient's life situation, it appears that the patient will tend to experience a greater intensity of pain, complain more about the pain, and react more intensely. These findings are well-documented more recently in the works of Craig 1978, pp. 73–109; Mersky, 1978, pp. 111–127; Pilowsky, 1978, pp. 203–217; Pinsky & Malyon, 1979 a; b.

The possible or actual threat that pain poses for the patient may take several forms. First, it may *threaten* the patient's very *life*. He may fear that the undiagnosed pain in his head is a brain tumor that will lead to his death. Or, he may know that the pain in his abdomen is from a malignancy that will cause his death in a few months. In other words, the pain may mean possible or certain death.

Second, the pain may not imply a fatal illness but may be *indicative* of an actual or possible *serious illness* that will threaten the patient's activities of daily living. Or, the patient may not associate his pain with a serious illness, but the pain itself may be severe enough to hamper daily living.

Third, pain may be associated with something that *threatens* his *body image*. Pain may remind the patient of the recent or impending loss of a leg, uterus, or eye. The pain from accidental lacerations of the face or from extensive burns over the body may mean possible scarring and additional body image disturbances.

Worse still, many patients with pain realistically are *exposed* to *all three* of *these types* of *threats* and their concomitant effects which are discussed in Chapter 7. These real or potential losses are accompanied by the emotions that are usually associated with loss and the patient may spend considerable time worrying about the things which are threatening to him.

A 35-year-old postpartum patient demonstrates how the threat and associated meaning of pain and the resulting anxiety can affect the patient's pain experience. Two weeks after the birth of her baby she called her physician and reported to the office nurse that she had severe diffuse pain in the perineal area that included cramping and burning sensations when she voided. An appointment was made for that day. She arrived in a wheelchair used to transport her from the car to the office. The patient said the pain was so severe she could not walk. While the nurse was with her in the examining room waiting for the physician, the patient asked, "What do you suppose this is? Do you think I'll need surgery? I don't know what I'm going to do about the baby." Her behavior indicated anxiety about the implications of the pain. She seemed to fear that she might have some serious illness that would threaten her mothering role and cause her to lose the pleasure of caring for her baby. The physician diagnosed her problem as cystitis, gave her prescriptions for medication, and explained that the sulfisoxazole would control the infection and the pyridium would alleviate the pain in the meantime. The patient told the nurse goodbye with a smile and started to walk out of the office. When the nurse asked if she would like her wheelchair, the patient replied, "I don't think I need it. The doctor says I'll be all right now." Her anxiety seemed to have disappeared, and she either did not perceive the pain as intensely as before or did not need to react to it any more. The patient's statement illustrated how a patient can bear pain more easily when hope is high, the end of the pain can be seen, and the reason for the pain is clear. Farnsworth (1956) demonstrated how pain responses are more intense when pain threatens the life situation.

Pain that continues beyond the point of being a necessary warning, may also be thought of as *beneficial pain* by some people. The benefit may be the meaning the patient attaches to the pain. For example, LeShan (1964) says that some patients with pain see it as having its own existence and believe that their experiencing the pain saved someone else from having to feel it. He also says that for other patients, pain clarifies the meaning of life. Such patients say they stop concerning themselves with trivial, unimportant things in life. Some of the patients interviewed in Copp's (1974) study voiced similar views. Although they said they would have avoided the suffering if possible, they nevertheless saw value in it. Thirty-nine out of 148 hospitalized patients saw pain as an opportunity for creative expression, self-searching, and self-testing; as enabling them to appreciate and improve their former good health; and as increasing their understanding of the suffering of others. Some patients regarded pain as a challenge and thought there could be emotional and spiritual benefits.

Assessment of the patient with pain needs to include determining what, if any, the meaning and values pain may have for him. Those values may assist him to endure the pain with less fear or depression.

It is hoped that both enjoyable and horrifying life experiences can be utilized by each of us in some beneficial way. We believe it is *possible* that pain can be a beneficial experience, but we believe it is more *probable* that most pain experiences will be characterized by much useless suffering and that most of the effects of pain will be detrimental to the person. With respect to most, but not all, pain, we agree with Leriche (1939) who says,

> Physicians too readily claim that *pain is a reaction of defense, a fortunate warning* [italics his] . . . . They would almost claim that, if pain did not exist, it would

be desirable to invent it. . . . But, as a matter of fact, the majority of diseases, even the most serious, attack us without any warning (p. 23).

He continues, "To regard it [pain] as a salutary warning, a reaction of defense, is surely a bitter jest" (p. 491). Regarding the benefits of experiencing pain, we also agree with him when he says,

> Philosophers and poets have imposed upon mankind a very inaccurate conception of physical pain. Oblivious of the many heart-rending cries . . . they have never ceased telling us, again and again, that pain is a blessing in the moral order . . . (p. 24).

And again, this sensitive surgeon of years ago says, "Not everyone has a soul of fire, and, in actual human life, even in the case of the great mystics, *the struggle against pain exacts a high price*" [italics his] (p. 26).

KNOWLEDGE AND UNDERSTANDING

This section refers to the extent to which a patient is able to obtain accurate information and then organize and process it to achieve an understanding of the pain experience. Nursing assessment should include asking the patient what he or she has been told about the anticipation and experience of pain, who told him or her, whether or not it is believed, whether or not it contradicts other information or his or her own experience, and what it is believed will relieve the pain. Finding out from other health team members what they have told the patient is useful only to the extent that it enables the nurse, after speaking with the patient, to assess that patient's ability to retain and understand what has been told. It is a mistake to assume that a patient possesses information simply because someone has told him or her. With young children who lack facility with language, the nurse's assessment must include observations of other behavioral responses to events, equipment, and people. These factors are discussed in Chapter 4 in relation to cognitive processes, and in Chapter 9, as they influence communication of the pain experience.

How much a person *believes* or *knows* about the cause, implication, and duration of pain will influence the response to pain, and perhaps even influence its intensity and existence. It is not uncommon for a patient to have unquestioning beliefs or preconceived ideas about pain. The adult patient may utilize what friends have said or what has been read or seen. Anyone who has ever mentioned illness to others is familiar with the wealth of free information and advice likely to be received from *well-meaning friends, relatives* and *strangers*.

One patient in a panic called for the nurse to report that he was having a heart attack. In actuality, he was experiencing referred chest pain from abdominal distention. Nevertheless this patient refused to ambulate until the physician arrived and listened to his heart. He later commented that a friend of his had had a heart attack and had warned him to be alert for chest pain.

In addition, the layman in this country is informed about diseases through the *mass media*. Some information may be accurate and helpful, while some is erroneous or incomplete.

Lack of information can also have a detrimental effect upon the patient's pain experience. For example, a patient had a regional anesthetic for excision of a growth on her foot. During the surgery she suddenly screamed, "I can feel it! Stop! It hurts!" After the patient had been calmed, the nurse discovered that pressure, which the patient could feel, had been misinterpreted as pain. The patient had not been told that pressure might be felt.

One area in which patients seem to have a gross lack of knowledge and understanding concerns the *relationship between organic pathology* and the *sensation of pain*. At the bedside physicians and nurses have used the ballpoint pen and the paper napkin to provide excellent visual aids regarding the anatomy of disease. This technique simply needs to be taken one step further to explain, for example, how swelling, a stone, or a mass can result in discomfort. Even a general idea of how the body functions is a mystery to most laymen. To many patients, pain means tissue damage, and they relate this to what is familiar to them—cutting and bruising. Each episode or increase in pain may mean to a patient that something is tearing and cutting away at the inside of the body. For example, unless it is explained to the patient, it may be difficult for him or her to appreciate that diminished blood supply to muscles or distention of an organ can be extremely painful.

Incomplete or inaccurate information not only influences the existence of a painful sensation and its meaning to the patient but such information also affects the level of anxiety, discussed in Chapter 7 and during the period of anticipation of pain, discussed in Chapter 5.

There are two kinds of information that patients have in varying degrees that appear to be especially relevant to the amount of anxiety experienced during the *anticipation* of pain:

1. One type of information is the information a patient has about *when* the pain will be felt. When the patient does not know how long he or she will have to wait before the painful sensation is felt, anxiety tends to increase. For example, if a patient is told he will have a spinal tap "sometime today" he or she is likely to be much more anxious than if told that the spinal tap will be done at ten o'clock that morning. It is also probable that the longer the period of anticipation, the higher the anxiety, unless this period of time is used to reduce anxiety.

Many patients remark that it is easier to endure the pain itself than it is to wait for it, not *knowing what it will be like or when it will occur.* Clearly, the period of anticipation of pain is a time when uncertainty may cause a great increase in anxiety. And when the pain occurs, this high level of anxiety as mentioned above tends to result in an increase in the intensity of the pain.

2. The other type of information concerns what the patient *knows* about the *intensity* and *duration* of *pain* and the *harmful effects* that may be *associated* with it. Anxiety tends to be particularly high when the patient anticipates that some of the pain felt may be indicative of harmful effects that are beyond the control of the physician. For example, if the patient believes that some of the pain associated with the spinal tap may mean that the physician has hit a nerve that will result in long-lasting or permanent back pain, anxiety will increase. The patient will tend to overestimate the intensity of the pain and be less tolerant of it. Also, if the patient is not told approximately how long the painful sensation will last, he or she may have a vague notion that the pain will last indefinitely or that once it subsides it could return at any time. Of course, this increases anxiety and heightens pain responses. The patient's anxiety is also increased if there is the anticipation that the pain will be severe.

The patient's information about pain may include ideas about pain relief. He or she may have been told by a friend that "shots are the only way" to get pain relief, or a home remedy handed down from one generation to another may be favored. A television commercial may have convinced him that a particular product is the most effective. For example, Jane, 11 years old, voiced her belief about pain remedies when she requested Alka-Seltzer for her headache which was associated with a possible brain tumor.

The young child cannot rely as heavily as the adult on verbal and written information. Observations of the *pain responses* of *others* and the *type of equipment* used in painful procedures are used as one source of information about pain. If a child sees another child cry with pain when the physician examines him, the observing child may ask, "Is the doctor going to do that to me?" The child also tends to anticipate pain on the basis of the equipment associated with it. Shining steel objects are frequently used in painful procedures. The child may anticipate pain whenever such instruments are seen. Merely being approached by a nurse or a physician may cause fear of pain.

Of course, regardless of the number of accurate facts a child or adult may have about pain, he or she may still be unable to be logical about them due to his or her level of cognitive functioning.

LEVEL OF CONSCIOUSNESS

The patient's level of consciousness may be lowered or altered due to such factors as head injury, infections of the central nervous system, sedatives, general anesthetics, anticholinergics, and conditions that decrease oxygenation of the brain. The patient's responses to pain will vary in accordance with the extent to which the level of consciousness is altered. Of course, the patient who is totally unconscious, regardless of the cause, will not respond to pain or any other stimuli.

Drugs such as scopolamine (an anticholinergic) and phenobarbital (a sedative) depress the central nervous system, causing drowsiness and sleep. A different reaction occurs if either of these drugs is administered alone in the presence of pain or in combination with a drug that does not provide adequate pain relief. Either drug may result in restlessness and confusion, and the patient may respond much more vigorously to pain than he would if he were fully conscious. In the aftermath of pain, the patient who received phenobarbital may be embarrassed that he had not controlled his behavior in his usual way, whereas when scopolamine is administered the amnesic properties of this drug may cause the patient to forget the pain experience.

Years ago a common method of obstetric analgesia was a combination of scopolamine and a barbiturate or analgesic. Mrs. Palmer demonstrated the possible effects of these medications. During the labor and prior to medication she was awake between contractions, crying quietly for a few seconds, and saying that the pain was terrible. She responded to the contractions with muscle tension such as clenched fists and clenched teeth, but she did not verbalize or vocalize. Within an hour after scopolamine and pentobarbital sodium were administered, she slept between contractions and screamed loudly during the contractions. In the postpartum period, she remembered nothing about this part of her labor. If someone had mentioned events that occurred during that time, she probably would have begun to remember.

Newer drugs are now being used with similar *anxiolytic, hypnotic*, and *amnesic effects*. For example, Ativan sometimes is used prior to chemotherapy. Patients often not only do not remember receiving the chemotherapy, they do not recall the undesirable side effects of nausea and vomiting. One problem of some of the newer amnesics is that the degree of *retrograde amnesia* may not be known. An anesthesiology resident reported using such a drug preoperatively on a school purchasing agent who had ordered eight school buses the day of his hospitalization. Sixteen buses arrived. When he had returned to work following his surgery the patient had reordered the buses and had no recall of his first purchase. Although one's cognitive level can be altered by many factors such as anxiety, the physician's feeling after reassessing this patient was that the amnesic effect of the drug was the cause.

General anesthetics depress the central nervous system in stages. The nurse may observe two stages of recovery from anesthesia in the immediate postoperative period. She or he may first observe the second stage of anesthesia, the stage of excitement. During this stage the patient may overreact to stimuli, especially noise. The patient then passes into the first stage of anesthesia, often called the stage of analgesia. This implies that the small amount of anesthesia retained in the patient's system provides some pain relief. The patient may awaken and complain of pain, but is usually drowsy and will fall asleep again. In some diseases, such as pneumonia or cerebral arteriosclerosis, the oxygen supply to the brain is depleted. Patients with these conditions may also complain of pain and then go to sleep.

It is very important to realize that *sleep* or *sedation may occur* in the presence of pain. That is, a patient may be both sedated and have pain. This point is frequently misunderstood. For example, nurses are often reluctant to awaken a patient for even a scheduled dose of an analgesic. But pain can exist and keeping on top of the pain may require that the patient receive his analgesics on a time-contingent basis. Although it may be necessary to awaken the patient to administer the analgesic, it is likely that he will go right back to sleep and when he awakens not be in severe or poorly controlled pain. A common example of trying to prevent a patient from having acute pain with serious consequences for his physical condition occurs in the recovery room and operating rooms. One current practice is to administer a narcotic prior to the time that the patient awakens so that he or she won't awaken in severe pain.

At the present time, the use of *marijuana* has not been decriminalized in the United States. However, it is now in the final stages as an investigational drug (Andrysiak, 1982), and it is smoked illegally by a large number of people. Nurses occasionally see patients under its influence. The patient may manage to smoke it unnoticed during hospitalization or may smoke it prior to admission. Marijuana is known to alter the level of consciousness, causing sleepiness, relaxation, and occasionally hallucinations (Dell & Snyder, 1977). Although it is reputated to provide pain relief, one of the few systematic studies available shows that it increases sensitivity to both painful and nonpainful stimuli and reduces tolerance for pain (Hill, 1974).

POWERLESSNESS

The concept of *powerlessness* has been defined as the individual's feeling that his behavior cannot determine the outcomes or reinforcements he seeks (Seeman & Evans, 1962). When a person is faced with a situation over which he believes he has little control he may cease to seek further information about his predicament. Why should he obtain knowledge about something he can do nothing about? Prior to becoming ill the patient may have a sense of powerlessness about all aspects of health and illness. Feelings of powerlessness may also be created by the illness situation and reinforced by health personnel who tell the patient that they will do everything necessary and that this is to be received passively. They give little information about the cause of illness or pain and what, if anything, the patient can do to help himself. This may well be one of the reasons a patient does not complain of pain since it is felt that the necessity for pain relief is determined and controlled by others. On the other hand, it could be the reason a patient complains frequently about pain since he or she has not been told of various pain-relief measures, such as positioning or distraction, that he could have utilized himself.

A prenatal class illustrates how *health team members* can *create* in the patient a *sense* of *powerlessness*. A physician in residency in obstetrics and a nurse from the prenatal clinic conducted this class of 15 members. During the class the physician listed on the blackboard three types of regional anesthetics that would be available to the mother during labor. Toward the end of the class, one expectant mother asked if she would have a choice of these anesthetics and a choice in whether or not she received one. The nurse replied that by the time she needed it she would not care which one she received and that the physician would decide. Further, no mention was ever made of anything the laboring patient could do for herself to alleviate discomfort, such as keeping her bladder empty, relaxing between contractions, trying various positions and having her husband rub her lower back. At the conclusion of the class one patient commented, "This sounds terrible. I guess all I can do is go home and practice my Lamaze." Although she had found her own resource for pain relief, her comment contained an element of doubt about its usefulness, a doubt that may have been generated by this prenatal class. For the other patients without their own resources for pain relief, one wonders about the extent to which this class engendered *fear* and *helplessness* and discouraged any attempt to obtain information about how to help themselves during labor and delivery.

The almost natural and spontaneous inclination of the nurse to help the patient with pain may take a form that engenders feelings of powerlessness. Crowley (1974) points out that severe pain, especially, emphasizes a person's weaknesses and that the spontaneous response to such patients may be to act on or for them rather than to assist them to use their own resources more effectively. Over time, this may cause the patient to feel that he or she is not very capable of helping, that he or she is in effect powerless and must rely upon others.

Bowers (1968, pp. 596–602) and Geer et al. (1970, pp. 731–738) report that suffering is more intense for individuals who believe that they are unable to avoid or relieve their pain (powerless and helpless) and stress than for individuals who believe that they can control the situation. *Feelings* of *powerlessness*, whether possessed by the patient initially or created by the situation, probably will *result* in the *patient's knowing little about how to achieve pain relief*, and it may also foster fantasies about the cause and meaning of pain.

Craig & Best (1977) have found that *personality characteristics* are less important determinants of pain behavior than *situational factors*. More importantly they found that even for individuals who believe they are powerless over situational factors it may be possible to provide some feelings of control. This would be consistent with Wolff's (1978, pp. 132–133) belief that consciousness and motor activity are a part of all voluntary responses under the individual's direct control. Fielding (1980, p. 706) says that activity and work help decrease the feelings of helplessness and hopelessness and distract the patient from pain, especially the compulsive patient. These findings are helpful in providing a rationale for the nurse to assess the extent to which the patient feels he can contribute to his own pain experience and help him identify possibilities which may minimize the suffering and pain behavior which the patient may have overlooked. This may also help the patient muster coping skills that he has but is not using at the present time.

PRESENCE, ATTITUDES, AND FEELINGS OF OTHERS

When a patient is in pain or fears pain, the simple *presence* of *another person may* influence his behavior and sometimes the perceived intensity of pain. Persons of different sociocultural groups may have different expectations of the people to whom they complain about their pain. Consequently, one patient may be more *expressive* about pain in the presence of a nurse or physician, whereas another patient may be more expressive with his family or friends. Or the patient may try to control all expressions of pain unless he is alone. In the United States, the patient who tends to be very expressive because of the expectations of culture may be influenced to behave in a more controlled manner because health team members with Old American attitudes, as described by Zbrowski (1952; 1969), convey to the patient that they find such expression of pain annoying. This seems to be a similar problem for patients in British hospitals. Bond (1980, p. 53) reports that "there are signs of a change toward a less tolerant attitude toward being in pain [and this change in attitude] may bring increased rather than decreased suffering for a person with pain."

Sometimes a patient is especially expressive in the presence of a certain person, often someone whom he is emotionally close to. In fact the patient's significant others usually become involved in acting on behalf of the patient by performing fairly specific functions. Strauss & Glaser (1976, p. 67) say that the efficiency to which the significant others assume these responsibilities may not only determine whether or not the patient gets better or worse, but may actually influence how long the patient survives.

Some of the types of *functions* that *significant others* may *fulfill* include supporting, assisting, protecting, controlling, rescuing, redesigning, and covering up in interactions for the patient. The following examples illustrate the more supportive, protective and, rescuing functions for patients experiencing pain. A woman may report pain to the staff matter-of-factly and only when she is asked, but when her sister visits, she may cry and describe her pain in detail. A similar situation often occurs with children. The child may cry only when the mother visits. With children, Salk (1973) suggests this probably is because the child has learned that his or her parents usually come to the rescue in the face of threat. The crying may be to persuade the parents to remove him or her from the threatening situation. The mother, sister, or other person who happens to be the one who elicits the crying, may very well misunderstand. Often the person feels that he or she should cease visiting the patient. This is not necessarily true. It may be that this is the only person who can provide an atmosphere of trust and safety in which the patient feels free to express more exactly and completely how he or she feels. Thus, it is important to identify the person who encourages *freedom of expression* in the patient and also how that person reacts to the patient's expressive behavior.

However, even during well-intended interactions, feelings of fear and anxiety in those who come in contact with the patient can cause or increase the patient's own fear and anxiety. This is especially important because fear and anxiety usually increase the subjective experience of pain. Some degree of these feelings almost always accompanies pain. However, as we have seen, a high degree of anxiety or fear may cause the patient to perceive a greater sensation of pain, or to intensify behavioral responses and make it even more difficult to utilize usual methods of coping with pain. This occurs in both the adult and the child patient. The following discussion focuses on the child as an illustration. It is easy to observe others *communicate fear* and *anxiety* to a child, and the effects on the child are rather remarkable.[1]

Nurses, doctors, and parents appear to experience a discomfort of their own when a child is in pain, particularly if they have had some part in causing that pain. The adult senses that the child depends upon him or her for assistance and protection. When the adult cannot provide this to the child's satisfaction, the adult sometimes feels helpless and inadequate. Since the child often cannot understand what is happening and cannot

---

[1] *The following material on the child is either a direct quote or adapted from McCaffery, M.: Brief episodes of pain in children. Current Concepts in Clinical Nursing, Vol. II, Bergersen, B.S., Anderson, E.H., Duffey, M. et al. (Eds.). St. Louis: C.V. Mosby Co., 1969, pp. 181–182.*

comprehend the therapeutic or diagnostic merit of a procedure or the reason for the illness, some responses may tend to increase the adult's feelings of failure. The child may strike out at the adult, blame the adult for the pain, scream for help, or cry loudly.

When the adult is concerned about the child and wants to help, this type of behavior in the child can be very disturbing to that adult. It is at this point that the adult, rather than continuing in a kind of caring manner, may become angry with feelings of failure and in turn become angry with the child. The adult may convey this to the child in many ways. For example, he or she may restrain the child more firmly than necessary, increasing the child's feelings of being punished and purposely harmed. The adult may tell the child to stop crying, showing very little understanding and acceptance of the child's point of view. In a way, the adult who tells the child to stop crying is merely attempting to erase the signs of inability to help the child. This expression of anger toward the child seems to be even more intense when the adult involved is unsure of his or her own competence in performing a procedure or giving care.

This can be illustrated by a nurse who packed an infected wound on Susan, six years old. She approached Susan pleasantly and explained very simply what she was going to do. As she proceeded Susan began to cry quietly. Very kindly the nurse said, "I don't mean to hurt you. Now don't cry." Susan attempted to stop crying by biting her lips. In a few seconds, the nurse became obviously embarrassed over having forgotten some necessary dressings and medication. Her anxiety was evident in her curt tone of voice when she asked another nurse to bring her the supplies. Susan immediately began to move her legs slightly and the nurse called an aide to hold the child's legs firmly. Then Susan began to cry loudly and another nurse was called to hold her hands and arms. In this example, the child's behavior became more intense and less controlled as the nurse's anxiety and anger increased.

A parent who is highly anxious about his or her child's illness and who has a strong need to prevent further harm to the child can sometimes increase the child's fear (Bandura & Menlove, 1968). In the child's presence, the parent may question the necessity of a procedure or cry about it. The parent can make the impending procedure seem even more ominous and punitive to the child. It has been found that the severity of the child's affective response is consistent with that of the parents' (Gordon et al., 1974), and the parents' expectation of how they should respond to pain (Craig, 1980, p. 47). On the other hand, when the parents are able to handle their own feelings, they can focus on helping their child.

With chronic pain patients, the significant others often "do" for the patient what he or she could do alone which serves to increase or sustain *pain behaviors, perceived pain intensity,* and further rob the patient of *self-esteem.* Further, it may make it difficult for him to increase his pain *tolerance* and progress in any rehabilitation efforts. Studies on the effect of marital partners of chronic benign pain patients have been done. In one study, it was found that when the patient's symptoms associated with pain were high, psychological distress scores were elevated for both the patient and the spouse (Shanfield et al. 1979, p. 349). In another study, patients whose spouse were solicitous to their pain behaviors reported significantly higher levels of pain (Block et al., 1980, p. 343). It becomes very clear that if the family is going to organize their lives around and cooperate with the patient's pain regimen, especially if the patient's pain is of a chronic benign nature, they must fully understand it and believe in it. If they do not or are not interested, they, in fact, may compound the patient's pain problem by actively or passively undermining his efforts.

PHYSICAL CONTACT WITH OTHERS

The patient not only responds to his own body with touch, position, or movement during the pain experience, but in the process of interacting with another person will indicate his interest in *physical contact* from a source outside himself. His use of physical contact with others reveals much about the meanings and emotions associated with his pain experience, such as varying degrees of anger, dependency and fear. In general, this physical contact can be observed as fight reactions, initiation of touch, or passive or active acceptance of touch.

Touch may be initiated by both adults and children. Many children want to be *held* during some phase of a pain experience. They may *cling* to any part of another person's body. An adult lying in bed helpless and in pain may *reach out* for the nurse the moment he sees her.

When the patient does not initiate touch, the nurse may offer it in the form of holding the patient's hand or rubbing some area of his body. The patient may accept this passively or actively. The patient demonstrates *passive acceptance*, for example, when allowing the nurse to hold a hand but does not actually grip the nurse's hand in return. *Active acceptance* would involve gripping the nurse's hand, or if the nurse is stroking the patient's forehead he or she might turn their head so that it could be reached more easily.

Secondary Gains and Positive Reinforcers

The *secondary gain* is used in several contexts. Here secondary gains of pain refer to any practical advantages that result from having the pain, especially *financial compensation* and *preferential treatment* at home and at work. *Positive reinforcers* refer to all those advantages or benefits, including secondary gains, that result when the patient expresses his pain or otherwise responds to his pain. The expressions of pain may vary considerably, depending upon the individual patient. The patient may state he has pain, merely grimace, or simply cease his activity or rest to reduce his pain. If cessation of activity and lying down to rest cause the intensity of the pain to decrease that is positive reinforcement for rest. However, decreased pain may not be the only positive reinforcer that rest provides. For some, rest may have the advantage of keeping the patient from working at a job he does not like; increasing the patient's time for pleasurable activities, or providing the patient with attention and concern from people who otherwise ignore him. These positive reinforcers usually are called secondary gains. It is obvious that a behavior such as rest can be a secondary gain. Chapman (1978, p. 177) says "the secondary gains associated with pain are [often] enough to make the patient *somatically hypervigilent.*"

In this way behavioral responses to pain may be reinforced and learned. They may persist and contribute to disabling the patient. But this is not inevitable. Some patients find, for example, that rest is undesirable as is the undesired use of time necessary to do so, and unsolicited extra attention from others. They want very much to resume their work, and they already have satisfactory ways of relating to other people. In these patients secondary gains are not present and the only positive reinforcements may be decreased pain. *Financial compensation* and *improved self-esteem* also are often additional *positive reinforcers.*

Presently there is much discussion about the use of *operant conditioning methods* to assist patients with chronic pain. These methods are based upon the general principles that: (1) pain behavior occurs not only because of the pain stimulus (*antecedent stimulation*) but also because of *environmental consequences*, and (2) that the frequency of a behavior may be increased by *positive reinforcement* or decreased by *nonreinforcement* or *aversive* consequences. Pain occurring in response to an antecedent stimulus (physical cause) is referred to as *respondent pain. Operant pain* most often involves respondent pain, but the most important component is that some environmental response or contingency occurs which makes it likely that the pain behaviors will be repeated. The pain helps the patient satisfy other needs which he has not otherwise been successful in getting met. Operant pain is considered for the most part to be counterproductive and efforts are made to extinguish it and the negative consequences it has on the patient's total life and that of others in his home, social, and work worlds.

When a program using operant conditioning methods is administered by a team of specially trained professionals to patients with chronic pain who have been carefully selected, fully informed about the program, and consent to participate in the prescribed methods, the results have been encouraging (Fordyce, 1973; 1974; 1976; 1978; and Pace, 1976). However, certain misconceptions and misuse have occurred in operant conditioning probably because the methods are still relatively new in their application to patients with pain and the information is not yet well disseminated. Therefore, it is important to clarify the relevance of these new ideas to general nursing practice and most specifically for the assessment of the patient with pain.

If a nurse believes that a patient may be helped by a *pain clinic* using *operant techniques* she should bear in mind several points as she proceeds to gather further data *before* suggesting such a referral. Obviously, not all patients are candidates for operant conditioning pain therapy programs. Only patients with *chronic pain, not acute pain,* are selected to participate. Information about the selection of patients for such a program is far beyond the scope of this book. Special assessment tools and screening methods are used. However, the nurse's observations and assessment may be very valuable in the initial assessment process prior to the referral.

Another point is that operant pain may not be psychogenic and it *definitely is not malingering.* "The *malingerer* does not feel pain but tries to make others believe that he does [through pretense in an attempt to avoid or gain something. His "pain behaviors" are] a conscious lie, for the malingerer by definition does not even 'imagine' pain or 'think' he has it" (McCaffery, 1979, p. 11). Fielding (1980, p. 706) says that the malingerer often has a very strong need to suffer and/or be taken care of but his symptoms usually disappear as soon as his ruse is discovered. Further, if one is tempted to negatively label a patient's motivation it may be helpful to bear in mind that none of us has not at some time used pain consciously. Malingering, to avoid or gain something, the "all-of-a-sudden" toothache, headache, other pain, or flu are common excuses.

Nor is the patient who responds to a placebo (*placebo responder*) the same as a patient with operant pain. A placebo refers to a medication, treatment, or other intervention which produces an effect in a patient because of its implicit or explicit therapeutic intent, not because of its physical or active components (McCaffery, 1979, p. 260). As previously mentioned when a person responds to a placebo a neurophysiological response occurs (most likely endorphin release) whether the intent is implicit or explicit and whether or not the intervention was inert or not. Moreover, Feather, et al. (1972) found that when a placebo is given, the patient's attitude changes but the sensitivity to pain does not. Patients become less willing to report pain.

Even though the patient with operant pain gains benefits from his pain, this is not on a conscious level. When assessing the patient for possible operant pain there are primarily two areas that the nurse should observe. First, the frequency and regularity with which a patient uses pain to manipulate others in an attempt to gain something from the interaction should be noted. What the patient gains must be something that would not otherwise be available to him. The nurse must be aware that what provides a secondary gain for one person is not necessarily what would be a desirable gain for another. For example, two patients may gain the "advantage" of keeping their television on late when they have pain. For one person it may provide a secondary gain if he enjoys the late night shows; for the other it may be used as a hypnotic, a type of sensory monotony to aid him in falling asleep. The nurse should also assess whether the patient is using his complaint of pain to avoid activities such as gainful employment, home responsibilities, or in the hospital, to avoid some part of his treatment that he dislikes.

It becomes very obvious that great care and sensitivity must be employed when assessing the patient who may have operant pain. Further, until it has been proven and the treatment plan has been changed, the nurse should treat that patient with the same positive responsive accepting manner that she would any other patient with pain. The patient's behavior must be validated because things are often not what they appear to be. Finally, if it is decided that the patient does have operant pain and could benefit from the use of operant conditioning techniques, the patient must be informed and have all of his questions answered before he signs a written consent to participate in a formalized program.

GENERAL PHYSICAL ENVIRONMENT

Laboratory studies show that the *social milieu* changes the basic quality of the pain experience. It may modify the sensory, affective, and cognitive components and the expression of pain. The affective component and the expression of the pain have a more important social function than do those of the sensory component (Craig, 1978, p. 104). We will now consider how the patient care setting and individuals in it may influence the patient's pain experience. In Chapter 9 the interplay of these variables in relation to communicating about pain will be considered.

The Health Care Setting as a Subculture

In addition to the patients' expressive style being greatly determined by the culture in which they have lived or in which they currently reside, the *health care setting* and its organizational structure in which they seek pain relief also has a *distinct culture*. It is a nonverbalized expectation that it is the patient's responsibility to adopt this new culture and assume the concomitant roles of the setting. Robinson (1976, p. 6) says that when a patient submits to medical care, there is a tacit agreement that he will "proffer his body" and deny expression of his personal identity including the emotional and intellectual components in exchange for treatment of his health problem. We are not suggesting that this is desirable, only that it is common.

Klein (1979, pp. 95–96) discusses the *patient's vulnerability* as he enters the hospital and leaves his role of "special" at home to "ordinary" in the hospital. He says that the *forced dependency* and *subordinated roles* make it highly unlikely that the patient and physician will be on equal footing. When the patient experiences conflict over the expectations that he be cooperative and compliant, alter his roles, responsibilities, power and prestige, he may respond in a defensive manner because of anxiety and fears, or because of perceived insults. The *patient's behavioral* response to the threats is likely to get him labeled the *bad patient*, compounding his pain problem and interfering with his quest for a solution to his pain problem. Further, the *staff* may *retaliate* or *withdraw*. The roles of the patient at home are contrasted with those of the patient in the hospital in Table 8.1.

Most of our discussion has focused on patients within health care settings without identifying differences between patients in *private health care settings* from those in *public health care* settings. Private or public indeed can be expected to influence care the patient receives for his pain problem. Milner (1980) says that the patient in the public setting usually has more severe health problems, yet, fewer resources, both personal and familial, to facilitate his recovery. Freidman (1981, pp. 14–18) adds that problems for the public clinic patient are significantly more exaggerated by the imbalance between demands and resources; the fact that the patient rarely sees the same physician twice; when the patient does see the physician, the average time, including time for questions and answers is five minutes, and the numbers of other clinic staff that the patient must interact with futher

TABLE 8.1. Roles of the Patient at Home and in the Hospital

Patient at Home	Patient in the Hospital
Uninhibited	Inhibited
Independent	Dependent
Secure	Air of apprehension
Doctor waits for patient	Patient waits for doctor
Doctor on call or can be changed	Doctor admits or discharges patient
Family, relatives and friends belong	Family, relatives or friends are visitors
Medication and treatments are prescribed	Orders are given
Led by explanation and persuasion	Pushed with little or no persuasion
Nurses hired and fired	Nurses are assigned
Nurses come and go	Patients come and go
Patients have tenure	Nurses have tenure
Patient sickest person in family	Patient may be "healthiest" patient on the unit
Habits, customs, social values well-established	Habits, culture and social values unique to hospital subculture

dilute his care and increase the possibility for distortions in communication, including inaccurate rumors.

Further, Schwartz (1975, pp. 167–171) says that one's waiting time may be equated as a component of one's social worth. Because waiting is such a source of extreme irritation, he believes that the extended waiting public patients experience both to get an appointment and when they arrive for scheduled appointments dilutes the benefit the patient derives from the care ultimately received. One must assume that directly proportional to all of the above variables confronting the public clinic patient may be the potential for increasing pain and suffering through decreasing the patient's pain tolerance.

Even a relatively noncomplicated well-handled (from the staff's perception) pain experience can be very threatening to the patient. This may be especially true for the patient who comes to the health care setting to have his pain relieved but in the process undergoes painful diagnostic and therapeutic processes. For example, Katz (1979, p. 2) found substantial generalization of the child's anxiety from the painful procedure itself to "hospital locations, personnel, both temporal and sensory stimuli (sounds, sights, and smells), and other stimulus discriminants."

Patients who are involved in either inpatient or outpatient *pain-treatment programs* may be especially fearful. One of the *goals of pain clinics* is to assist patients to endure pain and control their expression of it. To a large extent this reflects the desired pain response of the dominant Old American culture. All of these programs use *modeling techniques* of the desired pain behaviors by both the staff and other patients. It is very important that, when individuals are involved in such programs, they fully understand the goals and electively decide to participate. Lacking such information and commitment the patient may feel that he was being subjected to additional pain, possibly being ridiculed for his pain behaviors and being victimized in the situation, all of which could serve to increase the patient's pain perception.

Roles Ascribed to Patients

Harwood (1981, pp. 22–25) takes health care professionals to task for what he views as a unicultural view of patients which demeans their perceptions and concepts. He says that ascendency of health care professionals to a high status has contributed "to making a patient's own experience of his illness seem incorrect, irrelevant, and inferior" (p. 22). Other important points that he makes are that *although the health care professional, by occupation, chooses to focus on illness and disease, it is just one part of a patient's life*. Further, and especially important for the patient with pain, is that the *patient's* presenting condition has become the *focal point in his life* at this time and "has either totally or significantly inhibited the performance of valued or even essential life activities" (p. 24). Certainly it is not typical of his normal life.

Roles Ascribed to Health Team Members

The *patient's attitude toward a health team* member may be one of confidence or skepticism. The patient may value skill or bedside manner. In addition to these general attitudes, the patient may inaccurately ascribe various activities to members of the health team according to their occupational titles, age, or sex.

The patient may believe that the physician's role is broader and the nurse's narrower than is actually the case. For example, he may not believe that the nurse is competent to explain or relieve pain. If the nurse suggests that a change in position may relieve his pain, the patient may not do so until his physician suggests it. On the other hand, the patient may think that the nurse, the aide, and the physician all have comparable abilities to diagnose and treat pain. Sometimes the sex of the physician or nurse influences the patient's confidence; also, the age of the health team member may be important.

Robinson (1976, p. 3) sees the role of *childhood experiences* as very influential in how a patient will be able to adapt to the patient role and respond to health care professionals. She says that children who have grown up in a warm, loving, and accepting environment with reasonable parents are likely to perceive health care professionals similarly and expect the same treatment from them. Unfortunately, children who have had punitive or sadistic parents also are likely to expect similar treatment from health care professionals.

Other situational factors are concerned with the patient's general physical environment. For purposes of discussion, we have divided these into sensory restrictions and atmospheric conditions.

Sensory Restriction

Sensory restrictions may occur in any patient setting in or out of the hospital. There are three types of sensory restrictions: 1) sensory deprivation, 2) perceptual deprivation, and 3) perceptual monotony. The latter results in boredom. All three types of sensory restrictions may occur in any of the sensory modalities. *Sensory deprivation* refers to a complete absence, or the lowest level possible of sensory input through a sensory modality. An example is visual sensory deprivation for the patient who is wearing bilateral eye patches. The patient may be able to perceive some visual input but it is reduced to as low a level as possible. *Perceptual deprivation* is defined as the reduction in the patterning and meaningful organization of sensory input. For example, a patient in an intensive care unit may experience auditory perceptual deprivation because of the overriding noise from cardiac monitors, suction machines, oxygen equipment, etc. *Perceptual monotony* is defined as the lack of variation in stimuli. The stimuli are received at an adequate level and are understandable to the patient but are repetitive. This is by far the most frequent problem for most patients with chronic pain who are confined to bed or home. They may experience other types of immobilization further increasing the perceptual monotony depending on their pain problem. It usually involves the senses of hearing, sight, touch, and sometimes smell and taste (McCaffery, 168, pp. 161–168).

In patients with chronic pain, the major problems resulting from sensory restrictions seem to be an increased sensitivity to and perceived intensity of pain, an increased degree of anxiety, and a decreased ability to concentrate and think clearly with an accompanying inability to distract themselves from their pain (Blitz & Lowenthal, 1966 and Schultz, 1965). In addition, it has been found that people who were not experiencing pain may begin to complain of various aches and pain when they are subjected to sensory restriction. The patient reports more minor discomforts that would go unnoticed under conditions of adequate sensory input. Research on groups of 15 to 100 men confined together for several months in the limited area of a military base in the Antarctic showed a progressive increase in somatic complaints such as soreness of muscles, upset stomach, headaches, and chest pain related to perceptual monotony (Schultz, 1965).

Further, the patient is less able to tolerate pain. Again, this seems to be due to an effort to compensate for having inadequate stimuli upon which to focus his attention. The patient focuses upon the sensation of pain, and this attention makes the pain much more bothersome. It is a common observation that pain seems to be more severe at night. This probably is caused in part by the inevitable monotony that surrounds trying to go to sleep.

Avoidance of inadequate sensory input is involved in many pain-relief measures. Patient teaching, for example, provides information that reduces some of the perceptual deprivation in the health care setting. In other words, the patient is able to ascribe meaning to stimuli that otherwise might be meaningless. Other pain-relief methods help prevent or relieve boredom by demanding the patient's participation, such as rhythmic breathing patterns; or, the method attracts the patient's attention and interest, such as TENS, massage, music (audioanalgesia), and many others. Obviously, most pain-relief methods are based upon more than one theoretical possibility.

A roommate is no small part of a patient's sensory input. For many hospitalized patients, cost and bed availability necessitate having a roommate or several of them. When two or more strangers are suddenly together over 24-hour periods under stressful conditions, it is worth asking how they get along. Research has provided inconclusive but useful data. From one-third to over one-half of the patients preferred a private room (Reid & Feeley, 1973; Silvers & Harding, 1969). In one study, over half the patients said that a hospital roommate increased their pain (Copp, 1974). Too much noise was a factor adversely affecting the patient's response to a roommate. Noise was associated with visitors, television, equipment used in care, telephone conversations, unwanted attempts at conversation, and other disturbing noises. Bright lights, odors, and room temperature were also mentioned as sources of unpleasant stimuli caused by the presence of a roommate (Reid & Feeley, 1973).

In assessing the patient with pain, the nurse should be alert to the existence of any of the three forms of sensory restriction, including problems associated with having a roommate. Assessment of the patient with chronic pain should involve a typical 24-hour period, with special attention given to the variety and duration of activities engaged in by the patient.

Atmospheric Conditions

Solar radiation, extreme cold, wind, high altitudes, and air pollution are but a few examples of atmospheric conditions that may increase pain in persons with various diseases as well as cause pain in healthy individuals.

Exposure to rays from the sun in hot, cold, or cloudy weather may cause first-, second-, or even third-degree burns. The patient taking regular doses of certain drugs such as chlorpromazine may be photosensitive and develop dermatitis following relatively brief exposure to the sun. Radiation therapy may produce mild burns to severe necrosis.

Strong winds may excoriate unprotected areas of the skin. A very slight draft may cause severe pain in the patient with second-degree burns due to the exposure of nerve endings. Drafts may also stimulate trigger points and some pain syndromes such as trigeminal neuralgia.

Extremes in temperature and humidity may also affect some types of pain, as can the time of day. Both pain thresholds and pain tolerance levels have been shown to be higher in the early morning than in the evening (Rogers & Vilkin, 1978), or during the night (Robinson, 1976, p. 6). Strenuous exercise in hot weather may result in sudden muscle pain (heat cramps) by excessive loss of sodium chloride in perspiration. Very cold weather may cause frostbite, especially in people with poor circulation. It is first felt as numbness, but severe pain may occur as the part is thawed. Patients with musculoskeletal problems, such as arthritis, tend to experience increased pain in cold weather, particularly following chilling, possibly because the cold results in muscle tension. Many such patients, according to folklore, are able to predict changes in the weather because of increased pain. Underlying this pain may be muscle tension from slight decreases in temperature aggravated by increased humidity since water is a good conductor of temperature and can intensify the cold. These patients often seek a warm dry climate. Low humidity may increase the irritation of an inflamed respiratory tract. Some patients find that warm air increases efforts to breathe and thereby increases discomfort.

Low pressure of oxygen may result in pain in a healthy person as well as in patients with pathological processes that already endanger their oxygen supply. At high altitudes, the percentage of oxygen is actually the same as it is at sea level; however, since the barometric pressure is reduced at these altitudes, the partial pressure of oxygen is also diminished. Consequently, there may be inadequate delivery of oxygen to tissues, depending, of course, upon the altitude and the rate of ascent. Since the cabins in commercial airlines are pressurized, flight does not ordinarily present a problem. But rapid ascent into the mountains by car, for example, may precipitate a crisis in the patient with sickle-cell anemia or cause a migraine headache in a person with a history of vascular headaches. The patient with peripheral vascular disease is rarely affected by rapid ascent to high altitudes. But a patient with arteriosclerotic heart disease may experience anginal pain if he exerts himself at high altitudes. In the healthy person, the phenomenon of "mountain sickness" may occur with headache and other symptoms. In addition to the effects of low oxygen pressure, the low barometric pressure at high altitudes may cause abdominal pain from distension of the organs. Or, patients with chronic lung disease may experience increased chest pain because of the difficulty in expelling mucus. Coughing is less effective in dislodging particles and the respiratory tract is irritated even in the healthy individual.

Air pollution, which promises to become an increasing problem, may be another cause of pain. Large particules of pollutants such as sand, may cause minor irritation of the eyes. But a greater problem results from irritant gases such as oxides of nitrogen, sulfur gas, sulfate, and ozones which contribute to smog. These chemicals are thought to combine with water at the tissue level in the lungs, eyes, nose, and other areas, producing acids that irritate the tissues and cause pain. The resulting inflammation may be only mildly uncomfortable for the healthy individual, but it may be severely painful or fatal to the patient with chronic lung disease.

STRESSFUL LIFE EVENTS

Change, whether the person perceives it as good or bad, may cause stress and possibly may leave the person more susceptible to disease. Illness and any of its symptoms, including pain, are regarded by some as indicative of a need to reduce the amount of stress in one's life.

Benson (1975) defines stress as being the result of environmental conditions that require behavioral adjustment. According to Holmes & Rahe (1967), stress results not only from the death of a spouse, divorce, being fired, or going to jail, but also from marriage, retirement, or outstanding personal achievement. In other words, some of the things we value and strive for actually cause stress. This positive stress is called *eustress*. Negative stress is called *distress* though most frequently referred to as just stress. From personal experience, most people know that stress of any type can raise the blood pressure, cause muscle tension, affect digestion, or cause any one of a number of other physical signs and symptoms, including pain.

Avoiding stress or change is not always possible or desirable. It is the person's *reaction*, or the nature of the behavioral response, to stress or change, and not necessarily the stress itself, that concerns us here. In the assessment of some patients with pain it is pertinent to identify the existence of any change or stress in the patient's life that corresponds to the onset or increase in pain. However, the existence of stress does not in any way prove a cause and effect relationship. There are individual differences in responses to stress. What is stressful for one person is not stressful or as highly stressful to another. Some people prefer to live at a faster pace than others and seem to do so without detrimental effects. Perhaps the key factor is that they have adjusted already, that is, they are not in a period of adjustment and their life style, as stressful as it might be for someone else, does not require continuous adjustment for them.

Assessment involves identifying stress (a change in the person's life that requires behavioral adjustment), a corresponding onset or increase in pain, and the patient's style of responding to the stress. To identify stress, the nurse may rely upon a thorough psychosocial assessment, or simply, direct questioning. People often associate the word "stress" with distress, so other words may be more productive. The patient may be asked if anything different or new has happened in his life recently. He may be further questioned about sudden changes in his life and events he has found exhausting, exciting, or difficult. If a stress can be identified in the patient's life, he may be asked if the onset or increase in pain coincided with the timing of the stress. Here it is important for the nurse to convey that she believes the patient has pain—she is not suggesting it is "psychological" or "imaginary." She may explain that stress, or change, often results in bodily changes that affect pain and that coping with pain can be more difficult when there is also another stress requiring the patient's energy and attention.

What if we identify a stress that is associated with the occurrence of pain? Elimination of the stress is often not possible or desirable. Referral for appropriate counseling, for example marriage counseling, is one option. However, the nurse can make a more direct contribution to altering the detrimental effects of the stress. First, the nurse can assess the extent to which the patient has learned relaxation strategies to cope with stress. To identify relaxation methods the nurse should explore many possible means, referring not only to relaxation per se but also using other terminology such as "periods alone or just for yourself" and "times when you slow down and tune out." The frequency of relaxation must also be determined. Weekends are not enough. If stress is causing pain problems, relaxation needs to be done at regular intervals. Second, if assessment shows that the patient does not relax regularly, the nurse can help him learn some ways to do so.

In Chapter 9 we will consider how the patient communicates pain and need for pain relief.

REFERENCES

Andrysiak, T. Personal communication, Los Angeles, CA, May 27, 1982.

Bandura, A., & Menlove, F.L. Factors determining vicarious extinction of avoidance behavior through symbolic modelling. J Personal Social Psychol 8: 99–108, 1968.

Beecher, H.K. Relationship of significance of wound to pain experienced. J Amer Med Assoc 161: 1609–1613, 1956.

Benson, H. The Relaxation Response. New York: William Morrow & Co., 1975.

Blinchik, E.R., & Grzesiak, R.C. Reinterpretive cognitive strategies in chronic pain management. Arch Phys Med Rehab 60: 609–612, 1979.

Blitz, B., & Lowenthal, M. The role of sensory restriction in problems with chronic pain. J Chron Dis 19: 1119–1125, 1966.

Block, A.W., Kremer, E.T., & Gaylor, M. Behavioral treatment of chronic pain: The spouse as a discriminative cue for pain behavior. Pain 9: 243–252, 1980.

Bond, M.R. The suffering of severe intractable pain. In H.W. Kosterlitz & L.Y. Terenius (Eds.), Pain and Society. Report of the Dahlem Workshop on Pain and Society, Berlin, Nov. 26–30, 1979, Weinheim: Verlag Chemie 1980, 53–62.

Bowers, K.S. Pain anxiety and perceived control. J Consult Clin Psychol 32: 596–602, 1968.

Brechner, T. Personal communication, Los Angeles, CA, May 27, 1982.

Chapman, C.R. Pain: The perception of noxious events. In R.A. Sternbach (Ed.), The Psychology of Pain. New York: Raven Press, 1978, pp. 169–202.

Copp, L.H. The spectrum of suffering. Amer J Nurs 74: 491–495, 1974.

Craig, K.D. Social modelling influences in pain. In R.A. Sternbach (Ed.), The Psychology of Pain. New York: Raven Press, 1978, pp. 73–109.

Craig, K.D. Ontogenetic and cultural influences on the expression of pain. In H.W. Kosterlitz, & L.Y. Terenius, (Eds.) Pain and Society. Report of the Dahlem Workshop on Pain and Society, Berlin, Nov. 26–30, 1979, Weinheim: Verlag Chemie, 1980.

Craig, K.D. & Best, J.A. Perceived control over pain individual differences and situational determinants. Pain 3: 127–135, 1977.

Crowley, D.M. Chronic pain: Social aspects. In ANA Clinical Sessions. New York: Appleton-Century-Crofts, 1974, pp. 257–266.

Dell, D.D., & Snyder, J.A. Marijuana: Pro and con. Amer J Nurs 77: 630–635, 1977.

Farnsworth, D. Pain and the individual. 254: 559–562, 1956.

Feather, B.W., Chapman, C.R., & Fisher, S.B. The effect of a placebo on the perception of radiant heat stimuli. Psychosom Med 34: 290–294, 1972.

Fielding, J.M. Psychiatric aspects of pain. Med J Austral 2: 705–707, 1980.

Fordyce, W. E. An operant conditioning method for managing chronic pain. Postgrad Med 53: 123–128, 1973.

Fordyce, W.E. The office management of chronic pain. Minn Med 57: 185–188, 1974.

Fordyce, W.E. Behavioral Methods for Chronic Pain and Illness. St. Louis: C.V. Mosby, 1976.

Fordyce, W.E. Learning processes in pain. In R.A. Sternbach (Ed.), The Psychology of Pain. New York: Raven Press, 1978, pp. 49–72.

Friedman, M. The Public Clinic Patient: Situational Effects and Coping Efforts. Unpublished M.A. thesis, University of Southern California, Department of Sociology, 1981.

Geer, J.H., Davison, G.C., & Gatchel, B.I. Reduction of stress in humans through nonverbal perceived control of aversive stimuli. J Personal Social Psychol 16: 731–738, 1970.

Gordon, D., Terdal, L., & Sterling, E. The use of modelling and desensitization in the treatment of a phobic patient. J Dent Children 22: 102–105, 1974.

Harwood, A. Introduction. In A. Harwood (Ed.) Ethnicity and Medical Care. Cambridge, Mass.: Harvard Univ. Press, 1981, pp. 1–36.

Hill, S.Y., Schwin, R., Goodwin, D.W., et al. Marijuana and pain. J Pharmacol Exp Therapeut 188: 415–418, 1974.

Holmes, R.H., & Rahe, R.H. The social readjustment scale. J Psychosom Res 11: 213–218, 1967.

Katz, E.R. Distress Behavior in Children with Leukemia Undergoing Medical Procedures. Paper presented at the annual meeting of the American Psychological Assoc. Symposium on Psychological Strategies in the management of children with life-threatening illness. New York City, Sept., 1979.

Klein, N. Introduction: Patients and practitioners. In N. Klein (Ed.) Culture, Curers and Contagion. Novato, CA: Chandler & Sharp, 1979, pp. 95–96.

Leriche, R. The Surgery of Pain. London: Baillière, Tindall & Cox, 1939.

LeShan L. The world of the patient in severe pain of long duration. J Chron Dis 17: 337–340, 1964.

McCaffery M. Cognition, Bodily Pain, and Man—Environment Interactions. Los Angeles: Univ. of California Student Store, 1968 (out of print).

McCaffery, M. Brief episodes of pain in children. In B.S. Bergersen, E.H. Anderson, M. Duffey, et al. (Eds.), Current Concepts in Clinical Nursing, Vol. II. St. Louis: C.V. Mosby Co., 1969, pp. 181–182.

McCaffery, M. Nursing Management of the Patient with Pain. (2nd ed.) New York: J.B. Lippincott, 1979.

Merskey, H. Pain and personality. In R.A. Sternbach (Ed.), The Psychology of Pain. New York: Raven Press, 1978, pp. 111–127.

Milner, J.M. Unequal Care. New York: Columbia University Press, 1980.

Pace, J.B. Pain: A Personal Experience. Chicago: Nelson-Hall, 1976.

Piaget, J. Judgment and Reasoning in the Child. Paterson, NJ: Littlefield, Adams, 1959.

Pilowsky, I. Psychodynamic aspects of the pain experience. In R.A. Sternbach, (Ed.), The Psychology of Pain. New York: Raven Press, 1978, pp. 203–217.

Pinsky, J.J. Aspects of the psychology of pain. In B.L. Crue, Jr. (Ed.) Chronic Pain—Further Observations from the City of Hope National Medical Center. New York: SP Medical and Scientific Publications, 1979, pp. 301–314.

Pinsky, J.J., & Malyon, A.K. The intractable pain and suffering process— Facilitating change. In B.L. Cure, Jr. (Ed.), Chronic Pain—Further Observations from the City of Hope National Medical Center. New York: SP Medical and Scientific Publications, 1979, pp. 315–320 (a).

Pinsky, J.J., & Malyon, A.K. The eclectic nature of psychotherapy in the treatment of chronic pain syndromes. In B.L. Crue, jr. (Ed.), Chronic Pain—Further Observations from the City of Hope National Medical Center. New York: SP Medical and Scientific Publications, 1979, pp. 324–327 (b).

Reid, E.A., & Feeley, E.M. Roommates: To have or have not. Amer J Nurs 73: 104–107, 1973.

Robinson, L. Psychological Aspects of the Care of Hospitalized Patients. Philadelphia: F.A. Davis, 1976.

Rogers, E.J., & Vilkin, B. Duirinal variation in sensory and pain threshold correlated with mood states. J Clin Psychiat 39: 431–433, 1978.

Salk, L. What Every Child Would Like His Parents to Know. New York: Warner Books, 1973.

Schultz, D.P. Sensory Restrictions. New York: Academic Press, 1965.

Schwartz, B. Queueing and Waiting. Chicago: University of Chicago Press, 1975.

Seeman, M., & Evans, J.W. Alienation and learning in a hospital setting. Amer Social Rev 27: 772–782, 1962.

Shanfield, S.B., Heiman, E.M., Cope, D.N., et al. Pain and the marital relationship. Pain 7: 343–351, 1979.

Silvers, G., & Harding, W.G. Semiprivate rooms are not bad, these patients told surveyors. Modern Hosp 113: (July), 66, 1969.

Strauss, A.L., & Glasser, B.G. Chronic Illness and the Quality of Life. St. Louis: C.V. Mosby, 1975.

Webb, W.L. The therapy of psychosomatic pain. Curr PsychiatrTher 18: 73–84, 1978.

Wolff, B.B. Behavioral measurement of human pain. In R.A. Sternbach (Ed.), The Psychology of Pain. New York: Raven Press, 1978, pp. 129–168.

Zborowski, M. Cultural components in responses to pain. J Social Issues 8: 16–30, 1952.

Zborowski, M. People in Pain. San Francisco: Jossey-Bass, 1969.

SUGGESTED READINGS

Beecher, H.K. Limiting factors in experimental pain. Journal of Chronic Diseases, 1956, 4: 11–21, (July).

Endler, N.S. A person–situation interaction model for anxiety. In C.D. Spielberger & I.G. Sarason (Eds.), Stress and Anxiety, Vol. 1. Washington, D.C.: Hemisphere, 1975.

Jacox, A.K., & Stewart, M. Psychosocial Contingencies of the Pain Experience. Iowa City: Univ. of Iowa, College of Nursing, 1973.

Johnson, B.H. Before hospitalization: A preparation program for the child and his family. Children Today 6: 18–21, 1974.

Johnson, J.E. Effects of accurate expectations about sensations on the sensory and distress components of pain. J Personal Social Psychol 27: 261–275, 1973.

Johnson, J.E., & Rice, V.H. Sensory and distress components of pain: Implications for the study of clinical pain. Nurs Res 23: 203–209, 1974.

Kendall, P.C. Anxiety: States, traits—Situations? J Consult Clin Psychol 46: 280–287, 1978.

Langrehr, A.A. Social stimulation. Amer J Nurs 74: 1300–1301, 1974.

Levy, E. Children's behavior under stress and its relation to training parents to respond to stress situations. Child Devel 30: 307–324, 1959.

McCaffery, M. Sociologic effects of cancer pain. In J.J. Bonica & V. Ventafridda (Eds.), Advances in Pain Research and Therapy, Vol. 2. New York: Raven Press, 1979, pp. 99–102.

McMahon, M.A., & Miller, P. Pain response: The influence of psychosocial cultural factors. Nurs Forum 17(1): 58–71, 1978.

Mechanic, D. The influence of mothers on their children's health attitudes and behavior. Pediatrics 33: 444–453, 1964.

Melamed, B.G., Meyer, R., Gee, C., et al. The influence of time and type of preparation on children's adjustment to hospitalization. J Pediatr Psychol 1: 31–37, 1976.

Moss, F.T., & Meyer, B. The effects of nursing interventions upon pain relief in patients. Nurs Res 15: 303–306, 1966.

Neufeld, R.W.J., & Davidson, P.O. The effects of vicarious and cognitive rehearsal on pain tolerance. J Psychosom Res 15: 329–335, 1971.

Petrie, A., Collins, W., & Solomon, P. The tolerance for pain and for sensory deprivation. Amer J Psychol 73: 80–90, 1960.

Pizzo, P.D. When Your Child Goes to the Hospital. DHEW Pub. No. (OHD) 76-30092. Washington, D.C.: U.S. Government Printing Office, 1977.

Rasmussen, M., & Murphy, C.M. Hospital admission through a child's eye. Pediatr Nurs 3: 43–46, 1977.

Schachter, S. The Psychology of Affiliation. Stanford, CA: Stanford University Press, 1959, pp. 12–19.

Scott, D.S., & Barber, T.X. Cognitive control of pain: Effects of multiple cognitive strategies. Psychol Rec 2: 373–383, 1977.

Scott, D.S., & Barber, T.X. Cognitive control of pain: Four serendipitous results. Percept Motor Skills 44: 569–570, 1977.

Snyder, J. Psychiatric nursing in non-traditional settings. RN 5(2): 4–5, 1981.

Vaughn, G.F. Children in hospital. Lancet 1: 1117–1120, 1957.

West, A.R. Bringing the hospital to preschoolers: Teaching young children about hospitals and health care. Children Today 5: 16–19, 1976.

Wolfer, J.A., & Visintainer, M.A. Pediatric surgical patients' and parents' stress responses and adjustments as a function of psychologic preparation and stress-point nursing care. Nurs Res 24: 244–255, 1975.

Wolff, B.B., Cohen, P., & Greene, C.T. Behavioral mechanisms of human pain: Effects of expectancy, magnitude, and type of cross-modal stimulation. In J.J. Bonica & D. Albe-Fessard (Eds.), Advances in pain research and therapy, Vol. 1. New York: Raven Press, 1976, pp. 327–333.

Wolff, H.G., & Goodell, H. The relation of attitude and suggestion to the perception of and reaction to pain. Pain: Association for Research in Nervous and Mental Diseases Research Publications 23: 434–437, 1943.

Young, J.L. The pain of the terminally ill patient in the home. Nurs Clin North Amer 12: 653–662, 1977.

9

Communication of Pain

Generally, practitioners seem to believe that the assessment of pain is an easy matter. We tend to underestimate the difficulties the patient may have when he attempts to communicate his pain. Also, we often fail to realize the effects pain may have upon the patient. McMahon & Miller (1978, p. 67), report that

> patients who had nurses who viewed their complaint of pain only as a request for pain medication and talked with them in a stereotyped manner had much less pain relief than those patients having nurses who attempted to communicate meaningfully and assess and evaluate their pain response before attempting a nursing intervention.

Naturally, there will be times when pain can be assessed quickly and effectively. For us, one most unforgettable example of this occurred in an outpatient acupuncture clinic. We were present when a patient came for his first treatment. The acupuncturist met the patient in a busy crowded hallway, carrying under his arm many volumes of the patient's previous medical records. The acupuncturist was Chinese and spoke very little English. It is doubtful that he could have read the medical records himself, although it is possible that someone gave him a brief synopsis. In only a moment, the acupuncturist bridged the language barrier, assessed the pain, and conveyed a caring attitude by looking the patient in the eyes and asking softly, "Where hurt?" The patient responded by pointing. Acupuncture treatments began almost immediately, without further discussion.

FACTORS WHICH MAY PRECLUDE OR IMPEDE COMMUNICATION WITH THE PATIENT WITH PAIN

Studies by Jacox & Stewart (1973), Marks & Sacher (1973), McCaffery & Hart (1976), and Cohen (1980) presented in Chapter 1, indicate that pain is neither thoroughly assessed nor treated; that there is a lack of knowledge and/or use of available information in relation to pain and pain relief strategies resulting in patients being undertreated for their pain; and that most patients tend to deny or minimize their pain even when it is discussed directly. Further, more specific reports on transcultural communication by Harwood (1981), Klein (1979), and Spector (1979) and other documentation throughout previous chapters support these findings.

Misconceptions and Prejudices

Patients and practitioners frequently evade or "dance around" direct communication with and about the patient with pain as a primary problem for a variety of reasons. Some of these include misconceptions and prejudices about pain and pain relief as discussed and summarized by McCaffery (1979, p. 21) and extended in Figure 9.1.

Assumptions and Erroneous Conclusions

Unfortunately, both patients and staff may draw erroneous conclusions based on assumptions about the patient's pain and each other's motives. The patient may assume that the staff knows his condition and thus whether or not he or she has pain. On the other hand, the staff may misread or fail to validate the patient's verbal and nonverbal communication assuming that, if the patient had pain it would be reported. The feelings that the patient has about his or her own pain and those he or she believes others have about pain often result in quite complex communication and assessment problems both for patient and staff. Indeed, patients often are reluctant to communicate about their pain feeling that "If I tell the nurse about all of my pains and other symptoms, she'll think I'm exaggerating and won't believe me." Yet the nurse may also be reluctant to fully discuss the patient's pain fearing that "If I assess the patient's pain thoroughly, I may cause more pain than he already has through the power of suggestion."

This latter concern about possibly inducing more pain is justified to a certain extent. Pain and illness are stressful, and it is generally thought that stress increases a person's susceptibility to suggestion. Yet, Swanson & Maruta (1980, p. 565) say that "the patient's stated estimate of his suffering is somewhat fixed, an individual declaration that resists change." Our personal experiences also have taught us generally not to be as frightened of this possibility as we once were. As we have become more forthright in asking specific questions about the intensity, quality, and location of pain, we are increasingly surprised to find that patients will disclaim and discard a variety of suggestions until they find ones that accurately describe their pain. We see this even in working with young children under the stress of sudden accidental injury. Of the suggestions made to them about the possibility of existing pain with which they agree, we have found a remarkable positive correlation with what one would expect from the physical diagnosis.

We are also less concerned with the possible negative effect of the

Figure 9.1.

Misconception	Correction
1. Health team members are the authorities on the existence and nature of the patient's pain.	The patient is the authority on his pain. Pain is whatever the experiencing person says it is, existing whenever he says it does. The patient is believed.
2. The patient who uses his pain to obtain benefits or preferential treatment does not hurt as much as he says and may not hurt at all.	The patient who uses his pain to his own advantage may still hurt as much as he says he does.
3. The patient's pain can always be verified by the presence of certain behavioral and/or physiological expressions of pain.	Physiological and behavioral adaptation occur, leading to periods of little or no signs of pain. Lack of pain expression does not mean lack of pain.
4. All "real" pain has an identifiable physical cause.	Not all physical causes of pain can be identified. All pain is real, regardless of its cause. Calling pain imaginary does not make it go away.
5. Psychogenic pain does not really hurt and is almost the same as malingering.	A localized sensation does exist in psychogenic pain.
6. The severity and duration of pain can be predicted accurately on the basis of the stimuli for pain.	There is no direct and invariant relationship between any stimulus and the perception of pain.
7. All patients can and should be encouraged to have a high tolerance for pain.	Pain tolerance is the individual's unique response, varying between patients and in the same patient from one situation to another.
8. Health team members tend to make accurate inferences about the severity and existence of the patient's pain.	Health team members tend to infer less pain than the patient experiences.

(continued)

Figure 9.1. (Continued)

9. Infants and young children do not perceive as much pain as adults.	Research has shown that the younger the child, the lower the pain perception threshold.
10. If infants and young children do perceive pain, they will not remember it.	Research has shown that memory of pain may occur as early as 6 months of age. Pain may have long-term effects. Amnesia for pain does not assure lack of effect on behavior.

Figure 9.1. Misconceptions that hamper assessment of the patient with pain. *(Items 1-8 above from McCaffery M: Nursing Management of the Patient with Pain, 2nd ed. Philadelphia: J.B. Lippincott, 1979, p. 21, with permission.)*

suggestion of pain because we believe that most people are motivated not to have pain. We think this motivation leads them to reject suggestions of pain. Further, if a nurse believes that the assessment is resulting in an increase in the patient's perception of pain then the method of assessment should be modified.

Differing Focuses of Nurses and Physicians

Another factor which may preclude or jeopardize communication and relief for the patient with pain is sometimes overlooked. This is the different focuses of nurses and physicians. Nurses are *usually* more psychosocially oriented, focusing on the total patient, and physicians are *usually* more focused on the presenting signs and symptoms, making a definitive diagnosis, and establishing a treatment plan. Their corresponding different perceptions of the patient's problems carry with them a corresponding vocabulary to describe them.

Lynaugh & Bates (1979, pp. 129–137) say that the resultant communication gap between these two subcultures, nurses and physicians, is so serious as to exemplify another failure of two cultures to communicate. Further, specific areas in a hospital may be so specialized as to speak their own dialect. Even in relation to the more frequently discussed patient problems they suggest that it would be *helpful* for *nurses and physicians to become bilingual with each other.*

Preexisting Personality of Practitioners

Still another problem sometimes overlooked is that *practitioners may present any* of the *communication difficulties* that *patients do.* That is, they too may have similar preexisting personality characteristics, such as being very reserved or have emotional problems and have difficulty dealing with their own as well as those of others. The reality is these sometimes interfere with the best care for the patient. If a nurse is aware of a conflict with a patient that cannot be satisfactorily resolved for the sake of that specific patient and because of possible reverberating negative effects on other patients in the best interest of everyone the nurse should, if possible, ask to be reassigned. If this is not possible, she or he needs to be especially cognizant of anger that may be directed toward the patient.

Health Care Setting Related Problems—Outpatient Clinic

After it has been determined that the patient's pain problem is not of an acute or life-threatening nature, it is likely that most patients will receive the major portion of their further assessment and treatment in outpatient settings. Some of the special problems faced by patients in public hospital outpatient clinics which could potentiate pain and suffering were identified in Chapter 8. Here we will focus on the more frequent and specific communication problems that patients with pain in outpatient clinic settings are likely to encounter. The focus will be directed at public outpatient clinics because problems are likely to be more extreme for the patient there. This information is included in the hope that it may alert nurses working in these health care settings to potential problems in which they may intervene to minimize some of the pain and suffering for the patient. Further, nurses working in inpatient settings where the public clinic patient with a pain problem is likely to be admitted, need to be able to assess the patient to determine the types of experiences he or she has had and how they may influence inpatient pain experiences. The nurse may also have the opportunity to provide these patients with some clues on how to minimize future communication problems on subsequent visits to clinics. Some patients have had such negative experiences in attempting to communicate about their pain to practitioners that in one pain clinic patients attend classes to learn "How to communicate with your doctor" (Reeves, 1982).

PHYSICIAN-PATIENT COMMUNICATION

Studying physician and patient communications in a medical outpatient clinic, Pratt, et al. (1957) found that patients significantly lacked information that the physicians believed was necessary for them to have and different than what the patients' actually possessed. Physicians indicated that patients should be informed about the etiology, course, and prognosis of their condition, and the tests and treatments necessary to appropriately assume responsibility for these. However, in actuality, the information that patients had was very fragmented, often isolated facts, and often related only to such things as tests and treatments.

It was found that physicians were likely to give patients some information and this correlated with the information that the patients' possessed. Furthermore, the information was not what the physicians said they believed patients should know but rather was in relation to the physicians' immediate concerns such as treatments and tests. In spite of the already low level of knowledge that patients' possessed, the physicians who most seriously underestimated the patient's information were the ones who were less likely to discuss things with the patient. Their reasons being that they were afraid of frightening the patient. Moreover, physicians found it inordinately difficult to put things into language that the patient could comprehend, which is indicative of how a *highly specialized vocabulary* can result in exclusivity.

On the other hand, when communicating with physicians, patients seldom had expectations that the physician would provide them with information, did not make any direct demands or request anything, nor did they even direct the physician's attention to something which may be of concern to them. In spite of the patient's lack of direct communication through formulated questions, it was found that when the patients were interviewed, the majority of patients indicated a latent desire for information. This is most unfortunate because Svarstad as quoted in Freidman (1981, p. 18) found that not only does patient compliance depend on the adequacy of the communication with the physician but the amount of communication depends upon the questions that the patient asks. Patients with pain problems already are often suffering, feeling helpless and demoralized. Sometimes, due to their pain and suffering, they may find it even more difficult to ask questions hoping that they can depend on someone else to "take over" and allow them to be dependent at least until they are feeling better.

It seems that the patient's lack of knowledge is dysfunctional both for the patient and the physician in that patients are likely to receive poorer care and the physicians may be more frustrated by their noncompliance problems. The fact that physicians avoided communicating with patients, viewed them as poorly informed, even dull, and unable to handle information and that patients performed at even a lower level than the physicians estimated may be in part the physicians' self-fulfilling prophecy.

Brown (1962, p. 90) told of how very difficult it is for individuals of low status to ask for help and admit their inadequacies to those they perceive as their superiors, no matter how much in need of reassurance and concern they are. Further, "Higher status persons have the power to create either gratifying or depriving experiences for others." For the patient, this may be a tangible such as a prescription for an analgesic or an extension in deferment to return to work until pain problems are somewhat improved. Less tangible examples of the results of control exerted by the health team may include how well the patient is adhering to the prescribed pain regimen or how effectively he or she conceals expressions of pain to meet the practitioners' expectations. When patients do not qualify for such "rewards" from practitioners, they are likely to receive censure. It is hard to imagine what this might do to a patient who has a pain problem that has eluded the diagnostic talents of the health team. To add to the demeaning of patients is the fact that health care professionals often do not admit their own mistakes or errors of judgment, even to their own colleagues, let alone to the patients who may have been victimized by them. This certainly has been evident in the literature on reasons for malpractice. Poor communication, in the form of failing to acknowledge and apologize for errors, usually heads the list.

PATIENT COMMUNICATION WITH NURSE AND CLERICAL STAFF

Almost 25 years after Pratt, Seligman & Reader's study, Freidman (1981) studied the outcome of *situational coping behaviors* and *strategies* used by patients attempting to communicate with nursing and clerical staff to get their health care needs met in a public hospital outpatient clinic. Freidman also studied the *reciprocal coping strategies* of the staff communicating with the patients. She categorized the behaviors and strategies of both groups as either active quest strategies or passive acceptance strategies.

Active quest strategies most commonly were displayed by patients who were new to the hospital outpatient clinic, lacked knowledge, or were confused by the operational procedures of the clinic and the long waiting time. Initially, in attempting to obtain information, patients politely asked reasonable questions. When this failed to produce favorable results, the patients often became assertive, expressing their anger forcefully and dramatically directly to the staff or loudly enough for it to be heard by them. The content of these angry outbursts included expressions of dissatisfaction, disagreement, and/or the demands. When these tactics succeeded, other patients and their families who were waiting often verbally "cheered" the expressive patient on. Freidman found that patients who complained were less likely to be forgotten or miss their turn. Another active quest strategy that Freidman observed was that patients either "stormed" or walked out, even at times in the middle of a procedure. Sometimes these patients just did not return that day, more often they never returned to the clinic.

Passive acceptance as a coping strategy was used more frequently by the "oldtimers," those patients seasoned and experienced in the workings of a public hospital outpatient clinic. These patients nonverbally communicated their feelings of powerlessness, pessimism, and futility through a resigned, fatigued, and/or discouraged appearance. Another passive coping strategy used by these patients was to lower their expectations for medical care. The expection of receiving no information and discourteous treatment, and in a perfunctory manner, from the nursing and clerical staff allowed the patients to "be less upset" by their predicament. Other passive tactics included such things as defying the staff or breaking rules such as no-smoking. One patient, who used this later approach reported to Freidman that "it relieved his boredom, provided him with temporary pleasure, and communicated that the nurses could not run my whole life" (p. 31).

Some of the "newcomers" also used passive coping strategies. In fact, Freidman found that some of the patients were so passive that they arrived before the clinic opened and waited until the clinic closed before finding out that they had missed their turn or were waiting in the wrong area.

When interviewed by Freidman, patients who appeared more passive and less expressive about their negative feelings about the hospital clinic were those more likely to be the most negativistic and cynical. Pain and suffering while waiting were two of the most common reasons for the patients' negativity. Reasons they gave for continuing medical care in this clinic were that they were trapped and lacked other alternatives for care and/or urgently needed medical care.

Freidman also observed the nursing and clerical staffs' passive coping strategies. She found their tactics included maintaining a composed unemotional, yet unyielding, stance, rigidly adhering to sacrosanct rules; giving direct commands; providing little or no information; and ignoring or outright refusing to answer questions. Freidman found that the staff felt that the patients could expect to wait. Another observation that she made was that patients who were socially stigmatized such as drug addicts and the mentally ill were even further stigmatized by the staff in this clinic.

One clerk at that clinic described the waiting room as a setting for a "potential riot when 50–100 patients wait around hour after hour to be taken care of" (p. 29). Another stated that "patients learn that complaining does not pay off" (p. 29). From Freidman's observations and structured and unstructured interviews of patients and their families, she concluded that "patients who view their progress and prognosis more negatively had increased negative feelings toward the clinic and the converse was also true" (p. 33). It is difficult to imagine the impact of dependency on such a setting to have one's pain problem assessed and treated.

PATIENT SITUATION ILLUSTRATING MULTIPLE COMMUNICATION PROBLEMS

We will use one detailed patient example, interweaving patient reports with direct quotations from his medical records and our comments to illustrate a variety of possible communication problems. These are the problems we see with alarming and disheartening frequency in patients with pain. The necessity of the health team communicating with each other when they are consulting and treating a patient will also be apparent. However, the two points we hope will be most vividly illustrated are, first, the necessity of believing the patient about his pain, and, second, the suffering which may ensue when the subjective nature of pain is ignored and denied and the patient is not considered the authority about the presence and severity of his pain. (In reading this example be alert to the sequence of dates.)

The following referral for this patient with terminal cancer was made to a pain clinic by the patient's internist-oncologist on April 16, 1982:

> I first saw Mr. G in May 20, 1981 because of severe pain in his left anterior chest. Since that time, he has had multiple diagnostic studies performed, but there has been no definite evidence of recurrent neoplastic disease. The patient has been on large doses of Percodan for control of his pain. Recently, I have discussed this with him, because I believe that it may represent a problem for him since we have been unable to document any recurrence of his neoplastic disease.

The patient's radiation-oncologist report dated May 29, 1981, a year earlier, stated:

> This is a 53-year-old man who was referred because of known carcinoma of the lung and persistent pain. . . .
>
> The patient states that this pain is primarily in his left axilla and overlying his left pectoralis muscle and is present every day. This pain is quite severe. For this he is taking either Percodan tablets or Darvocet with one tablet every 60–80 minutes. He is frequently awakened at night because of this pain. For the past one week it has also involved his left scapula. Associated with this pain is numbness in his left fifth finger and partial numbness in his left fourth finger. In the past one week, he has also noted a similar pain on his right chest wall and right axilla. He states that this is quite mild but is similar to the left-sided pain when it first began.
>
> The patient states that this pain is a constant pain, it is not pulsating and pressure to this area or a heating pad gives him relief. He denies any tenderness in this area.
>
> The patient also complains of some left upper quadrant pain that has been present intermittently since October. This is quite tender and severe when it occurs but it occurs only infrequently. The etiology of this pain has not yet been found. It is not affected by food. . . .
>
> The patient was seen earlier today by the anesthesia department for consideration of a nerve block but was not considered a suitable candidate because the pain was not well localized. I would be concerned that this pain does represent tumor involvement of the brachial plexus or possibly, because he now has pain in his right anterior chest wall, of the cervical spine.

> Patients with tumors in the mediastinum or neck may develop severe pain which is difficult to relieve and which not uncommonly precedes the diagnosis of cancer by one to two years. I spoke with the patient regarding other modalities such as acupuncture and hypnosis but told him that in my experience, these have not been that successful in patients with pain due to malignant neoplasms. I told him that, after x-rays were obtained, if these were positive he may obtain significant relief from a radiation therapy program. I told him that if these were negative then I believe he should be given a trial of a transcutaneous nerve stimulator in an attempt to relieve his pain.
>
> I discussed with the patient that with his particular cell type it is likely that a significant response to a cytotoxic chemical therapy program would be small. In addition, the likelihood of response of his pain to such a program would be even smaller.

X-ray reports of the cervical and thoracic spine taken in September 1981 were forwarded with the patient's other reports. The x-ray report revealed no evidence of metastatic disease, however they were positive for compression fracture of C–5, and there was disc space narrowing at C5–6 with osteophytes posteriorly impinging on the foramen, especially on the left but also on the right. The request for pain consultation did not refer to these x-rays which were also done a year earlier.

The patient stated that when he first sought medical consultation it was for unrelieved pain in his chest. He said that he was told that he did not have cancer and that lung cancer did not initially cause pain. Five months later while he was in the hospital for diagnostic and potentially therapeutic lung surgery for cancer, his mother died of lung cancer in the same hospital and under the care of the same physicians this patient had. He reports that his mother's first symptom of lung cancer was chest pain. The patient said that he had come to the pain clinic feeling very fearful because his referring physician had refused to prescribe any more Percodan for his pain. The patient reports that this physician told him that if he now insisted on having a prescription for the Percodan, which he had prescribed for this patient for 1½ years, that he would report the patient to the "Police Department" to be registered as a drug addict because there was no cancer causing his pain.

During a four day hospitalization for pain management, this patient's reports of pain and pain relief were consistent on numerical, adjectival, and VAS scales on 24 assessments. Initially, to evaluate this patient's pain his medications were given on a PRN basis to get the baseline of pain estimate against which to measure pain relief. He consistently reported his pain as moderate to severe when requesting analgesia and also reported it was completely relieved within 30 minutes after taking the medication. He reported that when he did not take medication when the pain was mild that within 10–15 minutes it escalated to severe. (We have found this rapid escalation of pain very common.)

Additional information about this patient's pain was provided by having him complete a more extensive list of adjectives used to describe pain, "What Does Your Pain Feel Like?" (Melzack, 1975, p. 281). Figure 9.2 is this patient's completed form. Statistically, it correlates positively with other objective tests compiled by him.

Following a thorough assessment of his pain, titration of his analgesic, instruction in the continuation of time-contingent analgesics, and the use of TENS, this patient was discharged home. At the time of discharge he said that "this is the first time I have felt believed about my pain and not guilty. I think my pain problem was fully understood and I feel my pain relief is excellent. I can now see myself returning to work rather than lying in bed day in and day out as I have had to for the past year." This unfortunate patient died two months later with pain well controlled.

This patient's discharge pain regimen included time-contingent Percocet Tabs T̈T, q.4h. and TENS 30 mins. × t.i.d. His discharge diagnoses included: 1) myofascial pain syndrome causing left chest, shoulder, and axilla pain; 2) degenerative cervical osteoarthritis contributing to the pain of #1 and the paresthesias in his left third, fourth, and fifth fingers; 3) Pancoast's tumor syndrome; 4) S/P left thoracotomy; and 5) S/P radiation therapy. Each one of these separately is known to be capable of producing pain of high intensity.

If this patient's report of pain had simply been believed, his distress over being considered a potential addict and a liar about his pain could have been avoided. Further, had the patient been believed, a more thorough diagnostic attempt could have been made earlier and the cause may have been identified and treated earlier and more effectively.

Since many patients seem to be reluctant to communicate their pain or may not do so accurately or adequately, first we will consider some general conversation "rules" followed by general characteristics of the patient's communication of pain which need to be assessed. The patient may communicate pain with a variety of behaviors, discussed later in this chapter. Whatever these behaviors may be, the nurse needs to know the patient's ability and willingness to communicate pain and the other resources available to the nurse for assessing the patient's pain.

USE AND MISUSE OF COMMON CONVERSATIONAL CONVENTIONS

Parlee (1979, pp. 48–56) discusses the "rules" of conversation used to assert power and dominance. She says that these may be a product of the individual or of the environment. Common examples of *individual or people dominance*

What Does Your Pain Feel Like?

Some of the words below describe your present pain. Circle only those words that best describe it. Leave out any category that is not suitable. Use only a single word in each appropriate category -- the one that applies best.

1	2	3	4
Flickering Quivering Pulsing Throbbing Beating	Jumping Flashing Shooting	Pricking Boring Drilling Stabbing Lancinating	Sharp Cutting Lacerating
5	**6**	**7**	**8**
Pinching Pressing Gnawing Cramping Crushing	Tugging Pulling Wrenching	Hot Burning Scalding Searing	Tingling Itchy Smarting Stinging
9	**10**	**11**	**12**
Dull Sore Hurting Aching Heavy	Tender Taut Rasping Splitting	Tiring Exhausting	Sickening Suffocating
13	**14**	**15**	**16**
Fearful Frightful Terrifying	Punishing Grueling Cruel Vicious Killing	Wretched Blinding	Annoying Troublesome Miserable Intense Unbearable
17	**18**	**19**	**20**
Spreading Radiating Penetrating Piercing	Tight Numb Drawing Squeezing Tearing	Cool Cold Freezing	Nagging Nauseating Agonizing Dreadful Torturing

Figure 9.2. What does your pain feel like? *(Melzack, R. The McGill Pain Questionnaire: Major properties and scoring methods, Pain 1: p. 281, 1975, with permission.)*

include interactions between male–female, parent–child, and health care professional–patient. Common examples of *environmental or situational dominance* include those where there is a difference in race, class, job settings, in the health care setting, expressive styles, and even when two people meet for the first time. This is in contrast to the older view of communication which considered conversational habits more a characteristic of the personality, such as the obsessive-compulsive person.

Although there are general rules about *taking turns* on when to *initiate* and when to *listen* in conversation, in certain roles, under certain circumstances, and in different cultural settings these habits may vary, such as in the health care setting. There are certain *techniques* which are commonly employed *to assert power* and which violate rules of conversation. These include: using formal versus informal language; using nonverbal communication such as a formal demeanor or touch; using pauses including the length of the pause and the tolerance for silence; dominating the conversation by ignoring what the other person is saying, thereby not jointly developing the topic; interrupting, which is done by two people talking at the same time; ignoring the other's right to speak; asking more questions; and asking questions which demand an answer. *Prejudice* and *expediency*, perhaps are two of the reasons which most often *account for violation* of conversational rules and which can be most detrimental to communicating with a patient when assessing his pain problem.

Parlee says that *women's speech* which begins as early as age four, is sometimes considered almost different enough to be regarded as a separate dialect, a *genderlect* (p. 56). The rules and power characteristic of this type of speech include being more expressive and polite; less direct; less assertive; less informed; and less precise. By using women's language, individuals may abdicate power leading to a self-fulfilling prophecy. Women's language so often is characteristic of the patient-health care professional interaction. Although either the patient or the health care practitioner may set the tone of the conversation, most often the practitioner does so by virtue of his position behind a desk or "standing over" the patient who is in a bed, on an examining table, or seated.

ABILITY TO COMMUNICATE

The patient's verbal report is the only way to determine the presence, intensity, and quality of pain and is also obviously useful in assessing other aspects of pain. Lynaugh and Bates (1979, p. 135) say "words are currency for intellectual exchange" and they seem to be the most useful means of describing one's pain to another person. Hence, assessment of the patient's ability to communicate about his pain involves determining his facility with language.

If the patient is able to communicate verbally, this ability should be utilized to the extent possible. The nurse may begin assessment with general and open-ended questions to allow the patient to tell about his experience of pain in his own way.

Mental Image of Pain

Most people have mental images when they think of something although there are a few exceptions. Bresler (1976) once said that if he were allowed to ask a patient with pain only one question, he probably would ask, "What kind of picture do you have of your pain?" He has noted that even a physician may have a nonmedical or nonanatomical picture of his own pain. For example, one physician visualized his own low back pain as a dog chewing on his tailbone.

Assessment of the *image* or *mental picture* that a patient has of his *pain* serves several useful purposes. It reveals in many ways the meaning of the pain to the patient and often will significantly influence the degree of suffering that the patient experiences. A man who was dying of cancer of the stomach visualized his pain as a large rat eating a hole through his stomach. Reporting the image may give the patient another means of communicating about his pain. This may be very valuable if he has found the pain otherwise difficult to describe. One patient who was a real estate developer visualized his pain as being exactly 132 squares. He said that no matter what was done for his pain, two of the squares were never relieved. Mastrovito (1974) says that behind every significant pain there is almost always a fantasy that includes speculation about the body dysfunction that produces the pain. As an example, one patient with low back pain visualized his aching muscles as raw bleeding hamburger meat. Children especially may have very frightening and erroneous ideas about their pain.

The information obtained from the patient about the image he has of his pain may be used to identify sources of anxiety and areas of lack of knowledge. Anxiety may be relieved by providing accurate information. At other times the images can be used in assessing the severity of pain and in planning for successful pain relief methods. Some practitioners are skilled at incorporating the patient's image of pain in hypnosis or therapeutic guided imagery for pain relief.

Difficulty Describing Pain

If the patient has trouble finding the words to explain and describe his experience, the nurse should not hesitate to offer suggestions. In most cases, this will not "put words into the patient's mouth." Rather, the patient will be grateful for the assistance. The patient probably will choose carefully only those words that are most applicable. The patient with pain usually is very anxious for others to understand the pain as clearly and accurately as possible. Lewis (1978, p. 123) says "Apart from what is instinctive in the moves to ease, escape, or cry out the pain, there is a voluntary element in response which may well not seek to hide what is felt, but rather seek to alert and reveal how it does hurt." We too have found this to be true. Further, even patients who seem reluctant to verbalize about their pain will usually do so if encouraged.

As we have discussed before, pain is extremely difficult to describe. Virginia Woolf (1948) noted this when she said, "English . . . has no words for the shiver and headache. . . . The merest school girl, when she falls in love, has Shakespeare and Keats to speak for her; but let a sufferer try to describe a pain in his head to a doctor and language at once runs dry" (p. 11).

We are accustomed to wide variations in the adult's behavioral expressions of pain and in the ability and willingness to report pain to some people and not to others. Less well recognized is the fact that these variations may also occur in the young child. The child does not necessarily have the ability to clearly articulate the pain problem nor does he or she automatically report a sensation of pain (McCaffery, 1977). We have found this especially true if the pain has been present for a relatively long time or if the intensity of the pain has remained the same or increased gradually.

The child with ear pain, for instance, may not respond affirmatively when asked if his or her ear hurts. The word "hurt" may not seem applicable since, for the child, "hurt" refers to the sharp pangs of sudden scrapes and bumps. Further, the slow onset of pain probably has a significant effect; it seems to us that a gradual increase in pain may result in the child almost *incorporating* the *pain sensation* in his or her *body image.* The child simply may not recall a time when he or she did not have the pain. It may seem "normal" and yet it may disturb behavior in many ways, such as awakening him or her.

Thus, the young child may feel pain and react to it, yet may not seem to be consciously aware enough of its existence or location to communicate it. Rubbing or pointing at the pain may be as lacking as verbalizations. Contrary to popular opinion, the child with earaches will not invariably pull or rub his ear either. We have observed one of our own children from the age of 8 months to 3½ years who had countless ear infections resistant to all forms of medication and surgery. Never once was she observed pulling or rubbing her ear. Initially, the absence of this behavior was misleading to us as well as the physician, although the child did manifest her pain in many other ways.

A sudden onset or increase in pain usually evokes a behavioral response and enables the very young child to localize the pain, at least by pointing, if not with appropriate words. Even an infant may communicate pain, for example may refuse fluids if stomatitis or tonsilitis is present. On the other hand, minimal expression of pain may be learned by young children. Occasionally a young child is minimally expressive even when the pain is intense. Florman (1975) describes a young boy with toxic synovitis of the hip. In this condition, rotation of the hip is shown to cause considerable pain. However, when the child's hip was rotated he simply looked at the physician and gave no evidence of pain. The mother said he never cried with any type of pain. Pain in the child can be systematically assessed, however, by taking the time to understand the child's cognitive level and vocabulary and by formulating the right questions. With this approach the child may be able to mark his pain on a figure drawing and relate the intensity and quality (Isler, 1978).

Physical Limitations that Impede Communication

Language problems may also arise with patients with a variety of health problems including brain damage, those with an altered level of consciousness from various medications, those with hearing impairments, those who have had a mandibulectomy, glossectomy, or tracheostomy, and those with problems of the larynx, such as laryngitis. Behavioral expressions of pain other than verbalizations may also be limited in some ways. Paralysis of the face or parts of the body may prevent facial expressions or other body movements. Immobilization by casts, splints or traction may also limit certain types of nonverbal expressions. The patient who has had a massive cerebral vascular accident is an example of one who may have a major pain problem and multiple severe physical limitations resulting in communication problems. This patient may have a thalamic pain syndrome, paralysis of one side of his body, and have severely receptive and expressive aphasia. He or she may very rapidly also develop decubitus ulcers and contractures causing additional pain problems and physical limitations.

Language Difficulties

A variety of language difficulties may exist. Obviously, if the patient does not speak the language of the health team members or does not speak it well, verbal communication about pain will be virtually impossible without an interpreter. The use of an interpreter for pain assessment is discussed starting on page 339 of this chapter. One should not assume that if a patient was born in a non-English speaking country, that he or she will be unable to speak or understand the English language. Many countries are multilingual or the patient may have learned the English language since his or her arrival in the United States. On the other hand, the patient may not speak his or her native tongue, nor the language of the health care team, with ease. Some people have had a limited education or are inexperienced with respect to verbal communication. Such patients may talk very little, have limited vocabularies, mispronounce words, use poor grammar, any or all of which may make it more difficult to understand the patient. Since pain often is quite difficult to describe, these people are at a special disadvantage, in fact, may even be considered at higher risk in relation to having their pain accurately and continually assessed and in getting pain relief. Even though the nurse may not be viewed as prejudiced, the patient for some reason may feel discriminated against especially when having difficulty communicating about his pain. The patient will rarely ever volunteer a lack of comprehension. In fact, the patient may communicate the opposite. It is not uncommon for a patient to successfully mislead the practitioner with polite gestures used to acknowledge understanding or agreement such as eye contact and smiling or nodding one's head.

Limitations of the patient's ability to communicate about pain, verbally and/or nonverbally, must be noted. For each patient, the nurse should attempt to identify the behaviors that he is most likely to be able to use to communicate about his pain. Although nonverbal behaviors are very useful in the assessment of pain, the patient who cannot communicate verbally may pose tremendous assessment problems. In these instances it is very important to have current information on a nursing care plan and nursing history. Of particular importance will be the patient's physical status including physical stimuli that may be perceived as painful by the patient and psychosocial information to help anticipate the patient's possible response to his pain. Specific pain assessment forms are included in Chapter 10.

WILLINGNESS TO COMMUNICATE

In assessing the patient's pain, it is very helpful to know the extent to which we can depend upon the patient to provide us with information within the context of his or her ability to do so. The patient's *willingness* to *communicate* about pain may range from a *denial* that pain exists to a *readiness* to tell anyone all about the pain at any time. This will be influenced by the many psychological, cultural, and even physiological factors previously discussed.

Expressive Style

Part of the patient's willingness to communicate about his pain is concerned with his *expressive style*, defined as the way he presents his pain to others. Some patients are very expressive; others are not. Patients who are very expressive about their pain tend to be extroverts or members of demonstrative cultures (Sternbach, 1976). A high degree of expression may involve a variety of verbal and nonverbal behaviors such as many adjectives to describe the pain, moaning, crying, gestures, and frowning. A patient with a minimal expression of pain may present pain to others simply by saying he or she hurts and pointing to the area.

The patient's expressive style may complicate the matter of determining the pain intensity, pain tolerance, and degree of suffering. As we have seen, the patient's overt expression or physical pain may be totally unrelated to the severity of pain and suffering he is actually experiencing. We must remain constantly cognizant of this. American nurses, especially, seen, the patient's overt expression of physical pain may be totally unrelated to the severity of pain and suffering he is actually experiencing. We ior (Davitz & Davitz, 1975). However, the patient with severe pain may not even volunteer the fact that he hurts, but upon questioning him he may admit that the pain could not be worse. Klein (1979, p. 36) says that " 'Feeling' and 'communicating' have been promoted in this society in a way to make them seem appropriate for all. An individual's failure to show emotions is often interpreted as evidence that he or she does not experience the feelings of grief or pain."

However, the more expressive patient may be confronted with even greater problems through prejudice and outright stigmatization by the health team. Harwood (1981, p. 499) discusses the fact that we may be less likely to trust the more expressive patient and that this is unfair to that patient. He says that "florid narratives" and "lengthy recitals of symptoms with their accompanying emotional and social complications, should lead the clinician neither to *ignore* some of the *symptoms* in developing his problem list nor to *suspect psychosomatic etiology overhastily*. In fact, the [nurse] who is concerned with treating illness as well as disease may find patients who provide more elaborate histories easier to work with."

Patients with mild or moderate pain may freely tell almost everyone about it, giving detailed descriptions. Careful listening may reveal that despite the wealth of descriptive terms, the pain is mild in intensity, and the patient does not suffer from it nor may he necessarily want anything to be done about it. The patient simply may be intrigued by the pain or find it a good topic of conversation. One patient who had very limited experience with pain had an abscessed tooth of three days duration vividly and humorously described the moderate to severe pain she was experiencing. She refused medication for the pain saying I just needed to tell someone about it.

Readiness to Report Pain

Somewhat different from expressive style is the patient's *readiness* to report pain. In other words, regardless of the behavior used to do it, some patients seem to be more ready to report pain than others. Of special concern in assessing patients with pain is the patient who denies pain.

The patient may deny pain for any one of many reasons. Perhaps the patient takes pride in hiding pain from others. The patient may try to ignore the pain in the hope that it will disappear. Sometimes the patient is more afraid of the treatment for pain than of the sensation of pain. A very common reason for denying pain is fear of addiction when narcotics are used for pain relief.

In some instances, the patient does not deny pain but neither does he or she volunteer the fact that pain exists. The patient may report pain only if asked about it.

To illustrate how unwilling patients may be to communicate their pain we will use an example of one stoic, very active, retired 75-year-old Irish Catholic woman who used ignoring, minimizing, not volunteering, and denial with two different types of pain, both life-threatening, in two very different situations. In the first instance, this woman had "abdominal discomfort, you might call it mild pain" for two weeks. She noted rectal bleeding and finally went to her doctor because "two of my brothers died of cancer and I worked in medical records and know what it probably meant." After quickly undergoing diagnostic procedures her physician telephoned her and told her that she had cancer; it may necessitate a colostomy, and that she was to report to the hospital that afternoon for surgery. She told the physician "You don't understand. I am going on vacation with my cousin next week. If I don't go she will cancel her vacation and I don't want to frighten her. I can handle my pain." In spite of the fact that the physician told her that if she did not immediately enter the hospital he would not assume responsibility for her care. She persisted and went on the vacation. Later she told her daughters who were frightened and upset by her behavior that she thought "the physician seemed so unreasonable." Not only did she not tell her cousin until the afternoon they returned three weeks later, but she did not tell any of her family with whom she was very close. Again with the reason "I didn't want to worry them." When asked about the pain she said "It wasn't so bad."

The second instance occurred four years later and involved the same physician. This patient was even more of a challenge to the physician who was assessing her pain "which seems much better now." This patient lived in the same Boston neighborhood for 64 years. She had two widowed friends who were sisters and had lived in her same neighborhood for about the same number of years. One of the sisters died and the patient we are discussing became the "significant other," participating in making all of the funeral arrangements, helping prepare the food for after the "Rosary" and "Irish wake," cleaning up, running errands, and generally anything else which needed to be done, including shoveling snow from the front stairs. "You know, Catherine needed all the help she could get." That night she awoke with a classical picture of a myocardial infarction. "The pain was so severe, I couldn't get my breath so I sat at the kitchen table all night. I must admit now, I was a little frightened, but I knew God would take care of me because Catherine needed me." The next morning she drove Catherine to the church, to the cemetery, and then to pick up a few groceries. In the afternoon, she drove two other friends to a hospital 30 minutes away to visit their niece who had surgery, "Because I promised them." Her own physician was on staff so while they were visiting, without letting them know, she went to the emergency room to see "if my doctor might be there or in the hospital." Fortunately he was in the emergency room. After assessing her he told her that she had had a "heart attack" and he was having her admitted to the Intensive Coronary Care Unit. She again said "you don't understand, I can't stay right now. I brought two *senior citizen* friends in to visit here and they have no way to get home." Her exasperated physician said that they could take the subway or a taxi. The woman became very stern in tone and persisted in her determination. The physician said that he was going to call her daughter to come to the hospital immediately. The woman said "You can't do that. If you call, you'll frighten her. I'll drive my friends home and call my daughter and I promise I'll have her bring me back. Now I need to go upstairs and get my friends and I'll tell them." The physician insisted that she just rest and breathe some oxygen for awhile while he thought things over. He went and called the woman's daughter. When her daughter arrived the woman was admitted directly to the intensive care unit, finally admitting "the pain is very bad. I feel like I can't breathe".

ORIENTATION TO PAIN RELIEF

Without knowledge of how, when, why, and what a patient is requesting for pain relief, a major part of the assessment of the pain problem may be missing. Further, such information may be helpful to the nurse in knowing the extent to which the patient feels that he or she can influence his or her own pain experience so that the nurse may help identify possible methods of relief that may not have been considered by the patient.

Yet, the patient may not necessarily have much information about pain relief. He or she may not know whether or not pain relief is available for this particular episode of pain. The patient may have no idea of the type of pain relief, how to obtain it, from whom, or the degree to which it will alleviate pain. He or she may not even know to whom pain should be reported or when. On the other hand, the patient may have some very definite ideas about each of these points. Assessment needs to include what the *person knows, expects,* and *uses* with respect to *pain relief.*

Most people have had some experience with pain relief. Often it is in the form of medication such as "over the counter" products like aspirin or antacids. It is important to determine the type, amount, and frequency of medication the patient has taken for his current pain or other episodes, how effective it was, and what side effects, if any, he encountered. This kind of information is sometimes referred to as an *analgesic profile*. When patients are consulting doctors in pain clinics, they are usually asked to list all the medication and related information. Sometimes they are asked to bring all of the containers with them, especially if they have difficulty remembering the names or doses of the medications.

The patient may also have used strategies for pain relief other than medication. Copp's (1974) study revealed that such strategies were common, but that the patient often felt the health team would not find them acceptable. The remedies that patients used successfully, yet did not feel free to share with health team members, included baths, position changes, and a variety of self-control methods, such as distraction and imagery.

Patients with chronic pain may consult many physicians, at one time or one after another, "doctor shopping." This may have resulted in numerous different recommendations for pain relief, and the patient may have tried most of them. Medication, physical therapy, surgery and psychotherapy, are among the most common. Some patients with pain consult agencies or persons not associated with traditional or recognized health care, whose methods may involve anything from faith healing to reading horoscopes. Therefore, assessment needs to include determining the pain relief measures with which the patient is familiar, those which he has used successfully, and which ones he believes would be effective for the present pain. We have found it very valuable simply to ask the patient what has provided him with the most pain relief.

Assessment of how much pain relief the patient expects or desires is important since there are many differences between patients in relation to pain relief. This information helps the nurse assess the pain tolerance. It can be determined by ascertaining the intensity and duration of pain the patient is willing to endure. The patient may be proud of tolerating pain for long periods of time and not report his pain until it becomes severe. This may or may not be advisable; thus, it is important to know the patient's attitude. The patient may also have some idea of how much pain he "should" tolerate, or how much pain others can expect him to endure. When one is attempting to assist a patient to learn to control his expression of pain or increase his tolerance to it, how this goal is communicated to the patient is critical. For example, in a rehabilitation clinic, a kinesiologist became very frustrated with a patient who was arguing about not wanting to do a prescribed exercise because it increased his long-standing pain. In frustration the kinesiologist said to the patient "I don't care about your pain. You are here to increase your function and these exercises will help do that." Obviously, how the patient heard the communication was not what the therapist meant to communicate. However, the patient did not refute the therapist and became a "rehab dropout" for a considerable period of time until the communication conflict was resolved. During the resolution process the patient and therapist agreed that they had the same mutual goal. The patient was finally able to tell the therapist "You might not care about my pain, but that is the only thing I care about. It has totally destroyed my life."

When the patient does expect or desire pain relief, it is pertinent to determine what the patient would consider an acceptable level of pain relief since it is not always possible to eliminate pain entirely, although this may be the patient's expectation.

Sometimes patients may feel that intense brief pain or mild chronic pain is easier to endure than the measures required to relieve it. These patients may fail to complain of pain or they may state that the relief measures merely add to the pain or are not worth the trouble. For example, one woman with recurrent breast abscesses stated that the local anesthetic hurt as much as the incision and drainage, and expressed a desire not to receive the local anesthetic. Another woman complained of backache during the last trimester of her pregnancy. The public health nurse helped her with proper body mechanics and demonstrated pelvic rocking, suggesting that this be done for about 15 seconds five or six times a day. On the nurse's next visit the patient said these measures had alleviated the backache. However, on the third visit the patient admitted only upon questioning that her back still hurt and she said that the exercises were too much trouble.

In our culture, there is considerable concern about the possibility of becoming addicted to narcotics. This must be explored with patients who say they do not want pain relief or who claim they can tolerate pain that they rate as severe. Some patients who fear addiction simply will say they do not have any pain in spite of indications that they most likely are experiencing severe pain. Chapter 7 is devoted to behavioral parameters indicative of the effects of pain on the patient. The patient needs to know that *addiction* (psychological dependence) is very rare, less than 0.00034 percent (Porter & Jick, 1980).

In patients with prolonged pain who are terminally ill a rather common reason for denying pain and attempting to tolerate pain is the fear that the analgesia "won't work later when I really need it." The staff also undertreat pain because of their similar fear. Both the patient and the staff need to know that this rarely is a problem. If tolerance to the analgesic effect of the narcotic occurs, an increase in dose will increase pain relief (Trotter et al., 1981). If that is not adequate, consultation with a dolorologist, such as an anesthesiologist would be in order.

DIFFERENCES BETWEEN INDIVIDUALS

Upon repeated questioning, whether the patient volunteers information about his pain, denies his pain, or admits his pain, the information obtained may vary from one time to the next for several reasons. One important determining factor may be the person observing the patient with pain. Because the patient may deny pain to one person but summon another person to report the pain to, the patient's behavior may be confusing and misleading to all involved except the patient.

If great differences are observed in the patient's reports of pain, it may be assumed erroneously that the patient is being manipulative or is malingering. Often this is not the case at all. The patient may not trust certain practitioners with information about the pain, or may not want pain to interfere with his or her relationships with them. He or she may think they are not interested in the pain. But, the patient may have identified one person believed to be concerned about this pain. This may be the only person to whom he or she reports his pain. Other information in relation to this aspect of communication about pain was presented in Chapters 7 and 8.

No doubt the nurse's approach to the individual patient with pain will determine to a large extent her or his success in assessing the patient's pain. Feedback and general attitude are extremely important. In some way, the patient should know that he or she has been heard. So many patients say "No one listens." Conveying to the patient that *you believe him or her* and that you will assume some responsibility for assisting him or her are conducive to assessment.

A rather common problem is the patient who tells the nurse he or she "hurts a great deal of the time" but when the physician makes rounds and asks how the patient feels, the patient says "just fine." There are several possible reasons for the *differences* in patients' communication with *physicians* and *nurses*. For one thing, the physician's visit can elicit a positive placebo response. The physician's attention and concern may decrease the patient's anxiety and lead to decreased pain, or the patient may not want to discourage the physician by continual reports of pain. The patient may be less intimidated by the nurse than the physician and thus feel more comfortable about reporting pain to her or him. If the patient reports pain to the nurse and not to the physician, the nurse should note this problem and discuss it with the physician.

NURSING INTERVENTIONS AND RESOURCES FOR ASSESSING A PATIENT'S PAIN

The immediate verbal and nonverbal communication from the patient is not the only useful resource about the patient's pain. Information can be obtained from the patient outside the immediate situation by having him complete written questionnaires about his pain and by having him keep a daily diary about his pain. Such a diary is illustrated in Figure 9.3. Figure 9.4 illustrates a variation of this record devised and completed by a patient. If the patient is expected to report in writing, this requires thorough instruction. Valuable information also may be obtained from the medical record, nursing history and from the patient's family and friends. When others are consulted it should be with the patient's permission or it may be considered a breach of privacy and destroy the patient's trust and confidence.

Establishing Rapport

First of all, establishing rapport with a patient is of paramount importance and may significantly determine all of the nurses' successes or failures in

Daily Hourly Diary

Name____________________ Date__________

Time	Pain Rating 0 - 10 0=no pain 10=worst pain	Medication Type & amount taken	Other pain relief measures tried or anything that influences your pain.	Major activity being done: lying sitting standing/walking
midnight 12				
1				
2				
3				
4				
5				
6				
7				
8				
9				
10				
11				
noon 12				
1				
2				
3				
4				
5				
6				
7				
8				
9				
10				
11				

Figure 9.3. Daily hourly diary.

future communication with the patient. As with any other relationship, how a patient prefers to be *approached* can only be elicited directly from the patient. This is important if one acknowledges the necessity of a collaborative relationship with patients to provide optimal assessment and treatment of their pain problem.

One variable that will influence rapport with a patient is the *nurse's general demeanor.* A display of professionalism may be perceived by one

Medication Report
for Doctor

*= Medication given   Scale 0 – 10

6/ /82

time	Pain Level	Medication	Remarks
Pm-1:30	10	Meth 10mg fluid	
4:30	10	" 12" "	
5:40			Pain went from 10-7 - (Head full of cotton) upper part of leg feels bigger, fuller than right this happens often - makes the bed feel uneven 10 min later all of leg feels bigger and fuller. pretty nervous, Jittery
6:30	7		
7:00	10		
7:30	10	meth. 12 mg fluid	
8:00	10	Dilaudid 4mg	
9:00	9		
9:30	7		
9:40	6		(sudden decrease)
10:30	7	Methadone 12 mg, Percocet tab 1	
11:30	5		Remained at 7 until 11:30 then dropped 2 points in 5 min.
MN 12:00	5		Sign off time - Pain is at a firm 5 without threat of upward move (oh shut-up M and count your blessings!)

Note. Comb meth + Percocet = No head full of cotton

Comment - No drenching perspiration since 8:00pm. Hey! that's a record. Don't knock it.

—

Figure 9.4. Medication record. (Page 1)

time	Pain level	Medication	Remarks
6/9/82 1:00 AM	7	(so much for the firm "5")	
7:45 AM	6	Levo 2mg + Perc 1	Elavil or
8:25 X	6	Levo 2mg + Perc 1	Dilaudid worked
8:30	5		(last night
8:50	5		
9:10	2		
11:25 X	2		
2:15 PM	2		
2:30	5		
2:35	6		
2:40	7	Study Drug	
5:00	9	Levo 2 + Per	
5:20	10	Levo 2 + Per 1	
8:00	4	Levo 2 + Dilaudid 4	
8:25	4		
9:00	3	What?	
10:00	3	Yahoo!	
11:25	2	Hallelujah!	
6/10/82 2:25 am	2	4	

(6) A fluke?

Slept until 7:45 A. An Absolute "first" "2." The flat-footedness and physical gyrations involved in showering, have always sent the pain to a "10" - Not so this afternoon - Did not phase the pain - And to top it off - I'm not having nearly as much trouble with instant-memory-recall that I had ē 6 mg triavil

Figure 9.4. Medication record. (Page 2)

patient as impersonal, cold, aloof, or undesirable, where another patient may appreciate the seeming objectivity and efficiency of this approach. Similarly, some individuals value touch whereas others dislike "laying on of hands." The same applies as to how a person prefers to be addressed, first name, last, or a nickname. Age may command respect in some cultures. For example, Asians convey respect to an older individual by a slightly bowed head when talking to him. Direct communication may seem like an affront to one patient, yet indirect communication may be perceived as evasiveness and a need to conceal ominous information about his or her condition by another patient.

Another important aspect of establishing positive and helpful rapport with a patient involves establishing *trust*. Initially at least, this may be somewhat time consuming but in the long run it will usually bring results both to the nurse and to the patient. Establishing trust involves conveying a genuine concern for the patient through unhurried, attentive listening and politeness, not to be confused with being patronizing. One frequently used way of establishing trust is to establish a common tie in relation to something valued by the patient, such as discussing his child, pet, or something else of importance to him. Another way is finding something that you mutually enjoy such as the seashore or mountains. One value of such efforts is that it shows some of the nurse's willingness to share part of herself or himself and a more human side. This is of special relevance when one considers how much personal information we expect the patient to nakedly verbalize. It is also very different from reversing roles with the patient so he feels he has to assist the nurse to solve personal problems and certainly cannot burden the nurse with his or her own. Above all the nurse must convey mutual trust: that she or he can be trusted to believe the patient's statements and that the patient is regarded as trustworthy. Quite simply, the nurse must communicate "I believe what you say about your pain."

Identify Acknowledged Authority in the Family and Collaborate

As we have seen, compliance is very much influenced by the degree to which patients and families *feel free* to *decide* on the *course* of *treatment*. Therefore, it is very important to ascertain who is considered the health care authority and who is considered the head of the household. Remember, they may be two different people. In cultures where decisions are deferred to one person such as the husband or eldest son or are a family affair it is very unfair to expect the patient to make an on-the-spot decision. Moreover, such decisions may be doomed to fail completely or partially by the patient and his family. They may significantly alter the decision later through noncompliance. This may be evidenced in the patient's failure to return for follow-up care, failure to comply with the prescribed treatment, or "doctor-shopping". Also, the patient with pain who had acceptable and stabilized pain control in the health care setting may return with uncontrolled pain.

Practices in Relation to Privacy and Modesty

Individuals who have specific practices in relation to privacy and modesty including areas such as communication should be able to expect that every effort will be made to honor these practices insofar as they do not jeopardize patient safety. If a patient desires and/or due to cultural dictates expects a significant other present during embarrassing or painful procedures, every effort should be made to comply including making special scheduling arrangements. Further, when questions of a personal nature are asked the necessity of asking for such information should be explained prior to the asking of the question. Although the use of humor is sometimes very effective as a communication technique, it is unlikely to be of use when a patient's privacy is being invaded, and he is in pain unless in previous situations this has been found to be the patient's preferred coping style. Expediency may be the more valued skill at such times.

Medical Care Beliefs, Dietary Practices, and Treatment Preferences

Medical care beliefs and dietary practices are frequently inseparable especially during periods of illness. Previously pointed out was the possibility that the patient with a pain problem may suffer from significant *weight loss* or *weight gain* problems during periods of severe and/or prolonged pain. At such times the patient may consult or retreat to a folk healer or a "health food advocate." When medical care beliefs, dietary practices, medications, and treatments conflict, if appropriately handled, the problem may be converted into an ideal opportunity for the nurse to provide good patient teaching to reduce noncompliance.

Whenever possible, alternative treatments and dietary practices to which the patient subscribes should be incorporated into the overall plan of care. If the patient's pain regime involves taking medication and the patient prefers one form versus another, such as a liquid instead of a capsule, efforts should be made to prescribe the medication in the desired form. Occasionally, medications and treatments which have been medically prescribed or are self-prescribed may have a negative synergistic effect on the patient. When this occurs and one of these must be eliminated, every effort must be made not to blame, insult, or imply that the patient is not adhering in the desired manner with the treatment plan. An important strategy in such a situation is to attempt to convince the patient for the need of a specific medication or treatment. At times it is possible to negotiate a compromise with a patient and this is far more desirable than having the patient abandon using a medication or treatment altogether. Efforts also should be made to collaborate with folk healers and make allowances for "health foods" and megavitamins. This incorporates consideration of the patient as the responsible individual for himself and knowledge of the subjective nature of pain. When proposed treatments for pain interfere with the patient's roles and responsibilities, assisting the patient to find other ways of fulfilling these is very important.

Additional Considerations for the Hospitalized Patient

There are additional special considerations for the hospitalized patient. It is important to communicate hospital routines because they may vary significantly from the patient's cultural expectations and past experiences with hospitalization that he may have had. For example bedrest in many cultures is considered essential to regain one's strength during illness. In the United States, patients often are ambulated on the day of major surgery. This may seem very threatening or even sadistic to the patient and his family who have differing expectations especially if he has pain.

Fortunately, practices in relation to visitors in most hospitals are becoming more flexible. Visitors are allowed to remain for longer periods of time and to participate in the patient's care. In many instances this can be used effectively to minimize many potential anxieties, fears and conflicts which may influence the pain experience.

INTERPRETERS

For a variety of reasons, including minimizing suffering and pain and for safe patient care the use of an interpreter may be necessary when working with a patient with a pain problem. The *use of interpreters* is not confined to patients who do not have comprehension and fluency in the language of the health care practitioner; other patients may benefit from some type of an interpreter also. For example, the vocalizations and verbalizations of the very young child may sound like "jibberish" to the practitioner, but may be quite intelligible to the parent. Further, parents usually have become very sensitive to their child's nonverbal communications yet the nurse may be unclear about their meaning. Patients with vocalization, auditory and/or visual limitations, may, at times, need to be assisted by special interpretive services such as a lipreader, a person able to use sign language, or information in oversized print or printed in braille. The blind patient's seeing-eye dog and, more recently, the deaf patient's dog used as his "ears" may be of some help in communication for the patient in addition to serving as a source of comfort. Obvious things which minimize the need for an interpreter may include seeing that the patient's hearing aid is being worn and is in working order; that the patient is wearing clean eyeglasses when these are a part of his everyday needs; and that he is wearing dentures if their absence alters his ability to verbalize.

Unfortunately, the use of an *interpreter* has certain *limitations*. Additional time is necessary to translate questions and answers and to attempt to ascertain that the question that the patient responded to was indeed the one that was asked. Even then one cannot be certain that the patient received the message with the full intent it was sent. When time allows and the practitioner has a choice about who will be the interpreter, one, perhaps, can hope for more satisfactory communication. When there is no choice, the nurse must consider certain possibilities regarding the content of the translated communication. It may have been modified by the translator for a variety of reasons. The translator may interpret or filter the conversation and eliminate nuances which may change the meaning of the message. Sometimes this is done in an attempt to protect the patient from information that the translator knows the patient fears or will be upsetting, or the translator may believe that certain information that is being requested is not important or "any of the practitioner's business." The translator may rephrase a question which was asked in an informal or formal manner and although it may be more consistent with the patient's communication style, it may have altered the meaning. Another interpreter may be concerned with providing the practitioner with information that he or she believes the nurse should know. Or he may be attempting to establish rapport with the nurse himself. Still another may be trying to maintain his or her status with the patient and undermine that of the nurse.

In addition to these considerations there are other considerations that the practitioner must keep in mind when the choice of an interpreter is his or hers. Family members most often are the logical choice because of their investment in the patient; their understanding of his personal perceptions; and their understanding and ability to maintain many of the psychocultural variables which may come into play when evolving a treatment plan for pain relief and desired compliance. Children should not be used as interpreters because the health care personnel may feel that they have to filter their questions to protect the child. They may not, therefore, ask questions that may be very important to the assessment. Parents usually are the most likely interpreters for their children. Children respond to their siblings positively so they may be useful in helping with therapeutic modalities for pain. Sometimes there are "family secrets," thus for reasons of privacy the patient may not want a specific family member involved in his care. When it is necessary to select an interpreter who is not known to the patient, whenever possible the individual selected should be of the same sex, social class, and with as many of the other relevant variables important to the patient as possible. If the patient does not know the interpreter, for example, and has cancer pain, the patient may feel that another patient with a similar problem would be more understanding. The most important thing to consider when there is a choice of interpreters is to select one who will be known and most trusted by the patient and will most minimally interfere with the communication processes.

Finally, when working with the interpreter, if he or she is not experienced in interpreting with the health team, give some general guidelines. If the interpreter is known to the patient, explain how and why you will be asking certain questions; how you would like them to be communicated to the patient, that is, in your exact words and in the patient's exact words; and that when you are finished you will be asking some more questions both for the possibility of gleaning information that he or she is likely to have which may be beneficial to the patient. This acknowledges the interpreter's contributions and may minimize filtering of information by him. During the interview, ask the patient to ask you questions, and, perhaps, have him or her repeat back what he believes you said in an attempt to allow for clarification and minimize the understandable, natural proclivity that the interpreter may have toward reinterpreting information during the assessment. Also, remember, in some languages there may not be similar words for pain and suffering.

At other times, if there are any problems with the patient's ability or willingness to communicate about the pain, the patient's family or close friends may be especially helpful. For example, if someone knows the patient well, they may be able to detect indications of pain and alert the nurse to them.

Since neither an interpreter nor a significant other is likely to be available at all times, a system needs to be established that will maximize communication. For example, audiovisual aids can be used in the patient's language with the nurse doing the translating of common words. Such information can be done for common items, using word "flashcards," pictures, pointing, direct eye contact, nodding one's head for "yes" or shaking it back and forth for "no." A scale such as 0–10 for rating can be explained by the interpreter and used thereafter between the patient and health team.

TRANSCULTURAL NURSING COMMUNICATION

Ballard (1979) points out that "science belongs on the side of the people it studies, rather than aligning itself with a society that wants to control differences." Leninger (1970) asserts that patients have a right to have their sociocultural backgrounds understood and responded to in the same way that their physical and psychological needs are understood. In addition to the previously described physiological, cultural, and psychological factors discussed in more detail in previous chapters there are some points of a more general nature incorporating previous information that are helpful when assessing the patient's pain problem.

It seems likely that most individuals when they are in pain want quick answers to their questions and relief from their pain. Yet, the physician frequently finds it necessary to have a more protracted period of time for a more thorough assessment. "Wait and see" may be interpreted by the patient and his family as the physician does not know the cause of the pain, does not believe the patient about his pain, or that something very serious is causing the pain. If pain relief and other treatments are withheld during the assessment phase, the patient may view the practitioner as hostile or punitive, especially if the patient is from a different culture than the practitioner. Such individuals may be at special risk in getting their health care needs met, especially pain assessment and relief.

Busy and stressed health care practitioners may become impatient and embarrass the patient during the communication process. When such a patient feels stigmatized or uncertain, he is more likely to retreat to a folk healer or others in the lay-referral system who have had similar problems. It is encumbent upon the nurse to know the values and behaviors of the predominant cultures with whom she works frequently. Without such knowledge, it may be impossible for the nurse to respond appropriately to the patient and his family, intensifying the patient's pain problem. Although a social worker may be called upon to assist, Harwood (1981, p. 26) suggests that what we really need is a transcultural interpreter for both patients and health care professionals.

During the assessment process for the patient with pain, there are questions which the nurse may ask to ascertain a general idea of the degree of the patient's acculturation and how it may influence the patient's pain problem. The following questions have been adapted from Kleinman et al. (1978, p. 256), and Harwood (1981, p. 29) and transposed by us in an attempt to gain information about values related to pain, pain relief, and the effect of pain on the patients. Our questions for the patient with pain are:

1. What do you think has caused your pain?
2. Why do you think your pain started when it did?
3. What do you think that your pain does to you? How does it work?
4. How bad [severe] do you think your pain is? Do you think it will last a long time, or will it be better soon?
5. What do you fear most about your pain?
6. What are the chief problems that your pain has caused you?
7. What kind of treatment would you like for your pain?
8. What are the most important results you hope to get from your treatment?
9. If your pain is taken away adequately, what kinds of things that you did before would you like to do again?
10. If your pain is taken away adequately what other kinds of things would you like to do?

11. If we cannot take away your pain to your satisfaction, what will that do to your life?
12. What medications and/or treatments have you tried for your pain? (Itemize them and answer.)
13. Have they helped? How?
14. Do you still use them? Why or why not?
15. Do you agree or disagree with reasons given to you for the possible cause of your pain?
16. In addition with helping you with your pain is there anything else related to your pain that you feel we could do to assist you with it?
17. What other things can you think of that would be helpful for us to know while we work to find the cause of your pain and the best treatment for it?

In summary, no matter what the patient's culture, encourage the questions that he or she wants answered from the health team regarding his pain problem and general medical care. When patients have difficulty verbally communicating with their nurse or physician, encourage them to keep a running list of questions so that if they forget anything when the nurse or doctor visit, the next time they come they can ask the question. To help the patient become an active participant in his care, the nurse, at least initially, can offer to come when the physician visits the patient to facilitate the patient's getting his questions answered and his pain problem resolved. "Although different societies approach the problem of pain from many routes the aim of all is to relieve pain for the sufferers. If the sufferer says he feels relief then that is surely what counts" (Lewis, 1978, p. 122).

In the next and final chapter we will discuss tools for assessing the patient with pain.

REFERENCES

Ballard, R. An interview with Thomas Szasz. In N. Klein (Ed.), Culture, Curers and Contagion. Novata, CA: Chandler & Sharp, 1979, pp. 138–150.

Bresler, D.E. Therapeutic Guided Imagery. Paper presented at the Univ. of California at Los Angeles, Franz Hall, December 8, 1976.

Brown, E.L. Newer Dimensions of Patient Care: Improving Staff Motivation and Competence in the General Hospital, Part II. New York: Russell Sage Foundation, 1962.

Cohen, F.L. Postsurgical pain relief: Patient's status and nurses' medication choices. Pain 9:265-274, 1980.

Copp, L.A. The spectrum of suffering. Amer J Nurs 74: 491–495, 1974.

Davitz, L.J., & Davitz, J.R. How nurses view patient suffering. RN 38: 69–74, 1975.

Florman, A.L. Development and variables of pain in children. Cur Concepts Pain Analgesia 2: 1–3; 14–15, 1975.

Friedman, M.M. The Public Clinic Patient: Situational Effects and Coping Effects. Unpublished M.A. Thesis, Univ. of Southern California, Department of Sociology, 1981.

Harwood, A. Introduction. Ethnicity and Medical Care. Cambridge, MA: Harvard Univer. Press, 1981. pp. 1–36, 482–507.

Isler, C. The fine art of handling a hospitalized child. RN Mar.: 41–45, 1978.

Jacox, A., & Stewart, M. Psychosocial Contingencies of the Pain Experience. Iowa City, IO: Univ. of Iowa, School of Nursing, 1973.

Klein, N. Wake up and die right: Death in the age of feeling. In N. Klein (Ed.), Culture, Curers, and Contagion. Novata, CA: Chandler & Sharp, 1979, pp. 35–42.

Kleinman, A., Eisenberg, L., & Good, B. Culture, illness and care: Clinical lessons from anthropologic and cross-cultural research. Ann Intern Med 88: 251–258, 1978.

Leninger, M. Nursing and Anthropology: Two Worlds Blend. New York: John Wiley & Sons, 1970.

Lewis, G. The place of pain in human experience. J Med Ethics 4: 122–125, 1978.

Lynaugh, J.E., & Bates, B. The two languages of nursing and medicine. In N. Klein (Ed.), Culture, Curers and Contagion. Novata, CA: Chandler & Sharp, 1979, pp. 129–137.

Marks, R.M., & Sachar, E.J. Undertreatment of medical inpatients with narcotic analgesics. Ann Intern Med 78: 173–181, 1973.

Mastrovito, R.C. Psychogenic pain. Amer J Nurs 74: 514–519, 1974.

McCaffery, M. Pain relief for the child: Problem areas and selected non-pharmacological methods. Pediatr Nurs 3: 11–16, 1977.

McCaffery, M. Nursing Management of the Patient with Pain. Philadelphia: J.B. Lippincott, 1979, pp. 10–21.

McCaffery, M., & Hart, L.L. Undertreatment of acute pain with narcotics. Amer J Nurs 76: 1586–1591, 1976.

McMahon, M.A., & Miller, P. Pain response: The influence of psychosocial cultural factors. Nurs Forum 17 (1): 58–71, 1978.

Melzack, R. The McGill pain questionnaire: Major properties and scoring methods. Pain 1: 277–299, 1975.

Parlee, M.B. Conversational politics. Psychol Today May: 48–49; 51–52; 55–56, 1979.

Porter, J., & Jick, H. Addiction rare in patients treated with narcotics. N Eng J Med 302: 123, 1980.

Pratt, L., Seligman, A., & Reader, G. Physicians' views on the level of medical information among patients. In N. Klein (Ed.), Culture, Curers and Contagion. Novata, CA: Chandler & Sharp, 1979, pp. 119–128. (Reprinted from Amer J Public Health 47: 1277–1283, 1957.)

Reeves, J. Pain Classes. Lecture, Univ. of California, Los Angeles, Pain Management Center. February 19, 1982.

Spector, R.E. Cultural Diversity in Health and Illness. New York: Appleton-Century-Crofts, 1979.

Sternbach, R.A. Psychological factors in pain. In J.J. Bonica, & D. Albe-Fessard (Eds.), Advances in Pain Research and Therapy, Vol. 1. New York: Raven Press, 1976, pp. 293–299.

Swanson, D.W., & Maruta, T. The family's viewpoint of chronic pain. Pain 8: 163–166, 1980.

Trotter, J.M., Scott, R., Macbeth, F.R., et al. Problems of the oncology patient: Role of the liaison health visitor. Brit Med J 282: 122–124, 1981.
Woolf, V. On being ill. In V. Woolf, The moment and other essays. New York: Harcourt, Brace, 1948, pp. 9–23.

SUGGESTED READINGS

Baer, E., Davitz, L.J., & Lieb, R. Inferences of physical pain and psychological distress. I. In relation to verbal and nonverbal patient communication. Nurs Res 19: 388–392, 1970.
Brown, E.L. Newer Dimensions of Patient Care: The Use of the Physical Environment of the General Hospital for Therapeutic Purposes, Part I. New York: Russell Sage Foundation, 1961.
Brown, E.L. Newer Dimensions of Patient Care: Patients as People, Part III. New York: Russell Sage Foundation, 1964.
Cowherd, M. One child's reaction to acute pain. Nurs Clin North Amer 12(4): 639–643, 1977.
Diers, D., Schmidt, R.L., McBride, M.A.B., et al. The effect of nursing interaction on patients in pain. Nurs Res 21: 419–428, 1972.
Diller, A. Cross-cultural pain semantics. Pain 9: 9–26, 1980.
Dodson, H.D., & Bennett, H.A. Relief of postoperative pain. Amer Surg 20: 405–407, 1964.
Eland, J.M. Living with pain. Nurs Outlook 26: 430–431, 1978.
Eland, J.M. & Anderson, J.E. The experience of pain in children. In A. Jacox (Ed.), Pain: A Source Book for Nurses and Other Health Professionals. Boston: Little Brown, 1977, 453–473.
Graffam, S. Congruence of nurse-patient expectations regarding nursing intervention in pain. Nurs Leadership 4: 12–15, 1981.
Haley, J. The art of being a failure as a therapist. In N. Klein (Ed.), Culture, Curers and Contagion. Novato, CA: Chandler & Sharp, 1979, pp. 230–234.
Jones, A., Bentler, P.M., & Petry, G. The reduction of uncertainty concerning future pain. J Abnorm Psychol 71: 87–94, 1966.
Kauffman, R.E. Pain. In H.C. Shirkey (Ed.), Pediatric Therapy. St. Louis: C.V. Mosby, 1980, pp. 283–287.
Kelman, H.C. Was deception justified—And was it necessary? Comments on "self-control techniques as an alternative to pain medication." J Abnorm Psychol 84: 172–174, 1975.
Klein, N. Introduction. In N. Klein (Ed.), Culture, Curers, and Contagion. Novato, CA: Chandler & Sharp, 1979, pp. 1–8.
Klein, N. Patients and practitioners. In N. Klein (Ed.), Culture, Curers, and Contagion. Novato, CA: Chandler & Sharp, 1979, pp. 95–97.
Krieger, D. Therapeutic touch: The imprimatur of nursing. Amer J Nurs 75: 784–787, 1975.
Lenburg, C.B., Burnside, H., & Davitz, L.J. Inferences of physical pain and psychological distress. III. In relation to length of time in the nursing education program. Nurs Res 19: 399–401, 1970.

Lenburg, C.B., Glass, H.P., & Davitz, L.J. Inferences of physical pain and psychological distress. II. In relation to the stage of the patient's illness and occupation of the perceiver. Nurs Res 19: 392–398, 1970.

Leninger, M. Nursing and Anthropology: Two Worlds Blend. New York: John Wiley & Sons, 1970.

Leninger, M. Transcultural Nursing: Concepts, Theories, and Practices. New York, John Wiley & Sons, 1978.

Lloyd, J.W. The role of pain relief in terminal cancer. Nurs Mirror 137: 36–37, 1973.

McBride, M.A.B. Nursing approach, pain and relief, an exploratory experiment. Nurs Res 16: 337–341, 1967.

McCaffery, M. Cognition, Bodily Pain and Man—Environment Interactions. Los Angeles: Univ. of California at Los Angeles, Student Store, 1968. (Out of print.)

McCoy, P. Further proof that touch speaks louder than words. RN 40: 43–46, 1977.

McLellan, C.L. Herb badges mean more than courage. Pediatr Nurs 2: 7, 1976.

Moss, F.T., & Meyer, B. Effects of nursing intervention upon pain relief. Nurs Res 15: 303–306, 1966.

Rasmussen, M., & Murphy, C.M. Hospital admission through a child's eyes. Pediatr Nurs 3: 43–46, 1977.

Robinson, G., & Merav, A. Informed consent: Recall by patients tested postoperatively. Ann Thor Surg 22(3): 209–212, 1976.

Robinson, J. Anxiety and the control of pain: Highly illogical!! J Nurs Mirror 153: 46–47, 1981.

Robinson, L. Psychological Aspects of the Hospitalized Patients. 3rd ed. Philadelphia: Davis Co., 1976.

Robinson, V.M. Humans in nursing. In C.E. Carlson, & B. Blackwell (Eds.), Behavioral Concepts in Nursing Intervention. Philadelphia: J.B. Lippincott, 1978, pp. 191–210.

Salk, L. What Every Child Would Like His Parents to Know. New York: Warner Books, 1973.

Samora, J., Saunders, L., & Larson, R.F. Medical vocabulary knowledge among hospital patients. In N. Klein, (Ed.) Culture, Curers, and Contagion. Novato, CA: Chandler & Sharp, 1979, pp. 117–118.

Santopietro, M-C. S. How to get through to a refugee patient. RN Jan.: 43–48, 1981.

Simmons, O.G. Implications of social class for public health. In N. Klein (Ed.), Culture, Curers, and Contagion. Novato, CA: Chandler & Sharp, 1979, pp. 99–107

Swanson, D.W., & Maruta, T. Patients complaining of extreme pain. Mayo Clin Proc 55: 563–566, 1980.

Szasz, T.S. Language and pain. In S. Arieti, (Ed.) American Handbook of Psychiatry, Vol. I, Chap. 49. New York: Basic Books, 1959, pp. 982–999.

Tesler, M., & Hardgrove, C. Cardiac catheterization: Preparing the child. Amer J Nurs 73: 80–82, 1973.

Timmerans, G., & Sternbach, R.A. Human chronic pain and personality: A canonical correlation analysis. Adv Pain Res Ther 1: 307–310, 1976.

10

Assessment Methods and Tools for the Patient With Pain

In this final chapter, we organize the information presented in previous chapters into what we hope is the basis for workable assessment tools for nurses to use when working with patients with pain. Before we proceed, however, the nurse's role in the care of the patient with pain can be analyzed one step further by examining the dimensions of the staff's work with patients with pain. This actually serves as a summary of many points already discussed and as another "red flag" for the need for a thorough and ongoing assessment of the patient's pain problem. We will then discuss pertinent points relative to assessment and evaluation, and finally we will present specific tools.

PAIN WORK

Sociologists have observed the care of patients with pain and identified five types of "pain work" or tasks that are involved for health personnel (Strauss et al., 1974).

1. Diagnosing the Cause of Pain

The nurse's contributions to the assessment of the cause of pain primarily includes verbal and nonverbal communication of astute observations and recording of the characteristics of the pain sensation and pain-related behaviors and variables. For example, the nurse may be expected to assess the frequency of pain, the effect of the patient's visitors on his expression of pain, whether a patient sleeps after a specific pain intervention and awakens with or without pain. It is apparent that the health team usually does attempt to be accountable for diagnosing the cause of the patient's pain.

2. Controlling the Patient's Expression of Pain

Health team members are usually held accountable for getting the patient to be less expressive about his pain. The essence of this is a problem when the practitioner is held responsible for keeping the patient quiet without being responsible for helping the patient cope with his pain. In other words, the patient is made to suffer in silence. Unfortunately, the health team may convey to the patient "We are not responsible for relieving your pain. You are responsible for being quiet about it."

As was previously discussed, there are, of course, instances when helping the patient learn to control his expression of pain can be beneficial to the patient. This and other aspects of pain work will occasionally be involved with pain relief. For example, a legal secretary may acquire a painful disuse flexion contracture of his hand and splint it to minimize pain after the acute injury. For the patient to attain a rehabilitative goal of returning to his former position as a word processor, restoring both strength and motion to the involved muscles, tendons, and joints will be necessary. Physical therapy, often including painful exercises, usually will be prescribed, and the patient will be expected to endure some pain, often with the suggestion of "Hang in there." If the individual's employer is skeptical of rehiring the patient because of his injury, the demands of "pain work" for this patient may also involve controlling expressions of pain, "keeping a stiff upper lip."

Hence, the task of controlling certain carefully selected aspects of the patient's expression of pain is not always undesirable. Currently, however, its application tends to be for the staff's convenience rather than the patient's benefit, and it is inappropriate in acute pain.

3. Expecting the Patient to Endure Pain

Another frequent practice is that the staff expects that a patient will endure pain. Often this is related to the previous task of controlling the patient's expression of pain, but not necessarily so. The patient may be told that he can scream or cry all he wants during a painful dressing change, but implicit in this is the expectation that the patient will not refuse the dressing change. He or she is expected to allow the procedure and endure the pain. Of course, patients do sometimes refuse to undergo certain procedures because of the potential or inherent pain. In these cases, the staff may find it necessary to rely upon persuasion or negotiation to accomplish the task of getting the patient to endure the pain involved in the procedure.

Probably much more work goes into getting patients to endure pain than is needed, because practitioners are neither knowledgeable about nor accountable for pain relief. Misconceptions about addiction and a lack of knowledge about narcotics may lead to the nurse withholding a narcotic. Not being knowledgeable about noninvasive pain relief methods such as distraction strategies may lead the nurse to encourage the patient to "grin and bear it." Not being responsible for pain relief may also result in the nurse not having knowledge about noninvasive pain relief methods or not having time to teach them to the patient. For example, an approach that health professionals frequently employ is to put the patient on the defensive when he requests medications. Commonly asked questions and comments include "Do you think you really need your Demerol?", "Can't you see if you can wait just a little while longer before you take your medication?", or "We don't want you to become addicted." By embarrassing and/or making the patient feel guilty for requesting pain relief, we make the patient attempt to endure pain regardless of the cause and without a sound reason. Reports of the undertreatment of acute pain with narcotics by nurses clearly document this problem (McCaffery & Hart, 1976; Cohen, 1980).

Fortunately, not all undertreatment of pain is due to a lack of compassion, a hardened attitude, cynicism, a lack of knowledge or time, or other such negative reasons or "cop-outs." For example, a common dilemma that the nurse may face is that she or he feels powerless and guilty when medications prescribed are inadequate and is aware of this, yet becomes responsible for telling the patient that "It's not time for your pain medication." The nurse's feelings of powerlessness and futility may inadvertently compound the patient's pain experience with hopelessness if a nurse says something like "There's nothing else I can do. The doctor won't allow you to have anything else." The patient may feel abandoned if the nurse does not assume the responsibility she should for notifying the physician of the need for a modification in analgesic; helping with a noninvasive pain relief measure; or, even worse, if the nurse does such things as closing the door to the room or delays responding to the call light.

Another major problem resulting in undertreatment of pain is that the patient's underlying pathophysiology may be such that the most effective medications and/or treatments are contraindicated; for example, when the patient has had recent trauma or multiple conflicting medical problems. It is clear, however, that there are times when pain relief is possible, even prescribed, but no one is held accountable.

4. Minimizing or Preventing Pain

In this dimension of "pain work" efforts are made to avoid unnecessary pain. This may involve preventing an increase in existing pain, preventing the occurrence of pain or reducing the duration, frequency, or intensity of pain that must be inflicted in conjunction with some procedure. For example, taking the time to inject 1 or 2 ml of medication slowly via the subcutaneous route can result in little, if any, discomfort; whereas rapid injection of the medication may produce considerable stinging or burning pain. Unfortunately, "time" is often the criterion used by the nurse in whether or not this is done, and not the patient's comfort.

5. Pain Relief

This dimension of "pain work" is usually directed toward pain which already exists. It involves attempts to eliminate pain, decrease its intensity, or render the pain less bothersome to the patient. For example, most surgical patients are expected to experience some postoperative pain and analgesics are almost always prescribed in anticipation of this. Again, no one is specifically held accountable for relieving the patient's pain. It would seem that the fact that most analgesics are usually written on a PRN basis allows both doctors and nurses to defer this responsibility to the acutely ill patient, who may not only be experiencing pain but also many of the effects of pain and illness previously discussed, especially anxiety, sleep disturbances and a lowering of his cognitive abilities.

When an analgesic is ordered PRN, this means "as needed," and the nurse is supposed to use clinical judgment in determining when it is needed. Unfortunately, too often the nurse merely waits until the patient requests the analgesic, and may do little about noting its effectiveness. To be truly accountable the nurse would, for example, inform the patient of the need to prevent pain, encourage the patient to ask for analgesia as soon as pain returns, instruct him or her in the use of a rating scale, and keep a systematic record of the effectiveness and side effects of the analgesic and other pain relief measures used on a flow sheet, which will be described later in this chapter.

In summary, the specific dimensions of pain work may be appropriate in certain instances but some dimensions may occasionally be detrimental. Generally, it appears that diagnosing the cause of pain, minimizing or preventing pain, and pain relief are beneficial for the patient. Expecting the patient to endure pain is sometimes necessary for the patient's eventual well-being, but much pain is endured needlessly because of lack of knowledge about low-risk pain relief measures such as distraction. Controlling the patient's expression of pain is indicated in certain carefully selected situations but not in some cases of acute pain.

GENERAL GUIDELINES TO THE ASSESSMENT PROCESS

The assessment of pain is similar in principle to the assessment of other patient care problems. Problem solving is a circular process involving SOAPIE, discussed in Chapter 1. First, there is an overall assessment of the patient's pain problem, Subjective and Objective Assessment (SOA) identifying relevant characteristics of the problem and how it affects the patient. Then a plan (P) of intervention (I), including specific pain relief measures, is formulated and implemented. Finally, the effectiveness of these interventions is evaluated (E) with an ongoing assessment to determine whether or not the plan is acceptable to the patient and safe. A nurse may formulate and implement theoretically sound and appropriate nursing interventions for a patient with pain. Yet, what the nurse does may not be effective in relieving that individual's pain. The focus here is how to determine the effectiveness of nursing performance or activity designed to assist the patient with pain. There are only a few additional points to make about evaluation methods in comparison with the nurse's initial assessment.

Compare the Patient With the Patient

When the patient is assessed to determine the effectiveness of pain relief measures or for the evolution of two painful conditions in which treatment for the pain, especially analgesic, is being withheld, the assessment must be compared with the assessment of this patient either prior to the use of pain relief measures or at an earlier stage of the painful condition. This is not always realistic since the nurse may not have made the initial assessment. However, it may be possible for the patient to make the comparison. The important point is that the effectiveness of pain and pain relief measures cannot be assessed by comparing one patient's response with another patient's response. Sometimes it is tempting but it can be very misleading. Suppose individualized pain relief plans are made for several postoperative patients. The nurse may observe that one patient is doing much better than the others. This patient reports only mild pain and has ambulated twice, whereas the other patients are experiencing moderate pain and are unwilling to ambulate. However, the patient who is doing so well compared with the other patients may be doing very poorly compared with what he was able to do the day before. The reverse can also be true. A patient with pain may seem to experience very little relief compared with other patients with similar conditions, yet for him or her, what is being experienced may be an improvement.

It is important to remember to evaluate the chronic pain patient's progress in terms of the goals set by the individual, not the goals and values of others. As Sternbach (1974) points out, some practitioners believe that the only true indication of successful therapy for chronic pain is the patient's return to work, that is, gainful employment. This may be applicable to some patients, but to apply it to all patients is a clear imposition of the practitioner's own personal values associated with the work ethic. Some patients have already retired, while others have never worked nor have they ever wanted to do so. As Chapman (1976) notes, a *few* patients almost welcome pain as a device for gaining sympathy or for being excused from success, possibly retiring early but honorably. Other patients, however, might like to work but cannot realistically expect that degree of rehabilitation.

Clearly, we must recognize the importance of being realistic about our own abilities, evaluating the patients on their own terms, comparing present status with what it was before intervention, and considering the patient's values rather than ours.

Subjective Experience and Behavioral Responses

Pain is what the experiencing patient says it is and exists when he says it does and where he says it does. The patient says things about his pain through both his verbal and nonverbal behaviors. Pain is a sensation, as well as the effects of that sensation upon the patient's life. Pain results in both a subjective experience and observable behavioral responses. In evaluating the effectiveness of pain relief measures, it is not safe to ignore any aspect of what pain is. At the very least, we must consider both the sensation of pain and the patient's responses to it, that is, the effects of pain.

In an effort to make assessment and evaluation more objective, some investigators have tried to rely primarily upon the patient's behavioral responses to pain to measure the effectiveness of efforts to relieve or manage pain. This may inadvertently place an enormous value on stoicism. It also fails to consider the price a patient may pay in mental and physical energy expended simply to conceal the fact that pain is felt. Certain patients value stoicism, but to us it seems far from appropriate to impose this value upon patients who do not possess it. While some patients suffer considerable anguish when they are unable to control their expressions of pain, others suffer more when they are forced to control their expressions of pain.

We do not believe that it is at all productive to use observable pain-related behavior alone to determine the success of pain-relief measures. Under certain circumstances, almost any patient can be coerced, whether by threats, persuasion, or rewards, to act as if he does not have pain. Mothers can do this with children less than 2 years old. In other situations behavior can be controlled at an even younger age, for example, the "failure to thrive" infant. Eradicating the behavioral response does not eradicate the sensation. Actions do not always speak louder than words. Certainly, it is impossible to conclude that patients do not have pain simply because they do not act as if they have pain. Further, regardless of the patients' "improvement" in behavioral responses to pain, if they continue to feel the pain and to be bothered by it, it does not seem likely that behavioral changes will persist, especially if they do not value the behavioral change. This is particularly true of acute pain. However, as Sternbach (1974) noted, in patients with chronic benign pain, changes in behavior are sometimes followed by changes in the pain experience. In this instance, the behavioral changes are likely to continue.

Thus, an evaluation of the effectiveness of pain-relief measures or a patient's untreated pain problem must consider not only the patient's behavioral responses to pain but also his subjective experience.

ONGOING SPECIFIC AND OVERALL ASSESSMENT

Regular assessments focus on both the general and the specific. The presence of pain and/or the effectiveness of each pain relief measure is evaluated, and the combined and cumulative effect of all pain relief measures is also evaluated. Sometimes no single pain relief measure is of outstanding benefit, but the overall results of several measures may be quite successful.

Regardless of the type of assessment method used, it must be ongoing. One assessment is not sufficient. The patient and his pain are subject to change, and problem solving must continue in a circular manner.

A specific pain-relief measure or combination of measures may increase or decrease in effectiveness over a period of time. Daily use of relaxation techniques is an example of a pain-relief measure that may increase in effectiveness over a period of a few weeks. On the other hand, the nurse may find many instances where effectiveness of a pain relief measure seems to decline.

Interpreting Results of Assessment and Evaluation

Comfort versus Pain Relief This subjective experience is composed of the sensation and the effect of the sensation in terms of feelings of loss, discomfort, suffering, distress, and other emotions previously discussed. Evaluation following pain-relief measures may reveal some interesting changes in these areas that may or may not be regarded as favorable by the patient. The sensation may have lessened considerably, but the patient may remain just as distressed or bothered by it. Conversely, the sensation may remain the same, but the patient may be less bothered by it. The latter is generally considered a success by the patient, but the former is not.

This corresponds with observations made by Beecher (1956) many years ago. He found that following a pain-relief measure, four categories of response were possible: (1) no comfort, no pain relief; (2) no comfort, pain relief; (3) comfort, no pain relief; and (4) comfort, pain relief. In his opinion only the latter two categories of response represent the desired effect, either being acceptable to both physician and patient.

Two patients illustrate the differences between relief with no comfort and comfort with no relief. Following a cutaneous stimulation treatment for neck pain, one patient commented, "It still hurts just as much but I feel much better." This patient seemed to experience comfort without relief, that is, his pain sensation remained the same but did not seem to bother him as much. He seemed pleased with the results. For another patient in severe pain and extreme distress, evidenced by moaning and lack of sleep for 24 hours, a complex pain relief program was instituted. She was able to sleep through the night, the moaning ceased, she began talking with others, but she said, "I feel a little better but not much. I can still feel the pain some. No one understands." This patient's behavioral change seemed to suggest that the sensation had decreased considerably, and in a way her verbal statement also seemed to mean that the sensation had lessened. However, she did not *feel* much better. This seemed to constitute relief without comfort, or a decreased sensation of pain but about the same level of distress. This patient did not appear to be at all satisfied about the outcome.

Some perplexing results may occur following efforts to assist a patient with pain. Ultimately, it is the patient who labels them a success or failure.

Declining Success In some patients most pain-relief measures will seem to work initially, but rapidly decrease in success. Why? An example may be the use of TENS. This may relieve pain for a few days, but with successive treatments pain relief may decrease. The nurse's enthusiasm and the patient's motivation may combine to produce successful results initially with any pain-relief measure used. It may be essentially a placebo response. As time passes, however, a positive placebo response tends to diminish in most patients. Enthusiasm and motivation are invaluable, but they may result in multiple short-term successes. For the patient with short-term pain, this tends to be fortunate rather than problematic. For the patient with chronic pain, such enthusiasm and motivation increase the importance of ongoing assessment of the effectiveness of pain-relief measures.

In addition to obtaining a true positive placebo response that gradually fades, other problems associated with the placebo phenomenon may also occur in the evaluation of potentially effective and reasonably well-proven pain relief measures. In other words, results that obscure the true positive placebo response also obscure the results of proven or "active" measures such as TENS, methadone, and imagery. The patient may report pain relief following a placebo *or* an "active" method for the following reasons: (1) His pain was relieved but he has developed tolerance to the measure. (2) His pain is relieved by another pain-relief measure that has gone unnoticed. For example, the patient may have changed his method of weight-bearing on a joint because he fortuitously found it decreased the pain. (3) Pain relief is a result of a spontaneous fluctuation in pain intensity. (4) The patient is deliberately faking pain relief to please us or to encourage our continued efforts. Eventually, ongoing assessments help to determine whether or not a specific pain-relief measure will reliably, or repeatedly, produce pain relief for the individual patient.

Revising Goals Quite simply, the assessment should indicate the etiology and progress and status of the pain problem; that either the pain-relief measure should be continued in essentially the same way, or the plan for pain relief should be revised. If the pain-relief measures tried were not as successful as we had hoped, it may be appropriate to change the goal. Perhaps we expected total pain relief when that was unrealistic. Or the expectations may have been realistic, but to achieve them it may now be necessary to modify the pain-relief measures, discontinue certain ones, or add others. If the etiology is still unknown, the search will continue through meticulous assessment of all relevant variables.

Refusal to Use Effective Pain-Relief Methods An interesting and often misunderstood occurrence is the patient's refusal to use a pain-relief measure that is effective in relieving his pain and has no apparent undesirable side effects. Why would the patient refuse to use the method? His refusal may have nothing to do with any concerns about the measure itself. Rather, it may have to do with convenience. If a pain relief measure interrupts a patient's schedule or takes up too much of his time, he may simply omit it. Or, quite often, if it is a noninvasive method, he will take medication rather than use it. Some practitioners label this drug abuse or addiction, but we feel that often it constitutes an effort to lead a more normal life. It is less bothersome and time consuming to take a pill than to use guided imagery, for example. The patient may want to use his time for activities he considers more productive or important, such as working or being with his family. As one professional woman states it "I don't want my pain to become my career." Also, the pain-relief measure may be acceptable to the patient for some situations, but not for others. For example, a novelist had been stabilized on relatively high doses of time-contingent narcotic analgesics. She was able to do her daily five hours of writing and three hours of reading, referencing, and dictating on this regimen. About every two weeks she received "copy" back to proofread and edit. On these days, in spite of the fact she had become tolerant to the side effects, she took no medication prior to her work nor during it. However, the evening before, she took an additional hypnotic to ensure a good night's sleep. Her reason for eliminating her medications was her memory of the initial drowsiness encountered during titration of her narcotics and fear that if her sensorium were to become clouded that her accuracy would be impaired. For this patient pain and the concomitant anxiety were more likely to decrease her cognitive abilities. This was explained to the patient, nevertheless she elected to eliminate the narcotics saying "I'm not going to take any chances. Immediately following completion of the proofreading and editing, she would take a "loading dose" of her analgesics and return to her time-contingent narcotic analgesic regimen. That evening, she would retire earlier than usual and again take a hypnotic to accommodate what she referred to as the additional fatigue of being in pain and working without an analgesic.

Wouldn't it be nice if patients did not have to fear our censure for their creative solutions so that they could freely share these with us and experience the good sensations of a collaborative effort, an esprit de corps, with the health team. We, in turn, would add these to our "bag of tricks of our trade" and offer them to other patients who likewise might benefit and be encouraged to experiment for a better solution to their pain problems.

ASSESSMENT TOOLS

The assessment of pain is no different from the general problem-solving approach, nor is it necessarily complicated or time-consuming in all instances, though it may be. The problem has been that we have simply neglected, in most cases, to perform this logical task in relation to pain.

Even if tools such as these are not approved forms in a specific hospital, i.e., not a part of the official or legal record, the nurse may still use them at least to collect the data needed for the patient with pain. The professional nurse has both the right and obligation to use whatever forms are helpful in the systematic organization of data about a patient.

Two tools are described for the assessment of pain: (1) "Initial Pain Assessment Tool" and (2) "Flow Sheet—Pain." The latter is the ongoing assessment of pain, or evaluation of intervention for pain management.

Initial Pain Assessment Tool

As outlined in Figure 10.1, this initial assessment tool for pain has ten parts. When the nurse uses this in a specific clinical setting, no doubt alterations in this tool will be indicated. We are assuming that most nurses work in clinical settings where assessment tools for pain have not been developed, therefore, we offer this short and simple tool as a place to begin. We encourage nurses to use the tool and make changes appropriate for the types of patients they are dealing with in their own clinical setting.

I. Location On almost all pain assessment forms, the location of pain is shown with a figure drawing. When possible, the patient (child or adult) is encouraged to mark the location of pain on the figures. If the patient cannot do this or choses not to do so, the nurse can ask the patient to point on his body to the location of pain. The nurse can then make the appropriate marks on the figures. Some patients may be reluctant to mark the figures if they have experienced significant body image changes.

If there is more than one site of pain, the different sites can be labeled with letters, e.g., A, B, C. Further comments on the assessment form will need to be made in relation to each pain location. For example, the intensity of each pain site will have to be rated separately. It is also important to mark if the pain is internal with an I or external with an E.

II. Intensity The intensity of the pain sensation is, of course, rated by the patient since he is the only one who can feel it. It is helpful if the patient can use a numerical rating scale or a series of words such as none, mild, moderate, severe, and very severe. Some patients, however, are unable to do this and will only say that they are "comfortable" or "uncomfortable" or that the pain is "bad" or "OK." Whatever the numerical or word scale used by the patient, it should be noted on the Initial Pain Assessment Tool and used consistently with that patient by *all staff* caring for the patient. Obviously, it would be unnecessarily confusing if different people used different rating scales with the same patient.

It is useful to obtain pain ratings for the pain the patient feels at the time of the initial assessment including a rating for the most severe or "worst" the pain becomes, and for the least severe or "best" it becomes. It may also be helpful to add other ratings such as those following administration of specific medications or other pain relief measures. These serve as the basis for reassessment.

III. Quality The patient's own description is used. However, quality of the pain sensation is often difficult for the patient to describe. The nurse could ask the patient, "Can you tell me what your pain feels like?" If the patient cannot find a word that he feels is an adequate description of the quality of the pain, the nurse may offer words such as those from Melzack's (1975) pain questionnaire and which were seen in the patient example in Chapter 9.

IV. Onset, Duration, Variations, Rhythms This involves asking such questions as: When did the pain begin? How long has it lasted? Is it better or worse at certain times? Does quality or intensity of the pain change in relation to certain times or other factors such as eating or position?

V. Manner of Expressing Pain How does this patient respond behaviorally or physiologically to pain? Does he or she let others know that pain exists? If so, how? Information of this nature is especially important in patients who cannot or do not readily communicate about pain. If this is the patient's first experience with this type of pain, ask how pain was coped with in the past. If he or she has not had significant pain, sometimes asking what the usual response to stress is may provide some clue to how he or she might react or express the pain.

VI. What Relieves the Pain? In planning intervention, it is clearly helpful to identify whatever has relieved the patient's pain, especially the types of things that the patient prefers. If possible this should be included in the plan for pain management.

Date 1/20/83

Patient's name John C. Age 17 Room 360

Diagnosis Peri-stomal abscess, Crohn's Disease Physician D. H.
Ileostomy Nurse N. C.

I. LOCATION:

Mark on drawing,

E = external,

I = internal

E+I

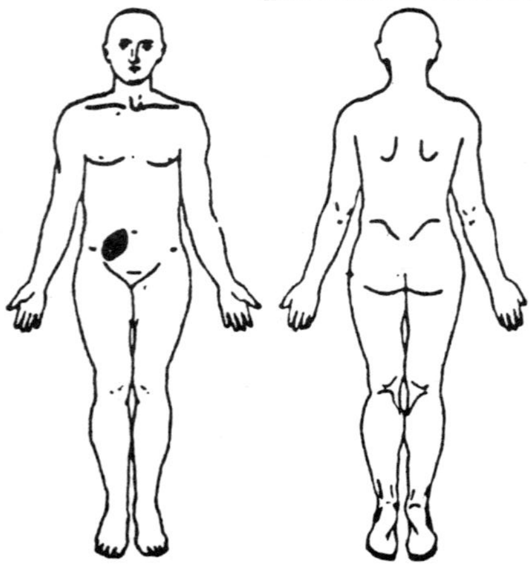

II. INTENSITY: Use rating scale, e.g., 0-10, 0= none, 10 = as bad as it can be.

Present 4 (Analgesic 2 hrs. ago)
Most severe 8-9; 10 c̄ dressing change
Least pain 3 - 45 min. after analgesic + at rest

III. QUALITY: Use own words (e.g., prick, ache, burn, throb, sharp, pull)
Deep ache "awful"

IV. ONSET, DURATION, VARIATIONS, RHYTHMS:

2 weeks ago; about the same all day, worst c̄ dressings bid

V. MANNER OF EXPRESSING PAIN:

Admits pain upon questioning; calls for analgesic

VI. WHAT RELIEVES THE PAIN?

Analgesic; Lying still; Keeping weight off areas

VII. WHAT CAUSES OR INCREASES THE PAIN?

Pressure, even slight movement of the legs or trunk
Dressing changes

VIII. EFFECTS OF PAIN:

Accompany symptoms (e.g., nausea) Slight when pain ↑ "7"
Sleep only dozes - not had full nights sleep in 2 wks.
Appetite Decreased due to pain
Physical activity Stays in bed because movement hurts
Relationships with others Doesn't want visitors
Concentration Alert
Emotions, attitudes (e.g., angry, suicidal) Seems despondent; tearful about pain,

IX. OTHER COMMENTS:

Tries to Cooperate with dressings; clenches fists and jaw, but eventually says "I can't stand it"

X. PLAN:

1. Assess response to analgesic - degree and duration of pain relief
2. Schedule dressing change approx. 30 minutes after analgesic given

M. McCaffery, R.N.

Figure 10.1. Initial Pain Assessment Tool. (The authors have devised this tool for use in assessing the patient's pain. It also has been helpful as a teaching aid for nurses and physicians. The authors encourage its duplication.)

VII. What Causes or Increases the Pain? Again, information elicited in what relieves the patient's pain should be considered, since it is helpful to know what should be avoided.

VIII. Effects of Pain Some of the most common adverse effects of pain on the patient are listed. These are discussed primarily in Chapter 7. It is usually necessary to ask specific questions to determine the effects of pain upon the patient. In other words, a general question such as "How do you feel?" or "How has the pain affected you?" does not elicit from most patients an adequate account of the detrimental effects of pain, such as sleep disturbances. Assessment of potential sleep disturbance can be used as an example of how specific the question must be: "Does pain keep you from going to sleep at night?", "Does pain awaken you?", "If so, how many times?", "For how long?", "How well rested do you feel when you awaken if you go to sleep when you are in pain?"

Assessment of the effects of pain upon the patient helps identify the extent to which pain may be interferring with recovery from an acute illness. With chronic pain, effects of pain indicate the degree to which pain decreases function and quality of life. The effects of pain can then be used to formulate specific goals of pain management. For example, if acute or chronic pain interferes with sleep, as it often does, an initial goal of pain management may be to relieve enough pain for the patient to obtain a full restful night's sleep.

IX. Other Comments Any other pertinent observations may be added here. It is also helpful to ask the patient a more general question such as, "Is there anything else you would like to tell me or that you feel would be helpful for me to know, to help you with your pain?"

X. Plan This refers to the immediate plan for relieving the patient's pain.

Flow Sheet—Pain

A flow sheet format is used to monitor the ongoing assessment or evaluation of many patient problems such as fluid intake and output or vital signs. The flow sheet quickly shows the patient's current status and the patient's responses to various types of therapy that may have been used to treat the problem. This same format is an efficient method of assessing the patient's response to pain-relief measures.

The flow sheet for pain in Figure 10.2 is an example of the application of the flow sheet format to the evaluation of the safety and effectiveness of analgesics. The only safe and effective way to administer narcotic analgesics is to observe the individual patient's response to the medication. A few patients will be at risk with even small doses of narcotics. The flow sheet does not have to be used every time the analgesic is administered, but

FLOW SHEET - PAIN - EXAMPLE

Date________________

Patient________________________________

Rx________________________________

Purpose: To evaluate the safety and effectiveness of the analgesic(s).

Analgesic order________________________________

Pain Rating Scale used________________________________

I. Time	II.* Pain rating	III. Analgesic	IV. R	V. P	VI. BP	VII. Level of arousal	VIII.** Other	IX. Plan & comments

*Pain rating: A number of different scales may be used. Indicate which scale is used and use the same one each time. Two common examples:
- 0 to 10 with 0 being no pain and 10 being as bad as it can be.
- Melzack's scale: 0 = no pain; 1 = mild; 2 = discomforting; 3 = distressing; 4 = horrible; 5 = excruciating.

Possibilities for other columns: respiratory depression, nausea and vomiting, bowel function, other pain relief measures, etc. Identify the side effects of greatest concern to patient, family, physician, nurses, etc.

Figure 10.2. Pain flow sheet. (The authors have devised this tool for use in assessing the patient's pain. It also has been helpful as a teaching aid for nurses and physicians. The authors encourage its duplication.)

probably should be used until safety and effectiveness have been established. Thus, the flow sheet would be indicated for the *initial doses* of an analgesic *any time* the *analgesic* is *changed*, whether this is change in drug, dose, interval between dose, or route of administration, and whenever the *patient's condition changes,* such as a decrease in level of consciousness or a new disease process.

The flow sheet is usually kept at the bedside as are flow sheets for other observations. Sometimes the patient assists in keeping the flow sheet. For example, the patient may write in hourly pain ratings in place of or in addition to his pain diary.

Column I is "Time" and is self-explanatory. Column II is explained in the footnote to the form. Column III is labeled "Analgesic." However, any other pain-relief measures, such as cold packs or massage, could be listed there if analgesics are not being used, or these methods could be added in Column VIII.

Columns IV, V, VI, and VII (Respiratory rate, Pulse rate, Blood pressure, and Level of arousal) may be important when analgesics are given. Respiratory rate is, of course, of special importance when narcotics are given. With nonpharmacological pain relief measures, these columns may not be necessary.

Column VIII, as well as additional columns, can be used for a variety of observations. This will depend upon the specific patient situation. Further examples are given in the second footnote to the form.

Column IX is used to note any additional information, such as the occurrence of an unexpected symptom, and to note a change in intervention. For example, if the analgesic is ineffective, a change should be made.

The flow sheet format can be altered in many ways. The columns that would be retained, however, would be I (time), II (pain rating), and IX (plan and comments).

Examples of Using Assessment Tools

Figure 10.3 is an example of how the assessment tool was used in caring for John who had pain related to a peristomal abscess. The initial assessment documents that, along with other things, the pain was having a detrimental effect upon his sleep, appetite, and ability to urinate.

A clearer picture of John's pain problem was obtained by starting a flow sheet to assess his response to the injectable analgesic. Immediately, as seen in Column IX, the nurse administering the injection noted that there was pain at the injection sites, a new observation that contributed to the decision to change to the oral route. Since pain returned to a significant intensity before the next dose of analgesic was administered, and since the current analgesic did not decrease pain intensity as much as was desirable, a regular time-contingent schedule of a longer-acting oral analgesic (methadone) was begun. The flow sheet shows total pain relief without respiratory depression but with some sedation and other side effects. Lowering the dose provided excellent pain relief without sedation or the other side effects encountered with the higher dose. As soon as safety and effective-

FLOW SHEET - PAIN - EXAMPLE

Date 1/20/83

Patient John C.

Rx Peri-ostomal Abscess - Crohn's Disease, Ileostomy

Purpose: To evaluate the safety and effectiveness of the analgesic(s).

Analgesic order Demerol 75 mg. I.M. + Vistaril 50 mg. IM q 3hr ATC (Not Prn

Pain Rating Scale used 0-10 0 = 0 pain 10 = worst pain possible

I. Time	II. Pain rating	III. Analgesic	IV. R	V. P	VI. BP	VII. Level of arousal	VIII. Other	IX. Plan & comments
1/20/83 0730	8	Dem 75 Vist 50 } I.M.	24			Awake		Painful injection sites
0900	3		16			Sleeps some	Screamed with Dressing	
1030	7	Dem 75 Vist 50 } IM	20			Awake		
1145	3-4		18			Awake		
1330	8	Dem 75 Vist 50 } i.m.	22			Awake		
1430	3		16			Sleeps some		
1530	4	methadone	18			Awake		change to
		20 mg q 4h po						po ATC
1630	0		16			Sleepy		
1730	0		16			Sleepy	Did own Dressing	
1830	0		20			Sleepy	Some nausea	
1930	0	meth 20 p.o.	20			Sleepy		
2100	0		16			Says "too sleepy"	nausea	↓ meth.
2330	0	meth 15 po	16			Sleepy		
1/21/83 0300	0		16			up to BR	Diff. urinating	Hold meth.
0500			14			Sleeping		
0800	0		18			Awake		↓ meth
1000	3	meth 10 p.o.	20			Awake	Did own Dressing	
1100	0		16			Awake	no nausea	
1200	0		16			not too sleepy		
1400	0	meth 10 po	20			Awake		

Figure 10.3. Sample completed pain flow sheet.

ness of the new analgesic order was established, the flow sheet was discontinued.

Figure 10.4 is an example of the flow sheet being used with Sue, a postoperative patient. Her IV narcotic order was discontinued and a new order written for a different drug by a different route. The flow sheet shows that the analgesic was safe but not effective for the interval ordered and that the interval between doses needed to be changed to 3 hours.

FLOW SHEET - PAIN - EXAMPLE

Date 1/29/83

Patient Sue J.

Rx Cholecystectomy, Post-op Day 1

Purpose: To evaluate the safety and effectiveness of the analgesic(s).

Analgesic order Demerol 75 mg. I.M. q 4° prn

Pain Rating Scale used 0-10 0 = No Pain, 10 = Worse pain imaginable

I. Time	II. Pain rating	III. Analgesic	IV. R	V. P	VI. BP	VII. Level of arousal	VIII. Other	IX. Plan & Comments
0850	8	Dem 75 IM	22			Dozing, Not sleeping		
1000	2		18			Dozing		
1100	3		18			"		
1230	7		20			Awake		
1300	8	Dem 75 IM	22					↓ interval
								to q 3h
1430	2		16			Has slept		
1600	4	Dem 75 IM	20			up sitting		
700	1-2					Has slept		

Figure 10.4. Sample completed pain flow sheet.

ONGOING ASSESSMENT AND FAILURES

Once the initial pain assessment is done and a plan of pain relief is implemented, ongoing assessment is necessary to evaluate the success of the plan. Unfortunately, the best of plans do not always work. A lack of success with either an assessment method or therapeutic intervention does not represent an invariant conclusion of failure, guilt, or need to blame either the patient or the practitioner. Such feelings are only likely to result in defensiveness and further delay or eliminate the possibility for the best solution for the patient.

When the patient with pain does not obtain as much pain relief as he or she or the practitioner had hoped, the patient very often feels some sense of guilt and failure. Nurses involved in teaching methods of childbirth were among the first practitioners to become alert to the sense of failure that may follow the use of pain-relief measures. These childbirth educators taught pregnant women various methods of coping with the discomfort of labor and delivery. When the methods did not produce the desired results, such as being able to go through labor and delivery without pain or without anesthesia or analgesia, the mothers often felt profound failure and guilt. In spite of the current emphasis upon each mother being different and the need to set personal goals rather than accept someone else's goals, many mothers who attend childbirth education classes continue to feel failure when they are unable to experience labor and delivery in the "normal" or "ideal" manner described in the classes or seen in the films.

Other nurses can learn much from this. Regardless of our attempts to individualize pain relief and our assessment of its success, the patient may tend to expect more than is realistic and may compare himself or herself with another patient who was more successful in achieving pain relief. The nurse must be alert to these feelings of failure and guilt. Rarely do they serve a useful purpose. Rather, they tend to depress and demoralize the patient further. The nurse may be able to assist such patients by using techniques that will help them in the assimilation of a painful experience. At the very least, we can avoid labeling the patient or ourselves as failures.

A very difficult situation that is often labeled a failure is the absence of improvement in spite of persistent efforts by a variety of competent health team members. Sometimes the patient, too, has been persistent, and other times the patient may not have cooperated with pain management. Regardless of what the patient does, when the practitioners have provided the very best health care known to be available and done all they know to do and the patient does not improve, it is discouraging and frustrating for all involved. Yet when the patient remains in pain and/or is disabled by it, it is tempting to blame the patient, especially if he or she did not cooperate fully. Sometimes, we also blame ourselves. It is far better, however, for the patient and the health team to acknowledge that no pain-relief method or program, no matter how good, is effective for all patients. Everyone concerned must realize that our knowledge of pain and its relief is very limited, although it is rapidly expanding. Sometimes lack of improvement seems to be largely a problem of not being able to motivate the patient to engage in all aspects of a pain-relief program. We wonder what we can do to motivate such patients to follow programs of pain relief. Again, motivation is an area of limited, but expanding, knowledge.

Patients with pain who do not improve following the use of the best known and available pain-relief methods continue to need assistance. Just as we do not abandon the uncontrolled diabetic, so we should not abandon the patient whose pain is not relieved despite our best efforts. It is extremely important to sustain a relationship with a patient under such circumstances and to continue to try to help. In one study of patients with chronic pain who entered a pain management program but did not improve and were dissatisfied with the treatment, the investigators emphasized that these unfortunate people still needed both treatment and understanding (Swanson, Swenson, Maruta, & Floreen, 1978). The patients were described as having repeated treatment failures, many hospitalizations, psychopathology, and some delusions. A few threatened to take legal action against the staff or agency. Compassion toward such patients is indeed admirable and warranted, although difficult. These patients are not easy to work with, but they continue to need our help.

For many varied reasons, ranging from the patient's lack of motivation to our limited knowledge of pain relief, the patient with either acute or chronic pain may not improve. Sometimes the only realistic goal, and perhaps the only one that is meaningful to the patient, is to keep the patient "out of trouble." In other words, the patient may continue to experience pain and/or to be disabled by it, but the goal is to keep him from getting worse. For example, with chronic pain it is important to help the patient find pain-relief measures that do not further disable him. This may include the more effective use of analgesics so that sedation can be minimized. It may also involve helping the patient avoid some "folk medicine" or surgical procedures that could be harmful, further disabling him. This is particularly relevant when pain is chronic.

For health professionals who value productivity or the work ethic, it may be very difficult to accept that a patient's simply staying out of trouble is the only reasonable goal. Such a goal may reflect insurmountable physical pathology, or it may actually be all the patient wishes to accomplish. Also, health team members who are cure-oriented may have difficulty accepting the lack of obvious change in the patient's condition. To those practitioners, maintaining the status quo may mean failure, but in reality it may be a success. Occasionally, it is appropriate to recognize that things could be worse.

Another problem that may occur and be erroneously labeled as failure is the appearance of a new pain problem once the original pain is relieved. This seems to happen with a significant number of patients with chronic pain. Too often the health team simply assumes that the patient wants pain for some secondary gain and that consequently it will not be possible to relieve pain in this patient. The patient himself is more or less judged a failure. However, at least two points should be kept in mind. First, either acute pain associated with acute disease processes or chronic pain associated with physical debilitation can decrease the patient's resistance to further injury or disease. In other words, many patients with pain probably have an increased susceptibility to further health problems. Each new symptom, including pain, should be thoroughly investigated and properly treated.

The second point is that once the original pain is relieved, the patient may become aware of another area of pain, perhaps near the site of the original pain. It may have been present all along, but the intensity of the original pain may have kept the patient from noticing it. Again, the pain must be investigated and treated.

In summary, the absence of improvement in the patient with pain is usually difficult and frustrating for both the patient and the practitioner. Care should be taken not to blame the patient or to label him or her a failure. Neither should the patient be abandoned.

In addition to sustaining a relationship with this patient and continuing to try to help, there are two specific nursing activities that may be beneficial. First, the entire problem-solving process may need to be repeated, with special attention to assessment of factors influencing the patient's pain. The nurse may also need to review all possible pain relief methods and ask herself or himself if any have been omitted that would be appropriate.

Second, the nurse may need to examine her or his attitude toward certain pain-relief measures being used. The nurse may not believe in the effectiveness of a pain-relief measure, or at least may not be enthusiastic about its usage. It is quite possible that the nurse's best efforts will not succeed in hiding a lack of confidence in a pain-relief measure. The patient may sense the nurse's attitude and a negative effect may occur. For example, in one study some patients did not receive pain relief from intravenous morphine when they were told it would be ineffective (Keats, 1956). This suggests that if the patient perceives that the nurse does not have confidence in the pain-relief measure, he or she may not benefit from it. It may be difficult for the nurse to overcome a disbelief that certain pain relief may be effective. She or he may have seen the pain-relief measure fail with several patients, or may have tried it personally without success. However, the nurse should try to appreciate the fact that every patient is different. Something that does not provide pain relief for one person may be effective with another. There are innumerable similar accounts of the relationship between the physician's enthusiasm and the results of the treatment.

REFERRALS

The more difficult pain problems often require a multidisciplinary approach if the patient is to be relieved of his pain or to be less disabled by it. Sometimes the patient can remain under the care of the same health team members and consultations can be requested. At other times the patient may be referred to an entirely new agency, physician, or health team. A list of resources regarding pain is seen in Figure 10.5.

Currently, there are three general types of referrals for patients with complicated pain problems. First, the patient may be referred to a pain clinic or center. Figure 10.5 provides the addresses of resources for locating pain clinics or centers throughout the world. Referral to a pain clinic may be very appropriate, but pain clinics should not be regarded as the final answer or the potential miracle. They, too, have limits. Each pain clinic is different, offering different approaches to evaluation and relief of pain. Therefore, referral to a pain clinic is an individual matter. Inpatient or outpatient care may be offered. Most pain clinics deal with chronic benign pain, but some also accept patients with pain associated with cancer.

Secondly, the patient with pain associated with a terminal illness may be referred to a hospice program. This may be an inpatient or outpatient program that provides palliative and supportive care for terminally ill patients and their families. These programs pay special attention to the relief of pain. Again, in Figure 10.5, under Hospice, there is an address for locating hospice programs, particularly in North America.

Third, the patient with pain may be referred to a holistic (wholistic) health center. Holistic health is difficult to define since it is a new label and changing rapidly. The concept of holistic health is sound and has long been recognized as valuable. Basically, holistic health centers focus on treating the whole person—the spirit, mind, and body. Preventive medicine is also stressed. Each holistic health center is different, but each tends to offer a variety of services including courses designed to help the layman stay well. These may include stress management, relaxation techniques, or diet therapy. Because of their preventive approach and their focus on the individual as a total human being, holistic health centers may meet at least some of the needs of the patient with prolonged pain.

A common referral for the anxious or depressed patient with pain is for consultation with a psychiatrist or psychologist. This may be an appropriate referral, but it is often threatening to the patient who may interpret it as meaning that his pain is "all in his head" or "imaginary." Indeed, this possibility may be why the referral was requested. As mentioned previously, however, psychogenic pain is quite rare. Most pain is best understood in terms of both physical and mental or psychological factors. It is also important to realize that the psychiatrist or psychologist to whom the patient is referred may or may not know much about the care of patients with pain. Thus, such a referral must be done carefully, with everything possible done to minimize the threat to the patient and to obtain the assistance of a psychologist or psychiatrist who has special training or experience in the care of people with pain.

Other types of referrals that may be appropriate include a hypnother-

RESOURCES REGARDING PAIN

IASP (International Association for the Study of Pain): Department of Anesthesiology, RN-10, University of Washington, Seattle, WA 98195. ($50 membership fee includes subscription to PAIN journal)

American Pain Society: 340 Kingsland Street, Nutley, NJ 07110. (201-235-0587) ($20 membership fee)

For *directions of pain clinics:*

1. Committee on Pain Therapy, American Society of Anesthesiologists, 515 Busse Highway, Park Ridge, IL 60068 ($15 (approximate) directory fee)
2. Pain, Medical World News, 1221 Avenue of the Americas, New York, NY 10020 ("Physicians' Referral Directory of Comprehensive U.S. Pain Clinics," 1980. McGraw Hill, $2)

For "Locator Directory of *Hospices* in America," ($25): National Hospice Organization, 1311 Dolley Madison Boulevard, McLean, VA 22101. (703-356-6770)

To locate *biofeedback* programs: Biofeedback Society of America, 4301 Owens Street, Wheat Ridge, CO 80033.

For free catalog of *tapes on relaxation and imagery*: Psychology Today Cassettes, P.O. Box 278, Pratt Station, Brooklyn, NY 11205.

Videotape or audio cassette programs on pain by McCaffery or Twycross. For information write: Scripps Memorial Hospital Cancer Center, 9888 Genesee Avenue, La Jolla, CA 92038.

Self-help group for patients with chronic benign pain. For information write: Chronic Pain Outreach, 8222 Wycliffe Court, Manassas, VA 22110.

Pain Research Nurses Forum: Department of Anesthesiology, B6/387 Clinical Science Center, 600 Highland Avenue, Madison, WI 53792. ($6 per year, bimonthly)

Hospice Nursing Newsletter (free): Hospice of El Paso, 1101 North Campbell Street, El Paso, TX 79902.

National Migrane Foundation: 5252 North Western Avenue, Chicago, IL 60625. ($10 membership fee includes excellent and informative newsletter)

Free copies of a fact sheet *for laymen on control of cancer pain*, 7 pages, ("Control of Cancer Pain"): Office of Cancer Communications, National Cancer Institute (NCI), Bethesda, MD 20205.

(M. McCaffery, 1982)

Figure 10.5. Resources regarding pain.

apist or biofeedback training in relaxation or stress reduction. Addresses of resources for locating these in your area are in Figure 10.5.

It is virtually impossible to make specific suggestions here about referrals or consultations for the patient with pain. A number of possibilities exist, but their appropriateness for the individual patient must be examined. There are no easy answers.

We hope that you will keep the following quote in mind about the necessity for objectivity in the assessment of the patient with pain, a quote attributed to Galen in the second century:

> All who drink this remedy recover in a short time, except those whom it does not help, whom all die. Therefore, it is obvious that it fails only in incurable cases.

Paraphrased in relation to pain: All who take this dose of narcotic are relieved of pain in a short time, except those who do not get relief, whom all suffer. Therefore, it is obvious that it fails only in those who wish to suffer. Or, it fails only in those in whom nothing would work. We continue to act as if we believe, erroneously, that equal treatment should produce equal results in all people, not allowing for individual differences in absorption, metabolism, degree of pain, and a multitude of other influences not yet even known.

This kind of absurd reasoning is not used with other conditions necessitating the use of such medications as antihypertensives or insulin. These are titrated to effect. For example, if the insulin is too much or too little, it is changed. If that simple logic were applied to analgesics, think how many more patients would receive adequate pain relief!

In summary, most of us were taught very little about pain and pain relief. Most of what we were taught over time has now proved to be erroneous. Consequently, practitioners all over are struggling to implement new and continually changing ideas about pain and pain relief that are contrary to what they were taught. The only thing we may gain by our errors is humility and compassion that can guide us in preventing such errors from occurring again.

REFERENCES

Beecher, H.K. The subjective response and reaction to sensation. Amer J Med 20: 107–113, 1956.

Chapman, J.S. Effect of auditory stimulation on gross motor activity of short gestation infants. Nurs Res Rep 11: 12, 1976.

Cohen, F.L. Postsurgical pain relief: Patients' status and nurses' medication choices. Pain, 1980, 9, 265–274.

Keats, A.S. Postoperative pain: Research and treatment. J Chron Dis 4: 72–83, 1956.
McCaffery, M., & Hart, L.L. Undertreatment of acute pain with narcotics. Amer J Nurs 76: 1586–1591, 1976.
Melzack, R. The McGill pain questionnaire: Major properties and scoring methods. Pain 1: 277-299, 1975.
Sternbach, R.A. Pain Patients: Traits and Treatment. New York: Academic Press, 1974.
Strauss, A., Fagerhaugh, S.Y., & Glasser, B. Pain: An organizational-work-interactional perspective. Nurs Outlook 22: 560–566, 1974.
Swanson, D.W., Swenson, W.M., Maruta, T., et al. Program for managing chronic pain. 1. Program description and characteristics of patients. Mayo Clin Proc 51: 401–411, 1976.

SUGGESTED READINGS

Cowherd, M. One child's reaction to acute pain. Nurs Clin North Amer 12(4): 639–643, 1977.
Dicken, A. Why patients should plan their own recovery. RN 41: 52–55, 1978.
Engelhardt, H.T. Ethical issues in pain management. H.W. Kosterlitz & L.Y. Terenius (Eds.), Pain and Society. Report of the Dahlem Workshop on Pain and Society, Berlin, Nov. 26–30, 1979. Weinheim: Verlag Chemie, 1980, pp. 461–480.
Epstein, M.H., & Harris, J. Children with chronic pain: Can they be helped? Ped Nurs Jan./Feb.: 42–44, 1978.
Gildea, J.H., & Quirk, T.R. Assessing the pain experience in children. Nurs Clin North Amer 12: 631–637, 1977.
Hackett, T.P. Pain and prejudice: Why do we doubt that the patient is in pain? Res Staff Phys 18: 100–109, 1972.
Jacox, A.K. Assessing pain. Amer J Nurs 79(5): 895–900, 1978.
Johnson, M. Pain: How do you know it's there and what do you do? Nurs 76 (6): 48–50, 1976.
Mahoney, E.A. Some implications for nursing diagnoses for pain. Nurs Clin North Amer 12(4): 613–618, 1977.
Maltbie, A.A., Cavenar, J.O., Hammett, E.B., et al. A diagnostic approach to pain. Psychosomatics 19(6): 359–366, 1978.
McGuire L. A short, simple tool for assessing your patient's pain. Nurs 81 (11): 48–49, 1981.
Mennie, A.T. The child in pain. In L. Burton (Ed.), Care of the Child Facing Death. London: 1974.
Munley, M.J., & Keane, M.C. Symposium on impressions of pain: A nursing diagnosis—Foreword. Nurs Clin North Amer 12(4): 609–611, 1977.
Schultz, N. How children perceive pain. Nurs Outlook 19: 670–673, 1971.
Smith, M.E. The preschooler and pain. In P. Brandt (Ed.), Current Practice in Pediatric Nursing: St. Louis: C.V. Mosby, 1976,
Storlie, F. Pointers for assessing pain. Nurs 78 (8): 37, 1978.
Wiener, C.L. Pain assessment on an orthopedic ward. Nurs Outlook 23: 508–516, 1975.

Glossary

Abuse liability: Likelihood of a drug being used for nonmedical purposes and/or in a socially unacceptable manner.

Abuse potential: *See* abuse liability.

Acupressure: Application of pressure or pressure and massage to acupuncture points.

Acupuncture: A treatment, originating in China, done by puncturing the body with needles to cure disease or relieve pain. It may be done with or without electrical stimulation.

Acute pain: Usually lasts less than 6 months, characterized by identifiable pathology that accounts for the pain; pain subsides as healing takes place.

Acute pain model: Includes expectation of observing visible signs of discomfort (physiological and/or behavioral signs).

Adaptation pain model: Includes realization that there is physiological and behavioral adaptation, leading to periods of minimal or no signs of discomfort.

Addiction: A behavioral pattern of compulsive drug use, characterized by overwhelming involvement with obtaining and using the drug plus a high tendency to return to this behavior after withdrawal from the drug.

A-delta pain: Fast pricking "first pain."

Algesia: Sensitivity to pain (*adj.* algesic, algetic).

Algesic types: A classification of responses to pain according to perceptual style, accounting for variance in estimation of the intensity of the stimulus. Three types are identified: reducers, augmenters, and moderates.

Algogenic: Causing pain.

Algology: The study of pain.

Allodynia: Pain due to a nonnoxious stimulus to normal skin.

Analgesia: Absence of pain during noxious stimulation.

Analgesic: A drug that acts upon the nervous system to relieve or reduce the suffering or intensity of pain without causing loss of consciousness.

Anesthesia: Without sensation.

Anesthesia dolorosa: Pain in an area or region which is anesthetic.

Anxiety trait: *See* trait anxiety.

ATC: Around the clock.

Autogenic training: Self-generated therapy; includes repetition of phrases about the desired state of the body, e.g., heavy limbs, especially those states that elicit relaxation.

Biofeedback: Return of physiologic information to the subject immediately after it is generated, often utilizes electronic monitoring equipment; feedback of information about the ongoing state of some body function, e.g., muscle tension.

Biogenics: Use of both autogenic and biofeedback training to achieve relaxation.

Cancer pain: Pain due to neoplastic disease or to the treatments which have cured or arrested it.

Causalgia: A syndrome of sustained burning pain after a traumatic nerve lesion combined with vasomotor and sudomotor dysfunction and later trophic changes.

Central pain: Pain associated with a lesion of the central nervous system.

C-fiber pain: Slow burning "second pain."

Chronic benign pain (CBP): Pain lasting six months or longer in which the pathology is not life-threatening or nonneoplastic, sometimes qualified to imply adequate coping of the pain by the patient.

Chronic cancer pain: Pain due to uncontrolled or progressive malignant, neoplastic disease.

Chronic intractable benign pain state (CIBPS): Chronic pain with which the patient seems unable to cope.

Chronic pain: Usually refers to any pain that lasts six months or longer.

CIPBS: Chronic intractable benign pain state.

Cognitive strategies: Pain-relief methods that require rather concentrated and active thought processes (thinking).

Counterirritant: An agent applied to the skin to cause superficial irritation for the purpose of relieving some other irritation or pain.

Cutaneous stimulation: Stimulation of the patient's skin for the purpose of relieving pain.

Depression: *See* endogenous; reactive.

Dermatone: A segmental skin area innervated by a particular spinal cord segment.

Desensitization: A form of treatment by reciprocal inhibition in which the stimuli that previously elicited unadaptive responses are reconditioned to elicit adaptive ones. A list is made of stimuli that cause anxiety and that list is arranged in order from those that produce the most anxiety to those that produce the least anxiety. The patient is taught a method of relaxation and then begins to imagine the stimuli, beginning with the item that elicits the least anxiety. If the patient begins to feel anxiety, he or she is taught to relax and start again.

Distraction: Focusing attention on stimuli other than the pain sensation.

Dolorology: The science of pain (a relatively new specialty).

Dorsal column stimulation (DCS): A technique for the relief of chronic pain, based on the gate control theory of pain. Internal electrical stimulation requiring a laminectomy to place an electrode that is activated by the patient resulting in paresthesia in the painful area of the body.

Double blind: When neither the patient nor the person administering the medication knows whether the medication is an active substance or a placebo (or when some other identifying factor, such as dosage, remains unknown).

Drug abuse: Use of any drug in a manner that deviates from the approved social and medical patterns in a given culture.

Drug addiction: Behavior pattern of overwhelming involvement with obtaining and using a drug for nonmedical purposes. It is an extreme form of drug abuse or compulsive drug abuse or compulsive drug use.

Drug tolerance: After repeated doses, a given dosage of a narcotic begins to lose its effectiveness. First duration of action shortens, then there is decreased analgesic effect.

Dynorphin: "Dynamite endorphin," a peptide fifty times greater than beta-endorphin.

Endorphin: Contraction of endogenous and morphine meaning "morphine within." Endorphins are opiod-like peptides found in the brain, spinal cord, and gut.

Endogenous (or psychotic) depression: Characterized by retardation or agitation, guilt, somatic disturbances. The person awakens early and the depressive mood is worse in the mornings. It is associated with a family history of depression.

Enkephalin: Weakly analgesic opiod-like peptide found in the brain and spinal cord.

Equianalgesic: Refers to the dose and route of administration of one drug that produces approximately the same degree of analgesia as the dose and route of administration of another drug. Equianalgesic dosages are only approximations.

Expressive style: The way a person presents his pain to others.

Extrovert: One whose style in reporting pain is expressive and outgoing. An extrovert probably complains of pain more readily and fully, and may tend to use more descriptive phrases.

"First pain": *See* A-delta pain.

Functional pain: Sometimes used interchangeably with the term "psychogenic pain." *See* psychogenic pain.

Guided imagery: See therapeutic guided imagery.

Hospice: An inpatient or outpatient program that provides palliative and supportive care for terminally ill patients and their families.

Hypalgesia: Decreased sensitivity to pain.

Hyperalgesia: Increased sensitivity to noxious stimulation.

- **Primary Hyperalgesia:** Excessive sensitivity of the pain receptors.
- **Secondary Hyperalgesia:** Facilitation of sensory transmissions.

Hyperesthesia: Increased sensitivity to stimulation, excluding special senses.

Hyperpathia: A painful syndrome, characterized by delay, over-reaction and after-sensation to a stimulus, especially a repetitive stimulus.

Hypoalgesia: Diminished sensitivity to noxious stimulation.

Hypochondriacal neurosis: A neurosis characterized by preoccupation with the body and a constant fear of disease and body malfunction.

Hypochondriacal pain: A form of "pure" psychogenic pain, that is, pain caused solely by mental events.

Hypochondriasis: The state of being preoccupied with one's body, afraid of disease and body malfunction, and/or being convinced that disease is present in spite of reassurance that it is not. There is a spectrum of hypochondriasis, ranging from healthy concern to delusion.

Hypoesthesia: Decreased sensitivity to stimulation, excluding special senses.

Hysterical neurosis: Conversion hysteria. A state in which there is loss or disturbance of body function resulting from unconscious emotional conflicts that have their origins in the past. The state may be precipitated by a recent emotionally charged event.

Hysterical pain: Pain that is a symptom of or results from an hysterical neurosis. Patients with hysterical pain appear calm and relatively unconcerned about their pain.

Hysterical personality: A lifelong character structure, a particular pattern of personality organization. The person tends to have a flair for the dramatic and to be responsive and warm, egocentric, impulsive, helpless, imaginative, and over-reactive. He or she may respond to organic pain in a more intense fashion, with more anxiety and greater demands for relief.

Ideosensory activity: The capacity of a person to develop sensory images that may involve any or all of the senses, that is, vision, hearing, movement, touch, smell and taste.

IM: Intramuscular injection.

Imagery: In this book, it refers to ideosensory activity, although quite literally the term refers only to the visual aspects of ideosensory activity. Used interchangeably with visualization. *See* ideosensory activity: *see also* therapeutic guided imagery.

Intractable pain: Pain that persists despite treatment.

Introvert: One whose style in reporting pain is less expressive as influenced by both culture and personality traits.

IV: Intravenous injection.

IVP: Intravenous push.

IVPB: Intravenous "piggyback."

Loading dose: An initial dose larger than the dosage that is estimated to be needed.

Malingerer: A patient who pretends to have pain.

Mantra: A preselected word, sound, or phrase that is repeated during Transcendental Meditation.

Meditation: Concentration; focusing attention on a single thought or task.

Modeling: In psychological studies on pain, this refers to subjects' observing a model, or person, who is responding to apparently painful stimuli in a predetermined manner, e.g., unresponsive to painful stimuli.

Motor point: That area of a muscle where a branch of a peripheral nerve innervates it.

Neural: Relating to nerves.

Neuralgia: Pain in the distribution of a nerve or nerves.

Neuritis: Inflammation of a nerve or nerves.

Neuropathy: A disturbance of function or pathological change in a nerve; in one nerve, mononeuropathy; in several nerves, mononeuropathy multiplex; symmetrical and bilateral, polyneuropathy.

Neuroticism: The amount of emotional lability, over-responsiveness and anxiety one has plus the frequency of reporting of minor aches and pains as measured by the Eysenck Personality Inventory.

Nociceptor: A receptor preferentially sensitive to a noxious or potentially noxious stimulus (adj. nociceptive; v. nociception).

Noninvasive pain relief methods: Techniques that can be used without physically invading or penetrating the body; no physical objects enter the body; the body's physical barriers of skin and mucous membrane are not breached; examples may include certain distraction strategies, relaxation methods, imagery, and cutaneous stimulation.

NPO: Nothing by mouth.

Noxious: A harmful or injurious stimulus. In relation to tissue it often refers to irreparable damage. In relation to the psyche it refers to offensive, insidious, or undermining stimuli.

Oral/parenteral ratio (o-p): That fraction of oral analgesia as opposed to parenteral analgesia. Used to determine what oral dosage probably is equal in analgesic effect to a given IM dose.

Organic pain: Pain sensations that result from physical stimuli.

OTC. (over-the-counter): Products, especially drugs, that can be bought and sold without a physician's prescription.

Pain (nursing definition): Whatever the experiencing person says it is, existing whenever he or she says it does, including both verbal and nonverbal behavior. (Medical definition) localized sensation of hurt or an unpleasant sensory and emotional experience associated with actual or potential tissue damage, or described in terms of such damage.

Pain behavior: Anything which a patient does or says which communicates that pain is being experienced.

Pain contingent: Treatment directed at pain but only provided if the patient reports pain, in contrast to a preventative approach to pain.

Pain experience: All that happens to and is experienced by a person who will have, has, or has had pain. Includes the three phases of pain: anticipation, sensation, aftermath, and the physical, social and psychological events and effects.

Pain expression: The way a person presents pain to others.

Pain language: The patient's way of communication about pain.

Pain mediators: Substances that can provoke pain, launched at the cellular level as an immediate response to acute insult to the cell. Mediators include histamine, kinins, prostaglandins, and serotonin.

Pain patient: A person who presents to a physician with a report of pain, seeking pain relief. In common usage, the label tends to be reserved for patients with chronic benign pain.

Pain perception threshold: The least stimulus intensity at which a subject perceives pain. That point at which graded exposures to noxious stimulation are reported as painful.

Pain-producing substance (PPS): The unequivocal single substance proven to cause pain. At this time, there is still no singly agreed upon substance.

Pain-prone patient: A person who suffers repeated or prolonged pain. The gist of the psychodynamic theories is that the pain-prone person is exposed to certain forms of abusiveness in childhood. As a result, the person adopts a lifestyle in which suffering is a major factor. Research indicates now that there may be a physiological basis such as endorphin depletion causing the pre-disposition to pain.

Pain reaction threshold: Point at which an individual first exhibits pain behaviors.

Pain threshold: Same as pain perception threshold.

Pain tolerance (level): The greatest stimulus intensity and or duration that the individual is willing to endure pain.

Phantom limb pain: Following surgical or traumatic amputation of the limb, severe burning, fiery, crushing, or cramping sensations. Pain or a sensation that the limb is edematous or being twisted or is in a distorted position.

Phantom limb sensation: Tingling, itching, or sweating in the illusionary limb following surgical or traumatic amputation.

Physical dependence: Withdrawal symptoms occur when a drug is not taken.

Placebo: *Any* medical, surgical or nursing procedure that produces an effect that was believed not to occur as a result of the physical or chemical properties of the procedure. Research now makes it seem likely that the result is endorphin-related.

PO: Oral.

Positive reinforcers: *See* reinforcers.

Potentiators: Drugs that increase the effectiveness of other drugs.

PPS: Pain-producing substance.

Practitioner: Any person involved in clinical practice who provides health care for individuals. This may be a physician, nurse, physical therapist, etc.

PRN: As needed.

Progressive relaxation exercises: Tensing and releasing specific groups of muscles while concentrating on the feelings of tension and relaxation.

Prolonged pain: A significant duration of pain that does not necessarily fit the accepted definitions of either acute pain (less than six months) or chronic pain (six months or longer). In this book, the term includes pain of varying durations, e.g., several weeks, several years.

Psychogenic pain: A localized bodily sensation of pain that is caused solely by mental events and is better described and understood in psychological rather than physical language. No physical findings exist to account for the cause and/or persistence of the pain.

Psychological dependence: The effects of a drug or the conditions associated with its use felt by the individual to be necessary to maintain an optimal state of well-being.

Psychological overlay: The involvement of intense mental processes such as worry or anxiety in a patient's response to the identifiable or organic pathology. Used in conjunction with a diagnosis of organic or somatic pain.

Psychological therapies: A fairly general term referring to those methods that rely upon the patient's beliefs, thoughts and emotions. Examples are placebos, relaxation responses, imagery, psychotherapy, spiritual healing.

Psychotropic drugs: Drugs that affect the functioning of the mind, e.g., alcohol, opiates, tranquilizers.

QS: Quantity sufficient.

Radiating pain (radicular pain): Pain that extends from the site of origin in known segments called dermatomes.

Radicular pain: *See* radiating pain.

Reactive (or neurotic) depression: Characterized by tiredness, loss of interest, hypochondriacal complaints, daytime depression with evening accentuation of mood. It is a persistent response to an environmental precipitant.

Recurrent (acute) pain: Pain which is episodic in behavior but more characteristic in nature of acute processes—periods of exacerbation and remissions.

Referred pain: Pain that is present in an area that is removed from its point of origin.

Reinforcers: Those advantages or benefits that result when the patient expresses his pain or otherwise responds to his pain.

Relaxation: Mental and physical freedom from tension or stress; a neutral state; freedom from both anxiety and skeletal muscle tension.

Relaxation response: Decreased autonomic nervous system activity, including decreased oxygen consumption, decreased respiratory and heart rate, decreased muscle tension, increased alpha waves, decreased arterial blood lactate (blood pressure decreases only in patients with high blood pressure).

SC: Subcutaneous injection.

"Second pain": *See* C-fiber pain.

Secondary gain: Practical advantages that result from having the symptom of pain, or advantages that can be achieved from using the symptom to influence others.

Self-control methods: Noninvasive pain relief methods that the patient can learn to do for himself. *See* noninvasive pain relief methods.

Slow push: May refer to IV administration of a total dose of drug over a three- to five-minute period.

Somaticizing: Handling emotional stress by focusing on body functioning and physical discomforts.

Somatogenic pain: Pain that is better described and understood in physical terms or in the language of physiology. Pain caused by a physical process.

Standardized image: A specific image that has been developed for a specific purpose and supposedly has fairly universal appeal; that is, it can be used with most people with some degree of success. *See* also imagery.

Stimulation-produced analgesia (SPA): Analgesia or pain suppression by electrical stimulation of specific areas in the brain. For treatment of CBP. The area of choice is the medial periventricular thalamic structure.

State anxiety: Subjective feelings of apprehension and fear in the presence or anticipation of a specific situation; present affect; transitory or situational anxiety.

Stress: Environmental conditions that require behavioral adjustment.

Subacute pain: Pain that is no longer of an emergent nature but which lasts for a few days to months and in which there is a known active pathological process being treated.

Substance p: A pain-producing substance.

TENS: *See* transcutaneous electric nerve stimulation.

Therapeutic guided imagery: Use of one's imagination in an especially designed manner to achieve a specific, positive effect in oneself. *See* ideosensory activity.

Tolerance: *See* pain tolerance; drug tolerance.

Trait anxiety: Anxiety as a persistent personality trait rather than anxiety that results from a specific situation.

Transcendental Meditation (TM): A form of yoga meditation involving the repetition of a mantra (word, phrase, or sound).

Transcutaneous electric nerve stimulation (TENS): External electrical stimulation of nerves through electrodes placed over the skin and activated by a battery-operated device to provide tingling or vibrating sensations in the area of pain.

Trigger point: Hypersensitive regions that may occur in muscles, connective tissue, ligaments, and joint capsules, especially in the neck, shoulder girdle and low back. When they are stimulated they cause patterns of referred pain that are fairly consistent. This referred pain does not follow a dermatomal or peripheral nerve distribution, yet the pattern of pain is fairly predictable.

Visualization: *See* imagery.

Yoga: An ancient art and science of total health care involving the physical, mental and spiritual aspects of life. Consists of meditation practices and physical postures and exercises.

Index